Documenting Occupational Therapy Practice

Karen M. Sames, MBA, OTR/L

*Associate Professor of Occupational Science
and Occupational Therapy
The College of St. Catherine
St. Paul, Minnesota*

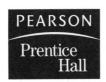
PEARSON

Prentice
Hall

Upper Saddle River, New Jersey 07458

Library of Congress Cataloging-in-Publication Data

Sames, Karen M.
  Documenting occupational therapy practice / Karen M. Sames.
      p. ; cm.
  Includes bibliographical references and index.
  ISBN 0-13-045214-9
  1. Occupational therapy--Practice. 2. Medical records. 3. Medical protocols.
  [DNLM: 1. Occupational Therapy--methods. 2. Medical Records--standards. WB 555
S187d 2005] I. Title.

  RM735.4.S264 2005
  615.8'515--dc22

                                                          2004000987

Publisher: Julie Levin Alexander
Assistant to Publisher: Regina Bruno
Senior Acquisitions Editor: Mark Cohen
Associate Editor: Melissa Kerian
Editorial Assistants: Mary Ellen Ruitenberg and
  Jaquay Felix
Director of Marketing: Karen Allman
Channel Marketing Manager: Rachele Strober
Director of Production and Manufacturing:
  Bruce Johnson
Managing Production Editor: Patrick Walsh

Production Liaison: Danielle Newhouse
Production Editor: Jessica Balch, Pine Tree
  Composition
Manufacturing Manager: Ilene Sanford
Manufacturing Buyer: Pat Brown
Design Director: Cheryl Asherman
Design Coordinator: Maria Guglielmo-Walsh
Cover Designer: Mary Siener
Composition: Pine Tree Composition, Inc.
Printing and Binding: Courier Westford
Cover Printer: Phoenix Color Corp.

Pearson Prentice Hall™ is a trademark of Pearson Education, Inc.
Pearson® is a registered trademark of Pearson plc.
Prentice Hall® is a registered trademark of Pearson Education, Inc.

Pearson Education, Ltd., London
Pearson Education Australia Pty. Limited, Sydney
Pearson Education Singapore Pte. Ltd.
Pearson Education North Asia Ltd., Hong Kong
Pearson Education Canada, Ltd., Toronto
Pearson Educación de Mexico, S.A. de C.V.
Pearson Education—Japan, Tokyo
Pearson Education Malaysia, Pte. Ltd.
Pearson Education, Upper Saddle River, New Jersey

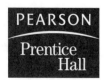

1 0 9 8 7 6 5 4 3 2
ISBN 0-13-045214-9

CONTENTS

▼ SECTION II ▼

ETHICAL AND LEGAL CONSIDERATIONS   37

▼ SECTION III ▼

CLINICAL DOCUMENTATION   57

PREFACE

For many years, I wished for a book that could be used by students to learn about documentation, while at the same time be used by clinicians to improve the quality of documentation in the field. Eventually, I realized that I could, and should, write that book. As a college professor, I spend a great deal of time reading written work produced by occupational therapy students. As a peer reviewer, I read client charts that insurance companies are unsure about; the charts that are so poorly written that the insurers cannot decide whether the services are medically necessary and appropriate.

For these reasons, I decided to begin the long and challenging task of writing this book. It has taken over three years from the time I started talking about writing it to the actual printing of the book. Federal rules and professional standards changed while I was writing this book, forcing me to revise and add topics as the book evolved.

During the process of writing this book, I learned even more about writing. I learned that I write better in the morning than in the afternoon. I learned that I have difficulty knowing when to use the word "that" (refers to a specific object) as opposed to the word "which" (not specific to an object). I learned the difference between "assure" (to convince or to promise) and "ensure" (to make certain). I learned about comma and semicolon placement in sentences. Just because I pause when I speak the sentence out loud does not mean that rules of proper punctuation call for a comma. I learned the difference between a hyphen, an em dash, and an en dash. Finally, I learned to say "finally," instead of "lastly."

My hope for this book is that it gets used; that it is not simply put up on a shelf. I want it to be written in, to have pages flagged, and to have the spine well broken from repeated use. Normally, I would be appalled at the vision of food-stained, rumpled pages in a textbook. But I think this book is different. If it retains its original pristine condition, then it hasn't served its reader well.

ACKNOWLEDGMENTS

This book would not have been possible without the help and support of several people. First, I want to thank the editorial staff at Prentice Hall, especially Melissa Kerian and Mark Cohen, for their persistence and willingness to let me write this book in my own voice. I owe many thanks to Jessica Balch and her team at Pine Tree Composition, Inc., for their work in copyediting the text. The drafts of this book were sent by Prentice Hall to many unnamed reviewers who were occupational therapy and occupational therapy assistant practitioners and educators. Because each reviewer read the draft from a different perspective, some of the feedback conflicted from one reviewer to the next. I did my best to accommodate as much of the feedback I was given as possible, but ultimately my revisions were based on what I thought was important. I'd like to acknowledge all the reviewers for this book whose feedback was critical in my revision. I appreciate the time it took each of them to read and comment on the text, their candor in criticizing it, and the overwhelming encouragement they provided.

Alma R. Abdel-Moty, MS, OTR
Clinical Assistant Professor
Occupational Therapy Department
Florida International University
Miami, Florida

Gail S. Bass, OTR/L
Instructor
Occupational Therapy
University of North Dakota
Grand Forks, North Dakota

Estelle B. Breines, Ph.D., OTR, FAOTA
Program Chair
Department of Occupational Therapy
Seton Hall University
South Orange, New Jersey

Catherine C. Brennan, MA, OTRL/L,
    FAOTA
Consultant
St. Paul, Minnesota

William R. Croninger, MA, OTR/L
Associate Professor
Occupational Therapy
University of New England
Biddeford, Maine

Anne E. Dickerson, Ph.D., OTR/L, FAOTA
Program Chair and Professor
Occupational Therapy
Eastern Carolina University
Greenville, North Carolina

Hahn C. Edwards, MA, MS, OTR
Assistant Professor
Occupational Therapy Assistant Program
University of Southern Indiana
Evansville, Indiana

Maria Hinds, JD, MS, OT
Assistant Professor
Occupational Therapy
Florida A&M University
Tallahassee, Florida

Joyce H. McCormick, MS, OTR/L
Fieldwork Coordinator
Occupational Therapy Programs
Pennsylvania State University—Mont Alto
Mont Alto, Pennsylvania

Deane B. McCraith, MS, OTR/L, LMFT
Clinical Associate Professor
Boston University
Sargent College of Health and Rehabilitation
    Science
Department of Occupational Therapy
Boston, Massachusetts

Nichelle L. Miedema, OTR/L
Program Coordinator
Occupational Therapy Assistant Program
Kirkwood Community College
Cedar Rapids, Iowa

Candice Jones Mullendore, MS, OTR
Assistant Professor and Academic
    Fieldwork Coordinator
Department of Occupational Therapy
Creighton University
Omaha, Nebraska

Kathy Nielson, MPH, OTR/L
Professor and Director
Division of Occupational Science
The University of North Carolina at Chapel
    Hill
Chapel Hill, North Carolina

Karen B. Smith, OTR/L
Program Director
Occupational Therapy Assistant Program
Stanly Community College
Albermarle, North Carolina

Kathy Clark Tuminski, MA, OTR/L
Assistant Professor
Occupational Therapy
Eastern Kentucky University
Richmond, Kentucky

Joanne Wright, Ph.D., OTR/L
Program Director
Division of Occupational Therapy
University of Utah
Salt Lake City, Utah

I was fortunate to participate in a writer's retreat while working on this book. I want to thank the leaders of the retreat, Cecelia Conchar Farr, JoAnn Cavalero and Gabrielle Civil for providing such a supportive environment in which to write. In addition, the other women at the retreat helped provide the right balance of privacy, encouragement, humor and food (especially sausage) to keep me writing. The retreat was sponsored by The College of St. Catherine and the Denny family.

I would also like to thank the faculty and staff of the Department of Occupational Science and Occupational Therapy of The College of St. Catherine for their continuous support during the course of my writing. I am so fortunate to work in an environment where people encourage each other and help each other out. In particular, I want to thank Linda Buxell, Nancy Flinn, Lisa Klein, Dawn Torrine-Micko, and Julie Bass Haugen for being sounding boards when I needed them to be and for the ideas they shared with me about writing in general, and writing this book in particular.

Finally, I want to thank my family. My husband Wayne, son Ethan, and younger daughter Emily provided quiet support. My older daughter Amanda provided very vocal criticism with just the right touch of humor to keep me going.

Karen M. Sames

INTRODUCTION: THE WHO, WHAT, WHERE, WHEN AND WHY OF DOCUMENTATION

As occupational therapists, we work with a variety of clients in a variety of settings. In every setting in which we use our skills as trained professionals, we are asked to document what we do in some way. We may do clinical documentation that becomes part of a medical record. We may contribute to the development of an Individual Education Program (IEP) for a grade school student. We may write a report summarizing our activity as a consultant to a company. It is imperative that our writing demonstrates a high level of professionalism.

▼ WHO ▼

The key to professional writing is knowing who we are writing for as well as who we are writing about. As indicated above, we write for multiple audiences. Some potential audiences include the intervention team, the client and/or surrogates (caregivers, family, or guardians), facility quality management personnel, third-party payers, peer reviewers, accreditation surveyors, administrators, and lawyers. Because the potential audience for our documentation extends far beyond our peers, it is important that we choose our words very carefully. I know of one occupational therapist who mentally says to herself before putting pen to paper, "Ladies and gentlemen of the jury . . ." then she begins her documentation. It forces her to think about how her words may be interpreted by others.

▼ WHAT ▼

On my first occupational therapy job, a director of nursing told me repeatedly, "If it's not documented, it didn't happen." It was like her personal mantra. As much as I got tired of hearing it, I have to admit she was right. It was good advice. If I had to be absent from work, and a substitute had to step in for me, I wanted the substitute to be fully informed about what things have been tried already and in what direction I wanted the intervention to proceed. In order for this to happen, there had to be accurate, complete, and clear documentation of what has transpired in occupational therapy thus far. Also, documentation that is written at the time of an event is stronger evidence in a court of law than one's memory. How many of you can remember exactly what you did last Tuesday at 10:00 in the morning? A month ago? Eighteen months ago? Who were you with? What were you doing? Were you successful at whatever you were doing? How much force did you use? You get the picture.

Not only do you want to document what was done, you want to document the client's reaction to the intervention. Think of it as painting a verbal picture of the occupational therapy session for the reader. You want to document what instructions were given (e.g., for a home program, splint use and care, adaptive equipment use and care, or instructions to caregivers) and whether the person receiving instructions appeared to understand those instructions. Finally, you want to document what the plan is for future occupational therapy service delivery.

With so much to document, it might become somewhat of a balancing act between working hands-on with a client and documenting that intervention. Most occupational therapists go into the profession because they want to help people. I doubt any become occupational therapists because they love to write notes all day long. In addition, increasing competition for health care dollars have pushed some clinics to develop productivity standards for the amount of billable services each clinician needs to provide each day. This results in less time available for doing documentation. Today, a clinician in a clinical setting will generally spend 6 hours or more (out of an 8-hour day) with clients. The rest of the time is usually for meetings and documentation. In educational or community settings, the time spent with clients may be 7 hours or more in an 8-hour day. However, needing to document so much of what we do does not mean we have to spend a lot of time doing it. Sections III and IV of this book will show you some ways of documenting in an efficient and effective manner.

▼ WHERE ▼

In clinical settings, each client has his or her own clinical record (chart). The chart may be electronic or paper based. Occupational therapists may document in a section of the chart dedicated to rehabilitation or therapies. In some settings, integrated notes are done, so that each profession documents progress in a progress note section of the chart that is compiled chronologically regardless of which professional is writing. It is important to follow facility standards for where and when to write in the client's chart, regardless of whether the chart is on a computer or is paper based. Standards for good documentation do not change when the format (electronic or paper) changes.

In educational settings, the Individualized Education Program (IEP) or Individualized Family Service Plan (IFSP) is written annually and reviewed every 6 months. The evaluation report, present levels of performance, and occupational therapy goals are integrated into those documents. The IEP or IFSP then goes into the student's educational record. If the school district is billing third-party payers for occupational therapy services, additional documentation may be required. The school district will have policies for the occupational therapist regarding where any other documentation will be filed and retained.

In addition to the official clinical or educational record, some occupational therapy departments retain copies of everything that is in the official record in a departmental file. These departmental files may also contain test forms, attendance records, and other nonofficial documents. Chapter 5 will go into more detail about records retention.

▼ WHEN ▼

Documentation is typically done as close to the time of service as possible. Some occupational therapists reserve the last 5 minutes or so of the intervention session to document in the client's chart. This works fine for contact or progress notes, but may not be sufficient for doing larger documents such as evaluation or discontinuation reports. These documents are usually done when there are no clients being treated such as at the beginning or end of the day or over the lunch hour. In some settings, the occupational therapist will dictate evaluation or discontinuation notes to be transcribed by secretarial staff. Others write them out longhand or on a desktop, laptop, or handheld computer.

The longer the time span from when the evaluation or intervention occurred to when the occupational therapist sits down to write about it, the more the chance that something will be forgotten. When possible, writing directly in the client's chart at the time of service delivery is best. However, this is not always possible. Some occupational therapists carry small notebooks or pieces of paper with them in their pockets, and jot quick notes about the clients they see during the day. Others use hand-held computers. This does help them remember more clearly what happened with each client. As you can imagine, if an occupational therapist sees 12 clients in a day, by the end of the day it can be difficult to remember who said or did what.

▼ WHY ▼

Occupational therapists document for many reasons. We document to show what has happened to the client in a chronological sequence. We want to show what happened first, then second, then the next thing, and so on. Some regulatory and accrediting bodies want to see that things happened in a clinically sound sequence. For example, if you were working with a client recovering from a severe head injury, you would want to show that the client is aware of safety precautions to take when using a knife before you work on how to use a knife. The client's chart will tell any third-party reviewer the story of that client's recovery following an illness or injury, or a client's development in the case of a developmental delay.

We document to show our high level of clinical reasoning. Someone walking by the occupational therapy clinic could see the occupational therapist watching a client make buttered toast. That person might think, "She went to college for how many years to teach that? I could do that without any training." If that person could read the chart, he or she would see that the occupational therapist was really working on sequencing a task, manipulating utensils, safety awareness, and/or energy conservation. The task of buttering toast represents many different learning opportunities for the client. There is often more to occupational therapy than meets the eye.

We document to inform others on the intervention team about what happened during an intervention session. Everyone is busy, we work different shifts, and there is not always time for each of us to talk to other caregivers about each client. By writing down the essence of what happened in the intervention session, others on the team can be informed in their own time. By the same token, we can read the chart and find out what happened that day in other therapy services, or in the lab, medical imaging, or nursing.

We document to demonstrate the effectiveness of occupational therapy for third-party payers. This is a critically important reason to document well, as payment is often based on the quality of the documentation. Third-party payers such as the government (Medicare, Medicaid, CHAMPUS, and other programs) and private insurers (managed care, worker's compensation, indemnity) want to be sure that they are getting what they paid for—results. A payer virtually never observes the client directly, but relies on the documentation of the services delivered to determine effectiveness. If the payers cannot see progress in the documentation, they will often terminate payment, which in effect terminates services, even if you believe the client could still benefit from further services.

Last, but not least, we document for legal reasons. As stated earlier, the medical record, anything written at the time, is stronger evidence of what happened than anything we can remember from a year or two ago. In many states, a client can bring forward a malpractice case up to 2 years after the incident occurred. In those 2 years, we could have treated more than a hundred other clients. Will we remember exactly what we did with that client on that day, or will all the other clients we have seen since then cloud our memory? Depending on what we write, and how well we write it, the clinical record can be used to protect, or to hurt, us as practitioners. There are ways to ensure that what we write is more likely to help than hurt us, and this book addresses them.

Section I of this book deals with some of the mechanics of writing. It includes tips on word usage, the use of frames of reference, abbreviations, and jargon. It also takes a broad look at how the language of the profession is ever evolving and describes both internal and external influences on the use of language.

The second section focuses on the ethical and legal issues around documentation, such as confidentiality, record retention, fraud, and plagiarism. This provides a different, yet necessary perspective on documentation: payers, reviewers, and attorneys.

Section III deals with the documentation of the occupational therapy process in a clinical setting. Clinical settings include all occupational therapy practice venues where third-party reimbursement is sought, such as in a hospital, nursing home, clinic, or psychiatric program. Usually, in a clinical setting, there is a physician order or referral, and services are billed for in some way. This is a very broad description of a clinical setting. It excludes services that are paid for with grant money or other funding sources that do not require physician oversight.

The fourth section is about documentation in school systems. While many school systems are now billing third-party payers to recoup the costs of some therapy services, there are also requirements for certain types of documentation that are unique to school-based services. This chapter addresses only the documentation requirements of school systems.

The last section deals with administrative documentation. Examples of administrative documentation include policies and procedures, incident reports, meeting minutes, and grant writing. Occupational therapy staff write some of these types of documents, while supervisors and managers generally write others.

If you are reading this book as a required text for a course in an occupational therapy educational program, do not be surprised if your instructor does not require you to read each chapter and do each exercise, in the order in which the chapters appear in this text. In an introductory course in occupational therapy, you may only be assigned the first three or four sections. However, I hope that at some point in your educational program, you will have a chance to work with chapters in the rest of the book. That means that you should hang on to this book even when the course is over. You will undoubtedly have opportunities to practice documentation in several courses in your curriculum, and this book will be a good reference to look back at as you draft your assignments.

If you are a clinician reading this book, I congratulate you on your dedication to the profession and to continuing competence. Depending on how long it has been since you were in school, some of the information in the book will be new to you, some merely a refresher. Each chapter of the book can stand on its own, and you can choose the chapter or chapters on which you want to concentrate. You will also find the material in the Appendices especially helpful.

Throughout the book there are exercises to help you develop your skills in documentation. Answers to the exercises are included in Appendix A. While comparing your answers to the answers in the book can be a good learning experience, it may be even more helpful to get feedback on your answers from an instructor or colleague. An experienced occupational therapist can provide feedback on the subtle nuances that different wording can have on a reader.

As you work through the sections of this book, you will become familiar with principles of good documentation in clinical and educational settings. You will also learn about other types of documentation that occupational therapists may be called on to write during their careers. People form opinions about you as a professional based on how well or how poorly you write. If you want to be thought of as a talented, competent, and skilled professional, you must write like one.

SECTION I

Use of Language

▼ INTRODUCTION ▼

Documentation requires the use of written words. To document well, one must write well. This involves selecting words that will have meaning to the reader and making the documentation clear, accurate, and relevant to the situation. In the first section of this book, general issues about writing are discussed.

How well you write is one way that others will judge your professionalism. If you write poorly, use outdated terms or excessive jargon, use too many abbreviations, or leave out words, people will think you are either careless or lacking in skill. Appendix B contains a review of general grammar and spelling considerations that may be a good review for some readers. The American Occupational Therapy Association has developed a framework for occupational therapy practice that can provide some guidance on the use of terms. Different frames of reference used in occupational therapy color the way occupational therapists write about clinical or educational progress.

▼ STRUCTURE OF THIS SECTION OF THE BOOK ▼

Chapter 1 will deal with use of language including buzzwords, jargon, and abbreviations. Lists of common abbreviations are included. This chapter is very specific to occupational therapy practice. Just as certain phrases used in everyday conversations can be trendier than others, so can certain phrases used in occupational therapy.

Chapter 2 relates the language used in documentation to the language used in the primary documents that guide the profession of occupational therapy. These documents are written by the American Occupational Therapy Association and the World Health Organization.

Chapter 3 suggests that the words chosen for documenting occupational therapy services will reflect the model or frame of reference used with a particular client. It includes a brief summary of several different models and frames of reference.

Finally, Chapter 4 includes a checklist for ensuring careful documentation. It deals specifically with documenting clearly and accurately, making the documentation relevant, and documenting any exceptions to the way the therapist expected things to go.

The lessons learned in these chapters will help improve documentation regardless of the setting in which the occupational therapy clinician or student works. What is important to remember is that you must always choose your words carefully.

CHAPTER 1

Buzzwords, Jargon, and Abbreviations

INTRODUCTION

The longer you write progress notes and intervention plans, the more you fall into certain patterns. You learn what words get the attention of reviewers in positive and negative ways. There are lists floating around, developed by experienced occupational therapists, containing words one should never use, and other lists with words that one should be sure to use. If your supervisor hands you such a list, she will expect you to use it. Go ahead and use these lists. Do not, however, depend on them as your sole source for good words.

▼ BUZZWORDS ▼

Buzzwords are words that are currently popular or trendy. They let the reader or listener know that you are up to date. Buzzwords in the early 21st century include "collaborative," "active learning," "function," "hands-on," and "community." Based on the proposed International Classification of Function (World Health Organization [WHO], 2002) language, I expect the phrases "activity limitation," "participation restriction," and "participation in life" to become buzzwords very soon. The problem with buzzwords is that as quickly as they become fashionable, they become unfashionable.

"Function" is a special buzzword. It is a necessary word to occupational therapy practice in the 2000s. Occupational therapy practitioners must show that their services result in functional changes in their clients. This is true of other providers such as physical therapists and speech language pathologists as well. Demonstrating improvement in function is essential to receiving payment for services. This means that as occupational therapists document their services, it is not enough to say that someone's range of motion increased. So what? Just because someone can bend more at the elbow does not automatically mean that person can do more because of it. Can the person now feed herself or button the top button on her blouse? Because a person can now follow three-step directions, what does it mean? Can this person now prepare a meal? Function is the difference between a client tolerating being in water for 3 minutes and taking a bath. Documentation must be explicit in its descriptions of functional activities.

Just as there are buzzwords, there are what I call "red-flag words." These words will cause the reader to stop and perhaps not read any further. They serve as big signs of trouble. An example of red-flag words are "continued" or "maintained" when read by a payer that only pays for occupational therapy services as long as there is demonstrable progress.

Some payers will also view documentation with an eye toward discontinuing service if they read that a client was "seen" in occupational therapy rather than "participated in" the occupational therapy session. If the writer says that a client was seen in occupational therapy today, the payer may interpret that as the client was seen in the room, but did not necessarily do anything while in the room. "Participated" implies some action on the part of the client.

For years, clinicians have refrained from writing goals that deal with the client's need to participate in cultural, religious, or spiritual activities. It seemed that culture, religion, and spirituality were red-flag words. Clinicians were hesitant to address issues of participation in cultural, religious, or spiritual activities, primarily because they were sure payers would not pay for such services (they may be viewed as diversionary activities, which are usually not reimbursable). One occupational therapist told me that even though she was working with an elderly priest who had had a stroke, the payer would not pay for her to work toward the goal that he be able to raise the offering as high as the ritual required for him to say mass, so she never tried to get any services involving religion or spirituality covered again. While raising his arms high enough to complete the tasks of the mass does relate to religion, perhaps if she had stated the goal in terms of regaining the skills required to return to work, she might have gotten paid for her services.

That was several years ago, and maybe things have changed since then. If what is important to your client is participation in religious or spiritual life, one strategy would be to find ways to dance around those words in setting goals. Instead of setting a goal that Mrs. Smith propel herself in her wheelchair to the chapel each week, the goal could be that she propel herself to all the places she needs to access in the building. Or instead of a goal that a client will be able to kneel on the ground to offer praise to Allah several times a day, the goal can be that the client be able to engage in activities that are personally meaningful.

That strategy can work, but there is something about writing vague goals that does not sit well with me. Instead of anticipating the reaction of payers to red-flag words, we should use them and then appeal the case if it is denied. We may find that we are no longer being denied coverage, we only think we will be, so we have been avoiding being totally honest and direct.

▼ JARGON ▼

Jargon is terminology widely understood by one profession or group of people, but not understood by others outside the group or profession (Lunsford, 2001). Occupational therapists are notorious for their use of jargon. As mentioned in the introduction to this book, occupational therapists need to consider the audience they are addressing. While occupational therapists know what bilateral integration is, most people do not. A look at *Uniform Terminology, 3rd Edition* (AOTA, 1994) or the *Occupational Therapy Practice Framework: Domain and Practice* (AOTA, 2002) will give you some idea of the kind of jargon that is frequently used in occupational therapy documentation.

Here is an example of a paragraph written with lots of buzzwords, jargon, and abbreviations:

> Patient seen for 3 units for ADLs. Patient sat at EOB with min assist. Patient told to perform upper body hygiene/grooming. Needed min assist and setup. Patient showed a poor bilateral integration due to left hemiplegia and left hemianopsia. Patient's significant other instructed by this therapist in compensatory techniques and cuing patterns. SO return demonstration not adequate. Will need additional instruction.

Here is the same paragraph written in relatively plain English:

> Patient participated in a 45-minute bedside session this morning for self-care activities. The patient sat at the edge of the bed with minimal assistance. With minimal assistance following setup, the patient washed his face and trunk, brushed his teeth, and combed his hair. He did not wash his left arm or the left side of his face. The patient's wife was instructed in ways to set up tasks and verbally cue the patient to compensate for left visual field cut. She tended to try to do the task for her husband; she will need more instruction.

Both paragraphs describe the same client doing the same activities. The second one is easier for most people to read and understand. Note that it does not eliminate every abbreviation or word of jargon. To do so would make it sound too simplistic and unprofessional. It is a question of balance and of which terms are likely to be understood by every professional in the program and by payers.

Exercise 1.1

Translate these paragraphs into plain English.

1. Jennifer attended three sessions this week. She needed encouragement to engage in the group discussion. She rarely made eye contact with the therapist or other group members. She mumbled incoherently and occasionally picked at something unseen in the air around her, possibly hallucinating. When given a task to do that involved generalizing and categorizing, she completely disengaged. Her attention span was less than 2 minutes. She appeared to respond positively to classical music, the mumbling and picking at the air ceased and she smiled. When asked specific questions at different times on different days, she was not oriented times three.

2. Chrissy was seen for a three-unit session today. She selected the 30-inch ball as the first thing she wanted to try. She positioned herself prone on the ball and proceeded to rock in a linear pattern. Then she went to the bolster swing and engaged in circular vestibular stimulation. Chrissy alternated between these two activities for 15 minutes. Next she asked to draw in the shaving cream on a mirror. She attended to this task for 10 minutes, then ran to the sink to wash and dry her hands. Next she retrieved the parachute and wrapped herself up tightly in it. Following that, she quietly played with puzzles. She is demonstrating improved tactile and vestibular processing. Plan is to continue working on sensory integration activities to improve sensory processing as outlined in plan of care.

▼ ABBREVIATIONS ▼

One way to shorten the time it takes to write notes is to use abbreviations. It takes less time to write "bid" than it does to write "two times per day." However, the problem with abbreviations is that not everyone knows what the abbreviations mean. Sometimes the same abbreviation can mean different things. In one setting "hoh" might mean hard of hearing, but in another it could mean hand over hand (as a form of assisting a client to complete a task). Most facilities have a list of acceptable abbreviations for use at that facility. It is important to use such a list if it exists, and not assume that other people understand your abbreviations.

Here is a paragraph written using abbreviations when possible and then rewritten using as few abbreviations as possible. Using abbreviations saved two lines of type, but made it harder to read.

Client partic. in OT bid 5x/wk. He partic. in a w.u. Ax consisting of ROM ex. for BUE including ✓/−, ab/ad, & IR/ER. Client shows ↑ in ROM and reps all directions. He worked coop. c̄ 2 other clients in a ball game, demonstrating leadership & teamwork. The ball game required him to use bilat integ. skills & social interaction skills. Client is showing ↑ in these skills & abilities. Plan to cont. per POC.

Client participated in OT twice daily for 5 days this week. He participated in a warm-up activity consisting of ROM exercises for both arms including flexion/extension, abduction/adduction, and internal/external rotation. Client shows increase in ROM all directions. He worked cooperatively with 2 other clients in a ball game, demonstrating leadership & teamwork. The ball game required him to use both hands together & socially interact. Client is showing an increase in these skills & abilities. The plan is to continue interventions as established in the plan of care.

COTA (certified occupational therapy assistant)
COTA/L (certified occupational therapy assistant, licensed)
FAOTA (Fellow of the American Occupational Therapy Association)
MOT (Master of occupational therapy)
MAOT (Master of Arts in occupational therapy)
OTA (occupational therapy assistant)
OTA/L (licensed occupational therapy assistant)
OTD (occupational therapist, doctor of [clinical doctorate])
OTD/L (doctor of occupational therapy, licensed)
OT/L (occupational therapist, licensed)
OTR (occupational therapist, registered)
OTR/L (occupational therapist, registered and licensed)
OTAS (occupational therapy assistant student)
OTS (occupational therapy student)

DC (doctor of chiropractic)
DDS (doctor of dental surgery)
DMD (doctor of medical dentistry)
MD (medical doctor)
OD (doctor of osteopathy)
PhD (doctor of philosophy)

DPT (doctor of physical therapy)
PA (physician's assistant)
PT (physical therapist)
PTA (physical therapist assistant)

SLP (speech-language pathologist)
CCC (certificate of clinical competence)

LPN (licensed practical nurse)
RN (registered nurse)

LMFT (licensed marriage and family therapist)
LP (licensed psychologist)
MSW (master's of social work)
RD (registered dietician)
RT (recreation therapist, respiratory therapist)

APE (adaptive physical education)
D/APE (developmental and adaptive physical education)
EBD (emotional or behavioral disorder)
LD (learning disabled)

FIGURE 1.1   Professional Credentials

In some instances, people expect abbreviations to be used. When signing your name on any formal documentation, it is common practice to identify yourself by putting your professional credentials after your name in the form of an abbreviation. Common abbreviations for professional credentials are listed in Figure 1.1. There are many others, but these are the most common.

Abbreviations are also used to document the frequency with which something occurs. Figure 1.2 shows a list of such abbreviations.

Abbreviations can refer to parts of the body, injuries, or illnesses. Figure 1.3 is a partial list, however, inclusion in this list does not guarantee that anyone who reads these abbreviations knows what they mean.

There are other abbreviations referred to in the jargon of the profession as the "x" abbreviations (Figure 1.4). These have varied use and acceptability in different parts of the country.

Occupational therapists and other medical professionals use a variety of abbreviations to identify types of range of motion, as shown in Figure 1.5.

qd (once a day)	1x/wk (once a week)
bid (twice a day)	2x/wk (twice a week)
tid (three times a day)	3x/wk (three times a week)
qid (four times a day)	(continues up to 7x/wk)
eod (every other day)	
	1x/mo (once a month)
i (once a day)	2x/mo (twice a month)
ii (twice a day)	3x/mo (three times a month)
iii (three times a day)	(continues)

FIGURE 1.2 Abbreviations Related to Frequency

Clinical procedures and common clinical terminology are abbreviated in letters and with symbols (Figure 1.6). The first part of Figure 1.6 contains those terms with letter abbreviations and the symbols follow.

Figure 1.7 shows abbreviations most commonly used when payment is being discussed.

Finally, Figure 1.8 contains a list of abbreviations related to education.

UE (upper extremity—arm)	CVA (cerebral vascular accident—stroke)
LE (lower extremity—leg)	DJD (degenerative joint disease)
BUE (both upper extremities)	DM (diabetes mellitus)
LUE (left upper extremity)	FTT (failure to thrive)
RUE (right upper extremity)	Fx (fracture)
BLE (both lower extremities)	GSW (gunshot wound)
LLE (left lower extremity)	HBV (hepatitis B virus)
RLE (right lower extremity)	HIV (human immunodeficiency virus)
	MI (myocardial infarction in some settings,
DIP (distal interphalangeal joint)	mental illness in others)
MP or MCP (metacarpal phalangeal joint)	MVA (motor vehicle accident)
PIP (proximal interphalangeal joint)	MVP (mitral valve prolapse)
	PNI (peripheral nerve injury)
AEA (above elbow amputation)	OBS (organic brain syndrome)
AKA (above knee amputation)	ORIF (open reduction, internal fixation)
BEA (below elbow amputation)	PDD (pervasive developmental disorder)
BKA (below knee amputation)	PNI (peripheral nerve injury)
	PTCA (percutaneous transluminal coronary
ADD (attention deficit disorder)	angioplasty)
ADHD (attention deficit hyperactivity	RA (rheumatoid arthritis)
disorder)	RSD (reflex sympathetic dystrophy)
AIDS (acquired immunodeficiency disorder)	SCI (spinal cord injury)
ASHD (atherosclerotic heart disease)	SLE (systemic lupus erythmatosus)
CA (cancer)	STD (sexually transmitted disease)
CAD (coronary artery disease)	TB (tuberculosis)
CABG (coronary artery bypass graft)	TBI (traumatic brain injury)
CHF (congestive heart failure)	THR (total hip replacement)
CHI (closed head injury)	TIA (transient ischemic attack)
CNS (central nervous system)	TKR (total knee replacement)
COLD (chronic obstructive lung disease)	TMJ (temporal mandibular joint)
COPD (chronic obstructive pulmonary	URI (upper respiratory infection)
disorder)	UTI (urinary tract infection)
CP (cerebral palsy)	
CSF (cerebrospinal fluid)	
CTR (carpal tunnel release)	

FIGURE 1.3 Abbreviations Related to Body Parts, Injuries, or Illness. *Sources: Borcherding, S. (2000) and Kettenback, G. (1990).*

```
Ax (activity)
Dx (diagnosis)
Fx (fracture)
Hx (history of)
PMHx (past medical history)
Rx (therapy)
Sx (symptoms)
Tx (treatment)
```

FIGURE 1.4   "X" Abbreviations

```
AAROM (active assisted ROM)
AROM (active ROM)
FROM (functional ROM)
PROM (passive ROM)
ROM (range of motion)
RROM (resisted ROM)
```

FIGURE 1.5   Range of Motion Abbreviations

```
Ⓐ (assist; assistance)                      ECG or EKG (electrocardiogram)
A (assessment)                              echo (echocardiogram)
abd (abduction)                             EEG (electroencephalogram)
ac (before meals)                           EENT (ears, eyes, nose, and throat)
add (adduction)                             EMG (electromyelogram)
ad lib (at liberty, at discretion)          eob (edge of bed)
ADL (activities of daily living)            eval (evaluation)
adm (admission)
ALF (assisted living facility)              f (female)
am or AM (morning)                          FCE (functional capacity exam)
ama or AMA (against medical advice)         flex (flexion)
amb (ambulation; ambulates)                 ft (feet; foot as in a measurement, not a body
amt (amount)                                   part)
ASAP (as soon as possible)                  FW I (fieldwork one)
assist (assistance)                         FW II (fieldwork two, also called affiliation
ATNR (asymmetrical tonic neck reflex)          experience)
                                            FWB (full weight bearing)
Ⓑ (bilateral or both)
b/c (because)                               G (good as in muscle strength)
b/4 (before)                                GM&S (general medicine and surgery)
BP (blood pressure)
B/S (bed side; blood sugar)                 H&P (history and physical)
                                            HEENT (head, ears, eyes, nose, and throat)
cc (chief complaint)                        HEP (home exercise program)
c/o (complains of)                          HOB (head of bead)
cont. (continue)                            HOH (hard of hearing or hand over hand)
                                            HR (heart rate)
D/C (discontinuation; discharge)            hr. (hour)
Dept. (department—may also be written with  hs (at night)
   a small d)                               ht (height)
DME (durable medical equipment)
DTR (deep tendon reflex)                    Ⓘ (independently)
                                            IADL (instrumental activities of daily living)
```

FIGURE 1.6   Abbreviations for Clinical Procedures. *Sources: Borcherding, S. (2000) and Kettenback (1990).*

ICD-9 (International Classification of Diseases, Ninth Edition)
ICU (intensive care unit)
ICF (intermediate care facility)
IM (intramuscular)
imp (impression)
in. (inches)
IP (inpatient)
IV (intravenous)

kg. (kilogram)

Ⓛ (left)
lb. (pound)
llq (left lower quadrant)
Loc (loss of consciousness)
LP (lumbar puncture)
LTC (long-term care)
LTG (long-term goal)
LUQ (left upper quadrant)

m (male)
max (maximum)
meds (medications, medicines)
mft (muscle function test)
mg. (milligram)
ml (milliliter)
min (minutes; minimum)
MMSE (Mini-Mental Status Exam)
mo. (month)
mod (moderate)

N (normal, as in muscle grade)
na or N/A (not applicable)
NDT (neurodevelopmental treatment)
neg. (negative)
ng (nasogastric)
NKA (no known allergy)
noc (nocturnal, at night)
NPO (nothing per mouth)
NSR (normal sinus rhythm)
nt (not tested)
NWB (non-weight bearing)

O (objective)
O₂ (oxygen)
od (once daily or right eye)
OH (occupational history)
OP (outpatient)
os (left eye)
ou (both eyes)
Ox3 (oriented times three [person, place, time])
oz. (ounce)

P (plan)
para (paraplegic)
pc (after meals)
per (by)
PFT (pulmonary function test)
p.m. or PM (between noon and midnight)

pmh (past medical history)
PNF (proprioceptive neuromuscular facilitation)
po (per mouth, orally)
P/O or post-op (after surgery)
POMR (problem-oriented medical record)
pos (positive)
poss (possible)
PRE (progressive resistive exercise)
pre-op (before surgery)
pro (pronation)
PRN or prn (per as needed)
Pt or pt. (patient)
PTA (prior to admission)
PWB (partial weight bearing)

q (every)
qt. (quart)

Ⓡ (right)
Re: or re: (regarding)
rehab (rehabilitation)
Resp (respiratory, respiration)
rlq (right lower quadrant)
r/o (rule out)
ruq (right upper quadrant)

S (subjective)
SBA (stand by assist)
sig (directions for use, give as follows)
SNF (skilled nursing facility)
SOAP (subjective, objective, assessment, plan; progress note format)
SOB (shortness of breath)
S/P (status post)
stat (immediately)
STG (short-term goal)
STNR (symmetrical tonic neck reflex)
sup (supination)

T (trace as in muscle strength)
TEDS (thrombo-embolic disease stockings)
TENS, TNS (transcutaneous electrical nerve stimulation)
t.o. (telephone order)
TNR (tonic neck reflex)
TPR (temperature, pulse, respiration)

UMN (upper motor neuron)
US (ultrasound)
UV (ultraviolet)

v.o. (verbal order)
VS (vital signs)

W/C or w/c (wheelchair)
WFL (within functional limits)
WNL (within normal limits)
wt. (weight)

FIGURE 1.6 (Continued)

y/o (year old, as in a 5 y/o girl)
yr. (year)

° (degree)
↑ (increased, up)
↓ (decreased, down)
→ (toward)
↔ (to and from)
+ (positive, plus)
− (negative, minus)
= (equal)
% (percent)
Δ (change)
♀ (female)
♂ (male)

\# (number, pound)
& (and)
@ (at)
~ (approximately)
< (less than)
> (greater than)
✓ (flexion)
/ (extension; per)
c̄ (with)
p̄ (post, after)
s̄ (without)
1° (primarily, primary)
2° (secondary, secondary to)
Ø (none)

FIGURE 1.6 (Continued)

CMS (Center for Medicare and Medicaid Services, formerly HCFA)
CORF (certified outpatient rehabilitation facility)
CPT (Current Procedural Terminology, a coding system used to bill for medical procedures)
DRG (diagnostic-related group)
DSM-IV (Diagnostic and Statistical Manual, Fourth Edition)
FI (fiscal intermediary)
HCFA (Health Care Financing Administration [part of the U.S. Department of Health and Human Services])
HCPCS (Health Care Procedures Coding System)
HMO (Health Maintenance Organization)
ICD-9 (International Classification of Diseases, Ninth Edition)
JCAHO (Joint Commission on Accreditation of Health Organizations)
MDS (Minimum Data Set)
OASIS (Outcome and Assessment Information Set)
OCR (Office of Civil Rights, U.S. Department of Health and Human Services)
OSHA (Occupational Safety and Health Administration)
PPO (Preferred Provider Organization)
PPS (Prospective Payment System)
RUGS (Resource Utilization Groups)

FIGURE 1.7 Abbreviations Related to Payment. *Source: Administrative and Management Special Interest Section (2000).*

APE (adapted physical education)
AT (assistive technology)
CFR (Code of Federal Regulations)
D/APE (developmental and adaptive physical education)
ECFE (early childhood family education)
ECSE (early childhood special education)
EI (early intervention)
FAPE (free and appropriate public education)
IDEA (Individuals with Disabilities Education Act)
IEP (Individualized Education Program)
IFSP (Individualized Family Service Plan)
LEA (local education agency)

FIGURE 1.8 Educationally Related Abbreviations. *Source: American Occupational Therapy Association (1999).*

LRE (least restrictive environment)
OHI (other health impaired)
OSEP (Office of Special Education Program, U.S. Department of Education)
PI (physically impaired)
PLEP (present level of educational performance)
SEA (state education agency)
SI (sensory integration)
USC (United States Code)

FIGURE 1.8 (Continued)

Exercise 1.2

Translate these notes into plain English.

1. Jacques is 4 weeks s/p surgical repair of tendons around his Ⓡ first MCP joint. He wears a thumb immobilizer splint, but is now allowed to remove it tid for 5 minutes of movement, within 20° of midline in ✓/ and ab/ad. Reports pain has decreased during Ⓡ thumb movements. No swelling evident, wound has healed nicely. He has begun to swing a bat, gripping it fully with his left hand and gripping with his fingers only, thumb immobilized with his right. Maintaining upper arm strength is important for him to be able to return to finish the baseball season (plays outfield for the Chicago Cubs). Plan to continue ROM exercises as prescribed, ice, and e-stim.

2. Andrea has been ref. to OT for work on ADLs, following a TBI, Fx Ⓛ clavicle and humerus, and fx Ⓛ pelvis. Visited Andrea in her room to introduce her to OT and explain the schedule of visits. She has no mem. of accident or first week in the hospital. In the 5 minutes I spent with her, she asked my name 6X. Knows she is married, but cannot remember the names of her 4 children. She appears to tire easily, yawning often. She is agreeable to tx, but states she has no idea what she'd like to accomplish in OT; does not know what would be realistic for STGs. For a LTG, she would like to go home and live life like she did b/4 her accident.

SUMMARY

Buzzwords, jargon, and abbreviations can give the appearance that you are on top of things, that you know what you are doing. However, they can also become barriers to effective communication. As with most things in life, using buzzwords, jargon, and abbreviations in moderation is fine, but do not overdo it.

In documenting occupational therapy practice, regardless of the setting, choosing your words carefully is a critical step in the writing process. There are words that are trendy or send positive messages to the reader, and there are other words that send up red flags to the reader. Sometimes occupational therapists get so involved in describing things so accurately that only another occupational therapist can make any sense out of it. Other times, occupational therapists use abbreviations to the extent that they make the note hard to read. Always remember who the readers of the documentation could be so that you write for all audiences.

REFERENCES

Acquaviva, J. (1992). *Effective documentation for occupational therapy.* Bethesda, MD: American Occupational Therapy Association.

Administration and Management Special Interest Section. (2000). *Occupational therapy administrative reimbursement algorithm.* Retrieved January 5, 2000, from *www.aota.org/members/area2/docs/industrial.pdf*

American Occupational Therapy Association. (1994). Uniform terminology (3rd ed.). *American Journal of Occupational Therapy, 48* (11), 1047–1059.

American Occupational Therapy Association. (1999). *Occupational therapy services for children and youth under IDEA* (2nd ed.). Bethesda, MD: Author.

American Occupational Therapy Association. (2002). Occupational therapy practice framework: Domain and process. *American Journal of Occupational Therapy, 56,* 609–639.

Borcherding, S. (2000). *Documentation manual for writing SOAP notes in occupational therapy.* Thorofare, NJ: Slack.

Kettenback, G. (1990). *Writing SOAP notes.* Philadelphia: F. A. Davis.

Lunsford, A. A. (2001). *The everyday writer.* Boston: Bedford/St. Martin's.

World Health Organization. (2002). *International classification of function.* Geneva, Switzerland: Author. Retrieved May 22, 2002, from *http://www3.who.int/icf*

CHAPTER 2

The Occupational Therapy Practice Framework and Other Documents

INTRODUCTION

The language of the profession of occupational therapy is ever evolving. As the leaders and great thinkers of the profession review and revise the documents that guide the profession, the terminology used to describe occupational therapy changes. In addition, organizations external to occupational therapy, such as the World Health Organization, change the way words are used to describe the human condition. In this chapter, we explore the changes occurring in the last 10 years.

▼ INTERNATIONAL CLASSIFICATION OF FUNCTIONING, DISABILITY AND HEALTH ▼

The World Health Organization (WHO) has changed the way in which it looks at disability and functioning. With this new look comes a new set of words to describe disability and functioning. Instead of looking at the source of the dysfunction, WHO is looking at the outcomes of the dysfunction; the body structures and functions, activities and level of participation in life, and the environmental factors affecting performance (WHO, 2002). Instead of a label of particular disease, WHO suggests describing the client's level of functioning. This will enable health professionals and payers to determine if progress is being made. The WHO intends this document to standardize the terminology used across health professions and across the planet. The document, *International Classification of Functioning, Disability and Health* (ICF), provides a numerical coding system for every possible body part, body function, activity one can participate in, and environments and personal factors that can affect a person's ability to actively participate in life situations. Without going into detail about the more than 1,400 terms that are identified and described, this document can help clinicians think globally while labeling the tasks and activities that their clients engage in on a daily basis. At the WHO website there is a sample checklist to aid in gathering data about a client's function (*http://www3.who.int/icf/icftemplate.cfm . . . checklist.html& mytitle=ICF%20Checklist*). The American Occupational Therapy Association (AOTA) used the *ICF* during the development of the *Occupational Therapy Practice Framework*, which helps illustrate the importance of this document.

▼ UNIFORM TERMINOLOGY ▼

For many years, the AOTA had a document called *Uniform Terminology for Reporting Occupational Therapy Services, Third Edition* (AOTA, 1994). This document was commonly referred to as *Uniform Terminology* or simply *UT*. It contained a list of the domains of concern for occupational therapy; it defined terms that outlined the scope of practice for the profession. However, by the late 1990s it became apparent that major revisions in the document were necessary. In 2002, AOTA officially rescinded the document.

Uniform Terminology was useful for teaching about the profession, and many occupational therapists grew up speaking about occupational therapy in terms recognized by the document (AOTA, 1994). One concept that was taught at many college and university programs was looking at occupational therapy in terms of performance areas, performance components, and contexts. Performance areas were observable occupations in which a person might engage, including those occupations necessary for the care of oneself, the care of others, work and productive activities, and play/leisure activities. Performance components were the skills and abilities needed to perform occupations such as muscle strength, self-esteem, sensory perception, reflexes, sequencing skills, and memory. Contexts were those environmental factors and internal characteristics that influenced performance of occupation such as age, living situation, point in the disease process, support systems, and the availability of tools and equipment. These concepts were useful because an instructor could ask students to summarize an evaluation, being sure to address performance areas, performance components, and contexts, or that students write goals addressing client needs in performance areas (AOTA, 1994).

It is likely that in some settings, *Uniform Terminology* is still used. This may be because not every occupational therapist or occupational therapy assistant is a member of AOTA and therefore might not know that *Uniform Terminology* has been replaced. Those who are members of AOTA may not read the *American Journal of Occupational Therapy* (AJOT) cover to cover each month. It may also be used because some occupational therapists really liked its clean delineation of the occupational therapy scope of practice.

The reason that AOTA replaced *Uniform Terminology* is that it had become outdated as the practice of occupational therapy expanded and new terminology was being incorporated into the profession. The most glaring deficit of *Uniform Terminology* was that the term "occupation" was not mentioned in the document, yet occupation is at the core of the profession (AOTA, 2002). In addition, it was silent on the concept of spirituality and the terminology was not consistent with ICF.

▼ OCCUPATIONAL THERAPY PRACTICE FRAMEWORK ▼

In 2002, AOTA withdrew *Uniform Terminology* as an official document of the association. It was replaced by a document called the *Occupational Therapy Practice Framework: Domain and Process* (AOTA, 2002). Often referred to simply as *The Framework*, the document describes the processes involved in interactions between occupational therapists and clients. It describes best practices for occupational therapy with an emphasis on the use of occupations as a therapeutic agent. *The Framework* begins with an understanding of the occupational needs of any client (a client can be an individual, a family, a group, or a community) and ends with achieving occupational therapy outcomes that are focused on the client's "engagement in occupations to support participation in context or contexts" (AOTA, 2002, p. 610).

While *The Framework* is summarized here, it is not a sufficient substitute for reading the original document. *The Framework* is available from AOTA through its online store (*www.aota.org*) and at some campus bookstores.

The Framework makes a distinction between occupations and activities (AOTA, 2002). Activities are defined as actions that human beings take toward a goal. Occupations, on the other hand, have inherent meaning and value. The choices a person makes about how to spend one's time is greatly influenced by one's choices of occupations. A person's sense of identity and competence are also influenced by the occupations in which that person engages. This distinction, while subtle at first glance, is a significant one. It is why the profession is called occupational therapy and not activity therapy. We do hundreds of activities each day that move us toward some goal, such as reading a textbook chapter in order to pass a course. This activity helps us reach a goal, but for some students, the act of reading that particular chapter may not have great personal meaning or value. Both activities and occupations are important to occupational therapy practitioners because of the effect each has on the state of a person's health and well-being (AOTA, 2002).

Domain of Occupational Therapy

The Framework uses the phrase "engagement in occupation to support participation in context or contexts" (AOTA, 2002, p. 610) to represent the domain of occupational therapy practice. There are six areas in the domain of occupational therapy and no one area is of greater importance than any other. The areas are illustrated in Figure 2.1. Each level of the domain influences performance for the level above it.

Areas of occupation are the observable acts that a person wants or needs to do (AOTA, 2002). Within these areas are seven categories:

- *Activities of daily living:* Those things we do to take care of ourselves, including bathing/showering, bowel and bladder management, dressing, eating, feeding, functional mobility, personal device care, personal hygiene and grooming, sexual activity, and sleep/rest.

- *Instrumental activities of daily living:* Those things we do to interact with the environment such as care of others, care of pets, childrearing, communication device use, community mobility, financial management, health management and maintenance, home establishment and management, meal preparation and cleanup, safety procedures and emergency responses, and shopping.

- *Education:* Those things we do as a student or to participate in a learning environment including exploring and participating in both formal and informal learning situations.

- *Work:* Those things we do to engage in paid employment or volunteer experiences such as identifying, seeking, and obtaining paid work, performance at work, preparing for and adjusting to retirement, and exploring and participating in volunteer experiences.

- *Play:* Those things we do simply for "enjoyment, entertainment, amusement or diversion" (Parham & Fazio, 1997, as cited in AOTA, 2002, p 621), including both exploration and participation in play.

- *Leisure:* Those things we do when we are not obligated to do anything else, including both exploration and participation in leisure.

- *Social participation:* Those things we do when we are interacting with others, whether that interaction takes place between friends/peers, family, or community.

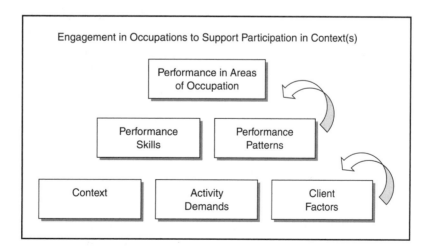

FIGURE 2.1 Domain of Occupational Therapy. *Based on the Occupational Therapy Practice Framework: Domain and Process by the American Occupational Therapy Association (2002).*

In *The Framework* (AOTA, 2002), performance skills and performance patterns enable a person's performance in areas of occupation. Performance skills are the building blocks of activities and occupations. They are small, observable, and purposeful. In *The Framework*, there are three categories of performance skills:

- *Motor skills* are those skills involved in moving including posture, mobility, coordination, strength and effort, and energy.
- *Process skills* are those used to manage or modify task performance such as energy, knowledge, temporal organization, organizing space and objects, and adaptation.
- *Communication/interaction skills* are those that are required for getting one's wants, needs, and intentions across to others, including nonverbal communication, giving and receiving messages, and appropriate relationships.

Performance patterns can be habitual or routine (AOTA, 2002). Habits are things we do without thinking. Some habits are useful in that they contribute to life satisfaction, like brushing one's teeth after every meal can prevent or delay the unpleasantness of having cavities filled. Others are dominating and interfere with daily life, as in obsessive–compulsive disorder. Impoverished habits either do not support daily life, or need practice to improve. Routines are "occupations with established sequences" (Christiansen & Baum, 1997, as cited in AOTA, 2002, p. 623). An example of this might be always putting the right shoe on before the left, or always taking a particular route to work, regardless of traffic delays.

Contexts are conditions that exist within or around a person that have an influence on the individual's performance (AOTA, 2002). *The Framework* names seven kinds of contexts:

- *Cultural contexts* represent the expectations of society and customs and beliefs of the community in which the client is a member. They can include political, legal, economic, educational, and employment opportunities.
- *Physical contexts* are natural and human-made space, objects, people, plants, and animals.
- *Social contexts* concern groups of people and the influences that they have on the performance of an individual. People can include relatives, friends, caregivers, and members of an organization in this context.
- *Personal contexts* are unique to the individual and include age, gender, financial status, employment status, educational status, and living situation.
- *Spiritual contexts* relate to the things that motivate and give meaning to a person's life.
- *Temporal contexts* include aspects of performance that relate to time, such as developmental age, life stages, seasonal considerations, and time of day.
- *Virtual contexts* are those where communication takes place without physical contact between people, such as via computers, radio, or telephone.

The demands of an activity are defined as those aspects of an activity that are needed to carry out that activity (AOTA, 2002). For example, some demands of the activity of grocery shopping include mobility enough to push a grocery cart, remove items from store shelves, and put them in the cart; money management to purchase items; and an understanding of social expectations for behavior in a public space. The aspects of activity demands identified by AOTA (2002) in *The Framework* include:

- Objects and their properties (things needed to carry out the activity such as tools and the inherent properties [weight, size, etc.] of the objects)
- Space demands (aspects of the physical environment such as temperature, lighting, noise, room size and color, etc.)
- Social demands (aspects of social and cultural contexts related to that activity such as rules for social conduct, social interaction, etc.)

- Sequence and timing (being aware of the order in which things happen, how quickly or slowly they happen)
- Required actions (the "doing" part of the activity, in terms of physical, process, and interaction skills; what any performer of the activity must do)
- Required body functions (what the body and mind do during the activity including mobility, cognitive processes, sensory functions, and functions of other body systems)
- Required body structures (parts of the body that are needed to engage in the activity)

The difference between activity demands and client factors is that activity demands are based on a particular activity and include conditions external and internal to the client. Client factors are identified regardless of the activity and are internal to the client.

In *The Framework*, there are two main client factors (AOTA, 2002). One client factor is body structures; anatomical parts and systems. The other is body functions; the physiological, cognitive, and psychological processes that occur inside a person. Specific examples of body functions include, but are not limited to, orientation, temperament, memory, proprioception, and muscle tone and reflexes.

Process

The process of occupational therapy, at its most simple, involves evaluation, intervention, and outcomes (AOTA, 2002). The process is intended to be "dynamic and interactive in nature" (AOTA, 2002, p. 614). While there is a fixed starting point (the occupational profile), the other parts of the process interact with and influence the other parts throughout occupational therapy service delivery.

The evaluation process has two substeps; the occupational profile and the analysis of occupational performance (AOTA, 2002). The occupational profile helps the occupational therapist understand "the client's occupational history and experiences, patterns of daily living, interests, values and needs" (AOTA, 2002, p. 616). The occupational therapist gathers information by interviewing the client or client's surrogate (i.e., a parent when the client is a child). The type of information gathered is influenced by the frame of reference and/or theories employed by the occupational therapist. Knowledge of disease processes, medical and psychiatric conditions, and human anatomy and physiology are also used to help guide the occupational therapist in gathering information about the client. While the occupational profile is the first step in the evaluation process, it is adjusted as the client moves through the process and new data comes to light.

The second step of the evaluation is the analysis of occupational performance (AOTA, 2002). In this step, more data is gathered about the client in relation to the domains of occupational therapy practice. The process of analyzing occupational performance includes identifying both barriers and facilitators to successful engagement in occupations. The frame of reference and/or theories used by the occupational therapist will influence the manner in which this data is gathered.

There are three substeps in the intervention process: the intervention plan, intervention implementation, and intervention review (AOTA, 2002). First, the plan is developed using the data gathered in the evaluation process. The intervention plan is influenced by the frame of reference and/or theories used by the occupational therapist and must be directed by goals established in collaboration with the client (AOTA, 1998, 2002). Other influences on the intervention plan include care for the well-being of the client, the setting, and the domains of occupational practice (AOTA, 2002).

The intervention plan requires identifying specific strategies to help the client achieve desired outcomes (AOTA, 2002). There are five strategic approaches to intervention that an occupational therapist could take in developing the plan (AOTA, 2002; Harvison, 2003):

1. Create or promote (health promotion)
2. Establish or restore (remediation, restoration, habilitation, rehabilitation)
3. Maintain

4. Modify (compensation, adaptation)
5. Prevent (disability prevention)

There are four main kinds of interventions that can be used to help the client achieve established outcomes (AOTA, 2002; Harvison, 2003):

1. Therapeutic use of self
2. Therapeutic use of occupations and activities (occupation-based activities, purposeful activities, and preparatory methods)
3. Consultation
4. Education

Intervention implementation involves putting the words of the plan into action (AOTA, 2002). Once the strategy and kinds of intervention are established, the occupational therapist or occupational therapy assistant works in collaboration with the client to execute the plan.

Periodically during the intervention implementation, the intervention must be reviewed to determine whether it is making a difference in the occupational performance of the client (AOTA, 2002). The plan is evaluated, and if necessary, modified to enable the client to most efficiently and effectively achieve the desired outcomes. During the intervention review, a determination is made as to whether or not to continue to provide occupational therapy intervention, or to make referrals to other professionals.

The last step in the process is the outcome (AOTA, 2002). Outcomes can be identified and measured in a variety of ways. One way of measuring the outcome of occupational therapy interventions is by measuring the occupational performance of the client. This can include looking at whether the client has improved (from some deficit in performance), maintained, or enhanced (when no deficit is present) performance in an area of occupation. Other types of outcomes include client satisfaction, role competence, adaptation, health and wellness, prevention, and quality of life.

▼ SPECIFIC OCCUPATIONAL THERAPY TERMS ▼

Occupational therapy practitioners often use terms they learn in school. This is usually a good thing. However, sometimes the way in which terms are used changes in official documents of the profession. If a practitioner is unaware of these changes, he or she may be using terms incorrectly in current practice. The following is a list of terms whose meanings have changed over the last decade (AOTA, 1998):

Assessment: The tools used in the evaluation process. It is sometimes incorrectly used interchangeably with the term "evaluation." Assessments can be written tests or performance checklists. They can be standardized or nonstandardized, criterion-referenced or norm-referenced. Some people use the terms "assessment" and "screening" interchangeably, with "evaluation" referring to a higher level of investigation and interpretation.

Evaluation: The process of gathering and interpreting data to establish the current level of function of a client. The evaluation can include the use of assessments, observations, chart review, and interviews of the client and caregiver, as well as the clinician's interpretation of the meaning of the data that is gathered.

Screening: A brief encounter with a client for the purpose of determining whether or not a full-blown evaluation is warranted.

Intervention: The act of providing services to clients. It is a broad term that can include direct and indirect services. It replaces the term "treatment." Intervention is an appropriate term to use in any setting, be it medical, social, or educational.

Treatment: Implies that the therapist is doing something *to* the client, not *with* the client, and as such, is falling out of favor.

Discharge: Also falling out of favor; describes the process of ending treatment (the word "treatment" was used then). It is used in some settings to refer to when the client is leaving a facility.

Discontinuation: Ending intervention with a client. The client may or may not be discharged from the facility. Rather than saying that one is "discharging a client," one now says "discontinuing therapy." It places the focus on the services provided and not on the client.

Other professions may use these terms in other ways, and they are not wrong. Each profession has its own standard. Some facilities may also use terms in certain ways. While it is very important to follow the standards established by your professional organization, it is also important to communicate clearly with coworkers in other professions. If there is any doubt about how a term is being used at a particular facility, ask a department head who has been at the facility for a few years or more. This will be an experienced professional who can advise you on how to best be understood by others at the facility.

Exercise 2.1

Using the following key, place the appropriate letter in the blank in front of each phrase.

A = Area of occupation
P = Performance skill
C = Client factor

1. _____ Combing one's hair
2. _____ Elbow range of motion
3. _____ Wheelchair mobility
4. _____ Making one's needs known
5. _____ Hand strength
6. _____ Career exploration
7. _____ Time management
8. _____ Understanding nonverbal communication
9. _____ Posture
10. _____ Endurance
11. _____ Knitting
12. _____ Balancing a checkbook
13. _____ Making eye contact

SUMMARY

The American Occupational Therapy Association has developed guidelines for the practice of occupational therapy, which in turn influences the words we use in occupational therapy documentation. The *Occupational Therapy Practice Framework* is a document that seeks to describe the process of providing occupational therapy services to clients across practice settings and to describe the domains of occupational therapy practice. The process begins with understanding the occupational needs of any client, and then an analysis of the client's occupational performance. Intervention is then planned and implemented in order to assist the client in achieving his or her desired outcomes. The outcome of any occupational therapy intervention is "engagement in occupation to support participation in context or contexts" (AOTA, 2002, p. 611). The *Practice Framework* describes seven domains of occupational therapy practice: (1) activities of daily living, (2) instrumental activities of daily living, (3) education, (4) work, (5) play, (6) leisure, and (7) social participation

(AOTA, 2002). This document also includes recommended language for discussing the work of an occupational therapist, including a glossary of terms.

Some facilities may still use the *Uniform Terminology* document that AOTA developed years ago. However, the AOTA has rescinded that document, and the terminology used in it is no longer considered correct. *Uniform Terminology* provided a system of organizing the domains of practice, but it did not address the process of providing occupational therapy services (AOTA, 2003).

In addition to AOTA, the World Health Organization has also developed a taxonomy for describing human function and dysfunction called *International Classification of Function* (ICF). The language of that document is also helpful in choosing words that members of other disciplines will understand. The language used by the *ICF* was influential in the development of the *Occupational Therapy Practice Framework.*

It is critical to use terminology that is understood and accepted by both others in the profession and those outside of the profession. The more consistent occupational therapy personnel are in using terminology, the more likely the documentation is to be understood by others.

Using the language of the profession can strengthen one's documentation. Your words carry the weight of the best minds in the profession. In addition, you show that you are current in your understanding of the profession by using the words of the professional association. The importance of staying up to date with the profession should never be overlooked.

REFERENCES

American Occupational Therapy Association. (1994). Uniform terminology for occupational therapy, 3rd edition. *American Journal of Occupational Therapy, 48*, 1047–1054.

American Occupational Therapy Association. (1998). Standards of practice for occupational therapy. *American Journal of Occupational Therapy, 52*, 866–869.

American Occupational Therapy Association. (2002). Occupational therapy practice framework: Domain and process. *American Journal of Occupational Therapy, 56*, 609–639.

Harvison, N. (2003). Overview of the occupational therapy practice framework: Part 1. *Administration and Management Special Interest Section Quarterly, 19*(1), 1–4.

World Health Organization. (2002). *International classification of functioning disability and health.* Geneva, Switzerland: Author. Retrieved May 22, 2002, from *http://www3.who.int/icf*

CHAPTER 3

Impact of Models and Frames of Reference

INTRODUCTION

In the last chapter we discussed the ways in which the language of the profession is changing. In addition to staying current on terminology, the words an occupational therapist uses while summarizing evaluation results, planning intervention, reporting progress, and planning discontinuation will also depend on the model or frame of reference being used for a particular client.

▼ DESCRIPTION OF MODELS AND FRAMES OF REFERENCE ▼

Depending on which textbook you read, the definition of a model and of a frame of reference will vary. Both models and frames of reference are based on theory and help organize knowledge so that it can be used to guide an occupational therapist in determining the cause of dysfunction and ways to assist a client to engage in occupations that are meaningful to the client.

According to Mosey (as cited in Christiansen & Baum, 1991), a model integrates theoretical assumptions for use in practice. Mosey describes a model as

> A profession's model is the typical way in which a profession perceives itself, its relationship to other professions, and its association with the society to which it is responsible. The model of a profession is characterized by a description of the profession's philosophical assumptions, ethical code, theoretical foundations, domain of concern, legitimate tools, and the nature of and principles for sequencing the various aspects of practice (as cited in Kielhofner, 1997, p. 325).

Christiansen and Baum (1991) describe a model as referring to ways of structuring or organizing information that is relevant to practice and for the purpose of guiding thinking.

A frame of reference is closely related to a model, but is typically more specific in terms of application of knowledge and information. A frame of reference is a bridge between theory and practice. It takes the knowledge we have and organizes it in such a way that it can be applied to working with clients (Christiansen & Baum, 1997). Frames of reference are based on theory and provide direction for evaluating, planning and implementing intervention, and discontinuing services. According to Mosey (as cited in Christiansen & Baum, 1991), frames of reference are the portions of models that are methodological in focus; they tell the occupational therapist how to use the information in practice. She goes on to say that frames of reference should provide the following: "1) information on the domain of concern; 2) the theories upon which their assertions are based; 3) the nature of function and dysfunction; 4) behaviors which reflect these states; and 5) the principles regarding intervention on how one can change from a dysfunctional to a functional state" (pp. 12–13).

Think of a frame of reference or model as being the lens through which you see your client. Just as different-colored lenses (i.e., sunglasses) change the way you see your surroundings and what parts of the environment stand out, so do different frames of reference change what parts of the client's situation stand out. For example, a biomechanical frame of reference (Hagedorn, 1997; Kielhofner, 1997; Neistadt & Crepeau, 1998) looks at structural enhancements such as strengthening, decreasing edema, and splinting to improve movement in an injured limb while a task-oriented frame of reference (Hagedorn, 1997; Kielhofner, 1997; Neistadt & Crepeau, 1998) looks at finding goal-directed functional behaviors to encourage use of the affected limb. In this example, the biomechanical approach has a focus on client factors and performance skills (AOTA, 2002) while the task-oriented approach looks at performance patterns and performance in areas of occupation (AOTA, 2002).

Some models or frames of reference focus on getting at the root cause of the dysfunction. Others focus on the level of dysfunction and ways to minimize it, regardless of the cause. Some use a developmental focus, others an environmental one.

In later chapters, we will discuss the mechanics of writing goals and completing different types of documents. This chapter focuses on identifying different models and frames of reference and how the word choices may vary between them.

▼ HOW MODELS AND FRAMES OF REFERENCE ARE REFLECTED IN DOCUMENTATION ▼

Table 3.1 summarizes different frames of reference used in occupational therapy and hints for how that frame of reference can be reflected in one's documentation. Please note that the summaries of these frames of reference are not intended to be comprehensive or all-inclusive. Because of the vast number of new and developing frames of reference, it would be impossible to cover every one. Memorizing this table will not tell you everything you need to know about each frame of reference.

The reader is referred to the sources used in developing this chapter for more information on each frame of reference. Note that the order in which the frames of reference are presented is completely random and should not be seen as hierarchical.

Having a good understanding of the frame of reference you are using will help you in writing reports and notes and in establishing goals. Often the frame of reference will suggest certain terminology.

People who work together at one facility tend to all use the same model or frame of reference, or the same mix of them. When you start working (or go on fieldwork) at a new place, be sure to ask which models or frames of reference are acceptable to use. Usually, but not always, more than one frame of reference is used at a facility or program. When multiple models or frames of reference are blended together, it is sometimes called an eclectic approach. Hopefully, this blending occurs in a thoughtful way, based on the collective experiences of the occupational therapy staff and the types of clients being served in that program or facility. However, sometimes occupational therapists say they are eclectic in their approach when they are unable to name a specific model or frame of reference.

Exercise 3.1

Are the following goals compatible with the frame of reference cited?

1. In the next 30 days, the client will increase range of motion of shoulder flexion from 40° to 60°. (Bobath)

2. Child will eat at least one meal per day, for 5 consecutive days, that contains at least three different textures without screaming, spitting, or turning away by June 15, 2004. (Sensory Integration)

3. Robert will consistently brush his teeth twice per day, without cues from his parents, by November 24, 2004. (Model of Human Occupation)

4. In 1 month, Sonja will independently ride the bus from home to work. (Behavioral)

5. In 6 months, DeNeda will demonstrate the self-care and home-maintenance skills necessary for her to return home to independent living. (Psychoanalytical)

6. In 6 weeks, Chris will word-process at a rate of 60 words per minute with two or fewer errors. (Cognitive Behavioral Therapy)

TABLE 3.1   Influence of Frames of Reference on Documentation

Frame of Reference	Description of Key Concepts	How It Is Reflected in Documentation
Biomechanical	Focus on "the body as a machine." Improve function through strength, endurance, and structural integrity. Use splinting, exercise, massage, biofeedback, and other physical means of intervention. Once range of motion, strength, edema, and endurance are regained, functional use will follow. Pain, loss of sensation, and poor coordination are not of primary concern.	Evaluation reports focus on performance skills/client factors. Progress notes reflect improvements in range of motion, strength, edema, and endurance. Range of motion, strength, edema, and endurance are easily quantified for goal setting. Functional goals would reflect new activities that increased movement will allow.
Contemporary Task-Oriented (Haugen & Mathiowetz)	Focus on the interaction between the characteristics of a person and the contexts in which the person exists. The personal and environmental characteristics have no hierarchy in terms of their influences on performance. The client's perspective is the focus of evaluation and intervention; it is client-centered. Intervention involves practice and experimentation.	Evaluation reports center on the client's unique characteristics, contexts, and motivations. Recording observations is essential in progress notes. Goals relate to functional performance.
Rehabilitative (Compensatory)	Emphasis is on what the client can do, the strengths. Through the use of compensatory techniques, a client can gain independence in self-care skills.	Evaluation reports emphasize both strengths and areas in need of improvement. Progress notes document what types of adaptations have been tried and the results of each trial.

(continued)

TABLE 3.1   Influence of Frames of Reference on Documentation *(continued)*

Frame of Reference	Description of Key Concepts	How It Is Reflected in Documentation
	A person's motivation and environments play a key role in the rehabilitative process. Intervention centers on the use of adaptive and assistive equipment, modification of environments, modification of techniques, and heavy use of teaching/learning techniques.	Goals do not specify specific techniques, tools, or equipment. Goals reflect functional outcomes, what the client will do.
Neurodevelopmental Treatment (NDT) (Bobaths)	Spasticity and hypotonia are the major barriers to normal movement. The trunk and proximal joints need stability to enable limb movement. The brain is plastic and capable of new learning. Work toward inhibiting abnormal reflexes and synergies to enable learning of normal movement. Bilateral focus; use positioning, handling, and sensory stimulation to facilitate normal movement patterns.	Evaluation reports focus on observations of movement patterns and barriers to normal movement. Progress notes need to reflect frequent clinical observations. Goals relate to patterns of movement that enable occupational performance.
Proprioceptive Neuromuscular Facilitation (PNF) (Knott & Voss)	Weakness and lack of voluntary control over movements are the main obstacles to normal movement patterns. Stimulating the proprioceptors promotes or hastens the response of the neuromuscular mechanism. Frequent repetition and stimulation support the learning of new motor abilities. Movements are more often diagonal than linear. Vision, breathing, and verbal commands all play a strong role in movement.	Evaluation reports emphasize observable movement patterns. Progress notes reflect client responses to inhibition and facilitation techniques. Goals relate to the client's movements during activities of daily living.

(continued)

TABLE 3.1 Influence of Frames of Reference on Documentation *(continued)*

Frame of Reference	Description of Key Concepts	How It Is Reflected in Documentation
Sensory Integration (Ayers)	Sensory integrative dysfunction is a result of a failure of the brain to properly organize sensory input. Dynamic systems process; a spiral of brain organization and adaptive behavior. There is interaction between brain organization and adaptive behavior. People have an inner drive to participate in sensory motor activities and seek out organizing sensations. Play is self-directed, within an environment carefully set up by the OT to meet that client's needs. Environment provides the opportunities to experience needed sensations in a safe, nonthreatening atmosphere, and includes access to sensory input to all sensory processing systems of the body, including vestibular.	Evaluation reports focus on identifying areas of sensory processing deficits and how these impact participation in everyday life experiences. Progress notes reflect the child's responses to different sensory experiences, qualities of movement, and changes in the child's participation in everyday life experiences. Goals focus on increased duration or repetitions of an activity, or the quality of movements during an activity.
Model of Human Occupation (Kielhofner, 1997)	Person viewed as an open system. Volition, habituation, and performance are hierarchical subsystems within a person that regulate choice, organization, and performance. Personal and environmental factors influence choice, organization, and performance. Change is a holistic process. Individuals are given the opportunity for guided participation in life tasks to improve organization, function, and adaptation as demonstrated by successful role performance. Occupations must be relevant and related to a person's roles, habits, and the environment.	Evaluation reports focus on the client's performance in areas of occupation. Progress notes focus on the client's performance during meaningful occupations. Goals relate to performance in occupations that are meaningful to the client.

(continued)

TABLE 3.1   Influence of Frames of Reference on Documentation *(continued)*

Frame of Reference	Description of Key Concepts	How It Is Reflected in Documentation
Person–Environment–Occupational Performance (Christiansen & Baum)	Many intrinsic (neurobehavioral, physiological, cognitive, psychological, and emotional) and extrinsic (physical, cultural, societal, and social support) factors contribute to occupational performance. Adaptation is the process used by people to meet challenges in daily living though the use of personal resources. The characteristics of the person, environment, and the nature/meaning of actions, tasks, and roles are considered when trying to understand occupational performance. Focus is on the person's wants and needs rather than on dysfunction.	Evaluation reports reflect the client's assets and limitations in relation to his or her occupational performance within environmental contexts. Progress reports demonstrate the client's occupational performance within environmental contexts. Short-term goals may relate to intrinsic factors inhibiting occupational performance. Long-term goals may relate to functional performance of daily life tasks and roles.
Developmental (Mosey)	Humans normally develop in a sequential fashion. Each new gain in structure enables a gain in function; each new gain in function enables further development. Physical, sensory, perceptual, cognitive, social, and emotional development are interconnected and affect the whole person. Stress can cause regression to earlier levels of adaptation. Focus on seven developmental areas: Perceptual–Motor, Cognitive, Drive–Object, Dyadic Interaction, Group Interaction, Self-Identity, and Sexual Identity.	Evaluation reports focus on comparing a child's performance to that of a typically developing child of the same chronological age to identify areas in need of intervention. Progress reports show the child has made gains in functional performance of daily occupations. Goals identify desired occupations to enable the child's maximum participation in life situations.
Spatiotemporal Adaptation (Gilfoyle, Grady, & Moore)	Movement and activity influence a person's development. Movement is important for physical, psychological,	Evaluation reports focus on the movements of the child in relation to environmental demands. Progress reports reflect the increasing complexity of the movement—

(continued)

TABLE 3.1   Influence of Frames of Reference on Documentation *(continued)*

Frame of Reference	Description of Key Concepts	How It Is Reflected in Documentation
	and social development of a child. Development occurs in an ever-widening spiral that represents increasing skills as influenced by experiences with the environment. Emphasis on integration of old behaviors with new ones.	environment interactions of the child. Goals can be structured to reflect prevention, remediation, and/or adjustment to dysfunction.
Ecology of Human Performance (Dunn)	Ecology is the interaction between a person and contexts (the environment). The person, the context, and task performance interact with and affect one another. Performance is improved by establishing/restoring the person's skills or abilities, or altering/adapting the context or the task to support performance in context.	Evaluation reports look not only at the person, but also contexts and tasks and the person–context match. Progress reports describe what interventions/alterations have been tried and their results. Goals reflect the person's performance in context.
Cognitive Disabilities (also called Cognition & Activity) (Allen)	Neurological problems lead to limitations in cognitive capacity, which lead to a performance deficit. Cognitive limitations occur as cognitive levels (6) on a continuum. Occupational therapy cannot change cognitive levels that are the result of brain pathology. Palliative treatment attempts to reduce symptoms by changing the tasks (adapting) a patient is asked to do. Expectant treatment means that nature takes its course, and the role of the OT is to document and monitor the patient's functional abilities. Supportive treatment is like maintenance treatment; the goal is to sustain strength during illness and recovery, using things like diversional activities.	Evaluation reports identify the current cognitive level as supported by descriptions of functional performance in everyday occupations. Progress notes describe the client's response to adaptations in the task or environment and any changes noted in cognitive level (based on observations). Goals are established to identify desired performance within the context of the client's environment.

(continued)

How Models and Frames of Reference Are Reflected in Documentation   **27**

TABLE 3.1   Influence of Frames of Reference on Documentation *(continued)*

Frame of Reference	Description of Key Concepts	How It Is Reflected in Documentation
	Tasks and activities are analyzed for fit with a person's cognitive level, they are adapted to remove obstacles to performance and use a person's available cognitive capacity.	
Psychoanalytic (Freud); Object Relations (Fidler)	Intrapsychic (unconscious) conflicts are at the heart of the problem. The major areas of concern are the psychodynamics, level of psychosexual and psychosocial development, and alterations of intrapsychic content. Goal is to resolve these inner-conflicts. Use of activity to resolve intrapsychic conflict and reality orientation such as psychodrama, projective art, creative writing and poetry therapy, and guided fantasy.	Evaluation reports focus on the affect of the client, symptoms of psychopathology, and how these interfere with daily life functions. Progress reports often reflect the client's subjective report of feelings as well as observations of client behavior. Goals are hard to define, but could reflect the client's self-expression of feelings.
Occupational Behavior (Reilly)	Active participation in tasks can lead to development of mastery and therefore, permit successful role performance. Focus is on activities of daily living, play, and work. Role fulfillment provides positive feedback to the person and enables that person to go on to new skills, more complex tasks. Skills become habits through repetition. Through the continuum of work–play, a person learns the roles needed to become competent in mastery.	Evaluation reports focus on activities of daily living, play, and work. Progress notes focus on the client's performance during meaningful occupations. Goals relate to performance in occupations that are meaningful to the client and address the different environments in which the client spends time.
Behavioral (Skinner, Pavlov)	Insight and personality are not considered. A person's behavior is the result of feedback from the environment.	Evaluation reports contain detailed observations of behavior including frequency of behavior and where and when behavior occurs.

(continued)

TABLE 3.1 Influence of Frames of Reference on Documentation *(continued)*

Frame of Reference	Description of Key Concepts	How It Is Reflected in Documentation
	One can unlearn maladaptive behaviors and learn adaptive ones through the use of participative techniques such as shaping, teaching, and reinforcement. OT works with others on the team to consistently work toward positive changes in behavior.	Progress notes document behavior modification methods used and the results of these interventions. Measurable goals specify the person, the observable behavior expected, and conditions for the behavior such as where, when, frequency, and any cuing that will occur.
Cognitive-Behavioral Therapy (Bandura; Rotter; Ellis; and Beck)	Maladaptive behaviors are the result of cognitive distortions and self-defeating thinking. People have automatic thoughts that they tell themselves internally. "Core schemas" are the thoughts people tell themselves that color the way they perceive themselves and their environment. Clients are taught to repeat positive "self-talk" to alter the core schemas. Clients are taught to challenge logically the core schemas and automatic thoughts they had.	Evaluation reports focus on client report of feelings and thoughts about oneself. Progress notes reflect client's report of feelings and thoughts. Goals suggest the positive statements the client will repeat to oneself, use of stress management techniques, and identify desired behavioral outcomes.

Sources: Christiansen, C. & Baum, C. (1997); Hagedorn, R. (1997); Kielhofaer, G. (1997); and Neistadt, M. S. & Crepeau, E. B (1998).

SUMMARY

Models and frames of reference are ways to organize one's thinking about how to approach a client, and guide the way an occupational therapist evaluates, plans and implements interventions, and determines when a client has achieved desired outcomes. Both models and frames of reference are based on theory.

The model or frame of reference that you choose to work from with a given client needs to be reflected in the way you document about that client. Often the words used in documentation are suggested by the model or frame of reference being used. A model or frame of reference is used to help you select an appropriate evaluation method, set goals, and describe progress. You can use Table 3.1 to help in ensuring that your documentation is reflective of the model or frame of reference being used. Some facilities or programs use multiple models or frames of reference.

REFERENCES

American Occupational Therapy Association. (2002). Occupational therapy practice framework: Domain and process. *American Journal of Occupational Therapy, 56*, 609–639.

Christiansen, C., & Baum, C. (1991). *Occupational therapy: Enabling function and well-being.* Thoroughfare, NJ: Slack.

Christiansen, C., & Baum, C. (1997). *Occupational therapy: Enabling function and well-being* (2nd ed.). Thoroughfare, NJ: Slack.

Hagedorn, R. (1997). *Foundations for practice in occupational therapy* (2nd ed.). London: Churchill Livingstone.

Kielhofner, G. (1997). *Conceptual foundations of occupational therapy.* Philadelphia: F. A. Davis.

Neistadt, M. S., & Crepeau, E. B. (1998). *Willard & Spackman's occupational therapy* (9th ed.). Philadelphia: Lippencott-Raven.

CHAPTER 4

Document with CARE: General Tips for Good Documentation

INTRODUCTION

If you have read the previous chapters, you know that careful wording in documentation is essential. There is a system for double-checking your documentation so that you can be assured that it will be well written. This system is called "Document with CARE" (Sames & Berkeland, 1998). CARE is an abbreviation for:

Clarity: The reader can understand what you are saying.
Accuracy: The documentation reflects what actually happened.
Relevance: The documentation relates to identified needs and purposes.
Exceptions: Any unusual occurrences, noncompliance, or changes are documented.

Let's examine each of these criteria one at a time.

▼ CLARITY ▼

In order for the reader to understand what you have written, it has to be written in clear, concise, unbiased language (Sames & Berkeland, 1998). Abbreviations and jargon need to be kept to a minimum, and when used, must be approved by the facility in which they are used. Grammar and spelling should not interfere with the professional appearance and intended message of the documentation. While computers are often used for formal documentation, any handwritten notes must be legible. These seem like common sense things, but you would be amazed at some of the documentation that is out there (Sames & Berkeland, 1998).

▼ ACCURACY ▼

Your documentation needs to be factually correct (Sames & Berkeland, 1998). Documentation is almost always done chronologically, that is, what happens first is written about first, and then events are recorded in the order in which they happen. Documentation also needs to be consistent with the protocols of the institution or agency involved. Documentation written away from the client's medical record or chart is placed in the correct file. Never document about another client by name in your client's record. For example, if Mr. Smith and Mr. Jones play checkers, and you are writing in Mr. Smith's chart, you may say that Mr. Smith played checkers with another client, but do not put Mr. Jones's name in Mr. Smith's note (Sames & Berkeland, 1998).

Another aspect of accuracy is distinguishing between what you observe and what you think it means (Sames & Berkeland, 1998). This will be addressed more completely in Chapter 9. In the meantime, think about the following. You observe a client with a plate of food in front of her and a fork in her right hand. She uses her right hand to scoop up the food and begins to raise the food to her mouth. The fork tips and the food falls off. She lowers her fork to the plate and scoops at the food, pushing the food off her plate. She then drops the fork and picks up the food with her fingers. If in your note you write, "The client made two attempts to feed herself with a fork, then proceeded to feed herself with her fingers," you are truly describing what you saw. If in your note you write, "The client is unable to feed herself with a fork. She gets frustrated and starts using her fingers," then you are interpreting what you saw. You are generalizing a short, one-time observation into applying to every time she eats. There are times when your interpretation is as important, or more important, than your description, but you must be careful to identify when you are describing and when you are interpreting a client's performance (Sames & Berkeland, 1998).

▼ RELEVANCE ▼

Based on what you write, the reader must see why occupational therapy was initiated, continued, and discontinued (Sames & Berkeland, 1998). In other words, the documentation must demonstrate the need for skilled service. By skilled service, I mean services requiring the expertise of an occupational therapist or an occupational therapy assistant under the supervision of an occupational therapist. The reader needs to see that what you are doing in occupational therapy is something that uses the unique skills and abilities of occupational therapy practitioners. When the occupational therapy practitioner is working in a transdisciplinary model (a model of service delivery in which several professionals from different disciplines all fulfill the same role, there is little or no differentiation between what each person does), then the documentation needs to reflect the client's need for the program's services (Sames & Berkeland, 1998).

When the chart is read from beginning to end, it should be clear that the results of the screening (if there is one), the referral, the evaluation, the intervention planning, the intervention, and the discontinuation have a common theme. In other words, if an adult with chronic schizophrenia is referred to occupational therapy to learn to live independently, then the evaluation summary should be centered on independent living skills, the intervention plan should address independent living skills, the progress notes should demonstrate work on independent living skills, and the discontinuation summary should also reflect the client's skills in independent living. If a child is referred to you to improve handwriting skills, then the documentation should reflect work on handwriting skills. This does not mean that you cannot document work on any other domain of concern, but other domains are documented only after demonstrating additional needs in those areas.

Documentation should always be timely (Sames & Berkeland, 1998). This means the documentation, in order to be relevant, needs to be done as close to the time as the event occurred. Generally, evaluation reports are done within a day or two of completing the evaluation; intervention plans are done according to the schedule of the facility (annually, bimonthly, or monthly); progress notes are often done at the close of each visit to occupational therapy; and discontinuation summaries are usually completed within 2 days of discharge. Each facility will have standards related to timeliness. These standards are to be taken seriously, not as general targets, but as deadlines (Sames & Berkeland, 1998).

Other relevant information needs to be available in the client's record. If there are precautions or contraindications that must be observed, they need to be documented (Sames & Berkeland, 1998). It is not necessary to include them on every piece of documentation, as long as they are easy to find in the client's chart. These can be very relevant to the activities and tasks selected during intervention (Sames & Berkeland, 1998).

There can be a tendency to overdocument. Out of fear of lawsuits, fear of forgetting something, or just plain verbosity, some people write very long documents. Time is precious, and time spent documenting is time spent away from clients. Eliminate all but the most necessary information (Sames & Berkeland, 1998). Ask yourself, is this relevant? If you are working with a client on managing a checkbook, is it necessary to document what the client is wearing? Is it necessary to document what the client says about the weather? Is it necessary to document about how the client holds the pen? The answers are no, no, and maybe. You would only document about how the client holds the pen if the act of writing was important to the case. If you were working on managing a checkbook because of cognitive deficits, then how the client holds the pen is not particularly relevant, unless the client used to know what a pen was and how to hold it and today he or she looked at it like it was a new and strange object (Sames & Berkeland, 1998).

▼ EXCEPTIONS ▼

Any unusual occurrences or events need to be documented (Sames & Berkeland, 1998). In the example above, if the client had suffered a traumatic brain injury, was progressing nicely, then suddenly did not recognize a pen, this would be unusual, and possibly indicate some bleeding on the brain. It would be essential to document this event, as well as inform nursing or the client's doctor verbally about what transpired. This might require immediate medical attention, and it is up to you to see that the proper people are informed as quickly as possible. It is also up to you to see that this critical event is documented in the chart. You are the one who saw what happened. It should be in your words. The doctor or nurse might also document what you told them, but when they do so, they are documenting secondhand information. In most courts of law, secondhand information is considered hearsay.

Client noncompliance is also something that should be documented (Sames & Berkeland, 1998). If you have prescribed a home exercise program, and the client reports not following through with it, you need to document that. It might explain why a client is progressing more slowly than you would like.

Since the clients we work with are human, unpredictable things can happen. New problems surface. When you deviate from your original intervention plan, there needs to be a brief explanation of why you are doing something new (Sames & Berkeland, 1998). In other words, you need to provide justification for deviating from the original plan. Many clients have multiple complications, for example, a person with schizophrenia may have a stroke, a person with rheumatoid arthritis may have diabetes and depression, and a child with Asperger's syndrome may suffer a traumatic amputation. This may mean that the intervention plan you develop may differ from your typical plan of action. A depressed client who rented an apartment could lose her lease and become homeless. This change in the client's environment would likely cause a change in plan.

Figure 4.1 is the Document with CARE Checklist. This is a handy, one-page document that you can use to help evaluate your report and note writing.

Exercise 4.1

Evaluate the following narrative progress notes using the Document with CARE checklist.

Case 1: This involves a 3-year-old child with cerebral palsy in a preschool setting. Her areas of concern are in hand use, balance, and using sign language.

Anoushka participated in three 30-minute sessions this week. She participated in group activities, snack, and playground activities each day. She played catch with another child on Monday. She signed "more" during snack. Anoushka loved balancing on the big ball. Wednesday she refused to go down the slide. Plan to continue seeing Anoushka per plan of care.

C:

A:

R:

E:

(cont. on p. 35)

```
┌─────────────────────────────────────────────────────────────────────────────┐
│                        ▼ DOCUMENT WITH CARE ▼                                 │
│                                                                               │
│                                                                               │
│  Clarity: The reader can understand what you are saying                       │
│  ❏ Free from jargon                                                           │
│  ❏ Only facility-approved abbreviations                                       │
│  ❏ Readable/legible                                                           │
│  ❏ Grammar and spelling do not interfere with the professional appearance     │
│    and the intended message of the note                                       │
│  ❏ Understandable to all readers                                              │
│                                                                               │
│  Accuracy: The documentation reflects what actually happened                  │
│  ❏ Concise                                                                    │
│  ❏ Chronologically, technically, and factually correct                       │
│  ❏ Instructions are specific and individualized                              │
│  ❏ Reflect the behavior observed, interpretations are labeled as such        │
│  ❏ Consistent use of terminology                                             │
│  ❏ Adheres to protocol of institution or agency                              │
│  ❏ Preserve confidentiality of all involved                                  │
│                                                                               │
│  Relevance: The documentation relates to identified needs and purposes        │
│  ❏ Clear why OT is initiated, continued, and discontinued                    │
│  ❏ Consistency between referral, evaluation, intervention plan, ongoing       │
│    intervention, discontinuation planning, and follow-up                      │
│  ❏ Documentation reflects the skilled service being provided                  │
│  ❏ Description of changes in function relates to treatment goals             │
│  ❏ Timely                                                                     │
│  ❏ Precautions and contraindications are clearly outlined for the individual  │
│  ❏ Include information necessary for quality management and research projects │
│  ❏ Eliminate all but necessary information                                    │
│                                                                               │
│  Exceptions: Any unusual occurrences, non-compliance, or changes are documented │
│  ❏ Deviations from original intervention plan are justified                  │
│  ❏ Deviations from evaluation, and intervention protocols are described and  │
│    explained                                                                  │
│  ❏ Client noncompliance is noted                                             │
│  ❏ Unusual occurrences and events are described                             │
│  ❏ Complications and responses are documented                               │
└─────────────────────────────────────────────────────────────────────────────┘
```

FIGURE 4.1   Document with CARE. *From Sames & Berkeland (1998). Copyright 1998. All rights reserved.*

Case 2: This case involves a teenager in a chemical dependency program.

Paul attended group as scheduled. He seems to be opening up and talking more. He still does not reveal much about his own feelings, but is identifying feelings in others. When confronted on any issue, he deflects the comments back to the person who made the comment. For example, when a member of the group accused him of being dishonest about the strength of his addiction, he shouted, "As if you people are saints! Your problems are way bigger than mine!" He recognizes that he had enough of a problem to land himself in this program, but he says that he really does not need any intervention; he can quit on his own anytime he wants. He says he is only here because it is better than going to jail.

C:

A:

R:

E:

Case 3: This case involves a 34-year-old man recovering from a massive hand injury from an on-the-job accident. He has had surgical repair of three tendons on the palm of his hand, and an amputation of the distal joint of his index finger.

Ivan has been receiving hard therapy for his injuries for 3 weeks. He is making steady progress. The post-surgical edema is almost gone. He has greater AROM in each finger than at this time last week. Refer to flow sheet for detailed ROM of each joint. Bruising has faded to pale yellow. He is able to squeeze lightweight putty and spread his fingers inside a ring of the same weight putty. Plan to continue therapy 3x/wk for 45–60 min to work on strengthening of hand and fingers, increased ROM, and functional use of hand and fingers.

C:

A:

R:

E:

SUMMARY

Documentation is a complex process; there are many things you must consider all at once when writing about a client. The *Document with CARE* checklist is one way to check to see that your documentation is on the right track. It can help you see if you are writing about the right things, and if you are writing them well. CARE stands for clarity, accuracy, relevance, and exceptions. If you document with CARE, you will be a good documenter of occupational therapy practice.

REFERENCE

Sames, K., & Berkeland, R., (1998). *Document with CARE.* Checklist and oral presentation at the Sister Genevieve Cummings Colloquia, June 19, 1998, St. Paul, MN.

SECTION II

Ethical and Legal Considerations

▼ INTRODUCTION ▼

If an attorney ever asks to see your documentation, it is usually because a client/patient is involved in some kind of litigation. The previous section of this book talked about general principles for good documentation. In this section, we will talk about ethical and legal considerations in documentation. If the records you write get called into court, the attorneys will likely tell the jury how they would like your writing to be interpreted. Your mistakes might be accidental, but an attorney may not see it that way. Table II.1 is a list of what your documentation might look like, and how an attorney could interpret it (Ranke, 1998).

▼ AVOIDING LEGAL ACTION THROUGH DOCUMENTATION ▼

Some, but not all, errors in documentation may be violations of laws, rules, or regulations. The best defense is to document appropriately and competently every day. Always be sure you are writing in the right chart (Fremgen, 2002). Be sure the client is named on every page of the chart; in larger facilities, there may be a stamp or sticker for this.

TABLE II.1 Ways an Attorney Could Interpret Documentation

What You Said or Did	What the Attorney Will Say About It
Erasures, cross-outs, or other alterations to original documentation	Writer was unsure of what to say, careless, or incompetent; writer is trying to cover up or hide something.
Poor grammar or spelling	Writer is not competent, is careless.
Negative statements by one provider toward another provider or toward the facility/administration	Providers not coordinated in care of client; blaming others might indicate decreased quality of care; client is caught in a fight between caregivers.
Negative statements toward the client	Words like "fat," "lazy," "abusive," "faking," "stupid," "goofy," etc., indicate that the provider disliked the client and therefore gave inferior service.
Gaps in documentation or documentation out of sequence	Writer is careless; problems in staffing, in adequate staff to care for client; writer is hiding something.

Sources: Fremgen (2002) and Ranke (1998).

Ranke (1998) lists three criteria for avoiding legal action. First, be careful and objective in your documentation. Base your documentation on firsthand information, things you see and hear. When you write that something occurred, you are identifying yourself as a witness in the eyes of an attorney. Do not assume something must have happened if you did not see it happen or write what someone else tells you happened. For example, do not document that the patient fell unless you saw the patient fall. Instead, you could say that you found the patient sprawled on the floor and that the patient said she fell. Documentation should never be derogatory toward the client or defensive in tone (Fremgen, 2002).

Be brief, but be complete (Borcherding, 2000; Fremgen, 2002). If you do something, but leave it out of your documentation, a court will determine that it never happened. Be sure to document the reason(s) for any missed evaluation, intervention, or follow-up sessions.

When you give instructions to a client, carefully document those instructions and whether the client was able to demonstrate understanding of the instructions (Ranke, 1998). The same is true when you are instructing family members or other caregivers in ways to follow through on an occupational therapy program for a specific client. Documenting that the client, or caregiver, nodded to indicate understanding is not enough (Ranke, 1998). Document any telephone conversations or other correspondence that relates to the client, as well as any actions you take as a result of those conversations/correspondence (Fremgen, 2002).

Second, Ranke (1998) says documentation should be timely, grammatically correct, legible, and correctly signed. All documentation should be done in chronological order and done as close to the time of service as possible (Fremgen, 2002). The longer the lag time between when the service was provided and when the documentation occurred, the less reliable it will be considered in court. In addition to recording the date of the entry into the record, many facilities require the time be recorded as well (Ranke, 1998). Only use facility-approved abbreviations (AOTA, 2003; Borcherding, 2000; Fremgen, 2002; Ranke, 1998). Use proper grammar and spelling to ensure understandability, accuracy, and clarity. Write legibly (printing is preferred to cursive) or word process documentation. Illegible notes can lead to improper care. Sign and date all documentation with at least your first initial, full last name, credentials (i.e. OTR/L, OTA/L) and the date it was written.

Finally, Ranke (1998) says your documentation should be tamper-free, which means you should not change, remove, add to, or write over any documentation. Always correct your errors with a single line through the mistake with your initials above or next to the error. Then make the correction. Never correct someone else's documentation in a client's record, only your own. Never sign anyone else's documentation. Do not leave blank lines or large blank spaces. Fill the blank areas with a line. Never use correction fluid or erasers. Always use ink in a permanent or official record.

▼ STRUCTURE OF THIS SECTION OF THE BOOK ▼

In this section of the book, we explore the ethical and legal considerations that impact documentation. For the purposes of this book, ethical considerations are defined as those actions that reflect doing the right thing. The principles outlined in the AOTA Code of Ethics (2000) will be the guide. While situations involving questionable ethics exist in many ways in clinical practice, we focus on those that involve documentation. Examples of these ethical considerations include, but are not limited to, confidentiality, fraud, plagiarism, and retention of records.

Chapter 5 presents considerations in confidentiality and records retention. This includes issues such as how to protect your client's confidentiality and where and for how long to retain client documentation. Specific standards from the AOTA Code of Ethics (2000) that apply to these issues as well as the Health Insurance Portability and Accountability Act (HIPAA), a federal law designed to protect the rights of recipients of health care services, are discussed.

In Chapter 6, situations that could be construed as fraud are discussed. There is an emphasis on Medicare fraud and abuse, since the government has recently been cracking down on this. You will learn what the penalties are for engaging in fraud. Standards that apply to these situations from the AOTA Code of Ethics (2000) are described.

The last chapter in this section, Chapter 7, takes us in a slightly different direction. While it is less about documentation and more about writing papers, plagiarism can be considered a form of fraud. As students, you will write numerous papers, and colleges seem to be paying more attention to issues of plagiarism these days. As a clinician, you will put together handouts for in-services, home exercise programs, and general information for your clients. In every case, you must give credit where credit is due. The AOTA Code of Ethics (2000) standards will be presented along with strategies for avoiding plagiarism.

REFERENCES

American Occupational Therapy Association. (2000). Occupational therapy code of ethics. *American Journal of Occupational Therapy, 54*, 614–616.

American Occupational Therapy Association. (2003). *Guidelines for documentation of occupational therapy.* Retrieved June 27, 2003, from *http://www.aota.org/members/ area2/docs/ra2.pdf*

Borcherding, S. (2000). *Writing SOAP notes in occupational therapy.* Thorofare, NJ: Slack.

Fremgen, B. F. (2002). *Medical law and ethics.* Upper Saddle River, NJ: Prentice Hall.

Ranke, B. A. E. (1998). Documentation in the age of litigation. *OT Practice, 3*(3), 20–24.

CHAPTER 5

Confidentiality and Records Retention

INTRODUCTION

Occupational therapists have access to very personal information about clients. There are rules that have to be followed in order to protect clients' rights to privacy. Confidentiality refers to keeping information to oneself, not releasing information about a client without the written permission of that client. Recently, the Health Insurance Portability and Accountability Act (HIPAA) has tightened rules concerning protection of client privacy. These rules include the kinds of information protected, when written consent is needed, and who may give consent (AOTA, 2003). In addition to issues of disclosure of information, in order to further protect confidentiality, how records are stored and who has access to stored records also need consideration.

▼ CONFIDENTIALITY ▼

When you write anything that identifies a specific client by name, you are ethically responsible for ensuring that the information remains confidential (AOTA, 2000). This means that you take all reasonable precautions to make sure that only the people who have permission to read the record actually read it. When sending confidential information via the mail, you first need permission from the client or responsible party to share the document, and then the envelope should be marked "confidential." When sending documents via fax, include a cover sheet marked "confidential" (Fremgen, 2002). In other words, no one except those who have written consent of the client or the client's guardian should have access to a client's medical record in any form (electronic or paper).

The client, however, does have a right to see what is written in his or her medical record (United States Department of Health and Human Services [USDHHS], 2002). This is another reason to choose your words carefully, to remain objective and nonjudgmental. Most facilities have specific policies and procedures for allowing clients to read their own records. In some cases, a physician or nurse needs to be present to provide immediate answers to any questions that arise. Other facilities will provide photocopies of medical records to the client (they may charge a fee for the copying). Again, find out the rules at your facility before you share the clinical record with anyone.

▼ ETHICAL RESPONSIBILITY ▼

The American Occupational Therapy Association (2000) has ethical standards that address issues of confidentiality. Occupational therapists are ethically responsible for protecting the confidentiality of all client information regardless of the format of the communication.

> Principle 3. Occupational therapy personnel shall respect the recipient and/or their surrogate(s) as well as the recipient's rights (autonomy, privacy, confidentiality).

E. Occupational therapy personnel shall protect all privileged confidential forms of written, verbal, and electronic communication gained from educational, practice, research, and investigational activities unless otherwise mandated by local, state, or federal regulations. (AOTA, 2000, p. 615)

▼ STATE LAWS ▼

Breaches of confidentiality can invite lawsuits. Many states have laws governing the protection of medical records. It is considered an invasion of privacy to allow unauthorized access to the clinical record or to disclose information about a specific patient/client in any way (Liang, 2000). Some types of information, such as HIV infection or drug/alcohol addiction, are protected to an even greater degree (Fremgen, 2002; Liang, 2000). For example, releasing HIV status of a patient without permission to release that specific information can result in both civil and criminal penalties. A client can make claims of "intentional infliction of emotional distress" (Liang, 2000, p. 51). Check the website for your state Department of Health or Department of Human Services for state regulations on confidentiality and release of information.

▼ HEALTH INSURANCE PORTABILITY AND ACCOUNTABILITY ACT ▼

Occupational therapists are required by law to comply with the privacy sections of the Health Insurance Portability and Accountability Act (HIPAA). This law covers many topics, including protections for American workers regarding health insurance, but also includes a section on protection of privacy rights of individuals (Centers for Medicare and Medicaid Services [CMS], 2002). HIPAA was enacted in 1996; however, the section on privacy did not take effect until 2003 (USDHHS, 2002). Violating the confidentiality statutes of HIPAA by disclosing information that should not be disclosed to another party without permission is punishable by fines of up to $50,000 or 1 year in prison (Liang, 2000).

Usually, when a client is seen in an institutional setting (e.g., hospital, nursing home, school, etc.), the institution has established policies regarding access to patient/client information. The occupational therapist must comply with these policies. These may vary somewhat from place to place, but generally all must be consistent with the language and requirements of HIPAA. Staff involved in direct caregiving, supervisors, medical records personnel, billing personnel, and insurance representatives usually are allowed access to a client's record provided it is necessary for "treatment, payment, or health care operations" (Office for Civil Rights [OCR], 2002, p. 8 [§ 164.502 (a)(1)(ii)]).

Clients must sign a form stating they have been informed of their rights, specifically how the health information will be used, what will be disclosed, and how the client can get access to this information (OCR, 2002). This form, called a HIPAA Privacy Notice, must be written in plain language so that it is readable by most adults, yet meets all the legal requirements of the law (Health Resources and Services Administration [HRSA], 2003). The required topics are (HRSA, 2003, p. 2):

- Header with specific language
- Uses and disclosures
- Separate statements for certain uses and disclosures
- Individual rights
- Covered entity's duties
- Complaints
- Contact

Figure 5.1 lists some suggestions from the HRSA (2003) for making the notice easier to read. The HRSA also has a thesaurus to aid in the translating of terms in the law into "plain language words and phrases" (HRSA, 2003, p. 9). For example, the HRSA suggests that "authorizing disclosures" can be translated into "allowing us to share information" (p. 9). Many of the principles for making the notice more readable, and the thesaurus, are also useful tools in creating any written materials for client education.

HIPAA requires that copies of documentation are not left on a therapist's desk where others can see them. Client charts or records should not be left where any identifiable information is exposed to public view (OCR, 2002). Documentation is also not left on computer screens when a therapist steps away from his or her desk. Computers, whether desktop, laptop, or hand-held, should be password protected for each user, again to protect the confidentiality of client information (Fremgen, 2002). Occupational therapists should not discuss clients in public areas of the facility (especially in hallways, the cafeteria, and in elevators) where they can be overheard. You can imagine what would happen if you were talking to a coworker in the cafeteria about Mrs. Johnson's rolls of fat getting in the way of her being able to clean herself while her daughter was at the next table listening in on your conversation! Or telling a coworker how sassy little Timmy is while his aunt is riding in the elevator with you. Besides being unethical and illegal, it is rude and unprofessional.

For health care providers, HIPAA stipulates that both the medical record and billing record of each client be protected (Federal Register, 2000). Under the act, disclosure is defined as "the release, transfer, provision of access to, or divulging in any other manner of information outside the entity holding the information" (Federal Register, 2000, p. 82489). Health information necessary for what the act calls "health care operations" do not require written permission of the client before being shared. Examples of health care operations include

> quality assessment and improvement activities, reviewing the competence or qualifications and accrediting/licensing of health care professionals and plans, . . . training future health care professionals . . . conducting or arranging for medical review and auditing services and compiling and analyzing information in anticipation of or for use in a civil or criminal legal proceeding. (Federal Register, 2000, p. 82490)

Individually identifiable health information is protected under the act (Federal Register, 2000; USDHSS, 2002). This includes any means by which a person could be identified,

---

Wording
- Translate the rules into a conversational style
- Use short sentences (15 words or fewer)
- Do not use hyphens or compound words
- Use examples to explain concept, category, or value-judgment words
- Use lowercase letters wherever possible
- Give context first, then giving new material

Appearance
- Allow white space (blank areas or wide margins)
- Break long lists into "chunks"
- Use visuals (pictures, drawings, and symbols)
- Use large fonts
- Use high contrast
- Do not use high-gloss paper
- Cue the reader (use arrows and captions for visuals)

FIGURE 5.1 Increasing the Readability of a HIPAA Privacy Notice. *Adapted from HRSA (2003).*

such as by name, social security number, address, phone number, and the like (OCR, 2002). Examples of prohibited activities include using a client's social security number as a client identifier (i.e., case number) on written or electronic documentation, and listing the full name of a client on a schedule hanging on a wall where anyone could see it. If the individually identifiable health information is included in an educational record, it is governed by the Family Education Rights and Privacy Act (Public Law 93-380).

▼ FAMILY EDUCATION RIGHTS AND PRIVACY ACT OF 1974 AND THE INDIVIDUALS WITH DISABILITIES EDUCATION ACT, 1997 REVISION ▼

The Family Education Rights and Privacy Act of 1974 (FERPA) identifies the confidentiality requirements of a student's educational record. The Individuals with Disabilities Education Act (IDEA), 1997 Revision governs the types of services provided to children with disabilities, and how those services are documented. An educational record includes material written by school district employees and contractors (AOTA, 1999; IDEA Partnerships 1999). If a student is receiving special education and related services (including occupational therapy), FERPA covers all documents that contain the student's name, address, phone number, parents' names, and any other identifying information. The file may be called a "cumulative file, permanent record, or official educational record" (AOTA, p. 128). These files contain documents such as the Individual Education Program (IEP) (see Chapter 16), the Individual Family Service Plan (IFSP) (see Chapter 15), and notice and consent forms (see Chapter 14) required by IDEA, as well as grades, samples of student work, and district- or state-wide test results.

The Individuals with Disabilities Education Act (IDEA), 1997 Revision (PL-105-117) also contains language about privacy of information. IDEA has separate sections that address early intervention services (birth through age 2) and school-age (ages 3–21) services. Both sections specifically define identifying information as including the name of the child, parent, or other family member; the address of the child; any identifier such as a social security number; or a list of characteristics or other information that would result in reasonable certainty of the identity of the child (34 C.F.R. § 303.401[a] and 34 C.F.R. § 300.500[b][3]). IDEA further provides for the opportunity for parents to examine the records of their child (34 C.F.R. § 303.402 and 34 C.F.R. § 300.560-576).

Exercise 5.1

Which of the following constitutes a breach of confidentiality?

1. A client was discharged from the hospital yesterday and was admitted to a transitional care facility. The occupational therapist at the transitional care facility calls to get more information about the client than you can usually find in a discharge summary, nitty-gritty things about the personality of the client and the supportiveness of the family. The transitional care facility has permission to get copies of discharge information from the hospital. Based on that, the occupational therapist at the hospital who has worked most closely with the client answers the questions of the occupational therapist at the transitional care facility over the phone.

2. You are working with a client at an outpatient clinic. The client has a work-related injury. As a result of participating in the worker's compensation system, this client is assigned a case manager. The case manager comes by the clinic and asks to review the client's record. The client did sign a release for you to share medical records with the insurer.

3. In a busy nursing home therapy room, a schedule is posted on the wall listing each client's full first and last name and room number. The schedule includes intervention sessions for physical and occupational therapy and speech-language pathology. The rehab aide who transports clients to and from their rooms can look at the schedule to see who needs to go where and when.

▼ RECORDS RETENTION ▼

Records, both educational and clinical, are retained for several reasons. One reason is to provide information about what happened in the past that could contribute to the client's present condition. Another reason is to provide comparative data that might enable a practitioner to identify trends toward improved function or loss of function. Records are retained in case legal questions arise after care is discontinued. Finally, we retain records for quality management purposes. By reviewing records of past clients, medical and educational professionals can learn which practices yield the best results.

Records are generally stored in locked file cabinets in a records office once the client has been discharged from the facility or program. The office is locked whenever it is unattended. Active client charts usually travel with the client (in hospitals), or stay in the nursing department (long-term care facility) or in a therapy office (outpatient clinic). In a school or community setting, records may be kept in a central office. Therapy departments often keep copies of client records. These should be kept in a secure area and be locked when not in use.

Each state has laws that govern medical records retention. At minimum, these laws require health care providers to retain records for at least as long as the statute of limitations for medical malpractice suits (Fremgen, 2002). A statute of limitation specifies how long a patient or the family of a patient has to file a malpractice claim against a health care practitioner. The statute of limitations may be different for physicians, nurses, and therapists, but generally range from 2 to 6 years.

Records for adult patients are usually kept for 5 to 10 years after discharge, although some records may be stored off-site when storage space is limited (Fremgen, 2002). Records for children are kept until the child turns age 21 plus the number of years that state statutes require records to be retained. These are generalities, and some facilities may keep files for as little as 2 years or as long as 15. The American Health Information Management Association (AHIMA) has adopted standards for recommended retention of records (Fremgen, 2002). AHIMA recommends that records be retained for 10 years beyond the last encounter for adult patients, until the age of maturity plus the length of the statute of limitations for a child, and that Medicare and Medicaid records be kept for at least 5 years (Fremgen, 2002; Liang, 2000). The key is that there is a policy and the policy applies to all clients.

When the required length of time for records retention has elapsed, the records must either continue to be retained or be destroyed. Duplicate records need not be retained after the client is discontinued unless facility policy requires it. Because of the sensitive information in the records, destroyed means that the records are shredded and/or burned. Simply putting them in the trash or in recycling would violate the client's right to confidentiality, since a good gust of wind could blow them into someone's path, or the trash collector could read them.

SUMMARY

Confidentiality is a major concern of all health care providers. As health care providers, we are obligated to protect the confidentiality of our clients. This applies to all settings, to all types of documents, and to spoken words as well. A new federal law, HIPAA, limits the kind of information that can be shared without written permission and protects clients from public disclosure of any information. FERPA protects the educational records of students. Our clients deserve to have their privacy protected to the furthest extent possible without interfering with intervention.

Records are retained for at least the length of each state's statute of limitations, and often longer. These records are also protected and stored where they will be safe and secure. Access to stored records is limited to only those who absolutely need access to them. Once the statute of limitations has expired, the records may stay in a secure and locked site, or be thoroughly destroyed by burning or shredding. Never toss old records into the garbage.

REFERENCES

American Occupational Therapy Association. (1999). *Occupational therapy services for children and youth under the Individuals with Disabilities Education Act* (2nd ed.). Bethesda, MD: Author.

American Occupational Therapy Association. (2000). Occupational therapy code of ethics. *American Journal of Occupational Therapy, 54,* 614–616.

American Occupational Therapy Association. (2003). *Fact sheet: HIPAA privacy rule web links.* Retrieved March 15, 2003, from *http://www.aota.org/members/area5/links/LINK07.asp?PLACE=/members/area5/links/link*

Centers for Medicare and Medicaid Services. (2002). *HIPAA insurance reform.* Retrieved March 15, 2003, from *http://cms.hhs.gov/hipaa/hipaa1/content/more.asp*

Federal Register. (2000). *Final privacy rule.* Retrieved March 5, 2003, from *http://www.hhs.gov/ocr/hipaa/finalreg.html*

Fremgen, B. F. (2002). *Medical law & ethics.* Upper Saddle River, NJ: Prentice-Hall.

Health Resources and Services Administration. (2003). *Plain language principles and thesaurus for making HIPAA privacy notices more readable.* Retrieved July 15, 2003, from *http://www.hrsa.gov/language.htm*

IDEA Partnerships. (1999). *Discover IDEA CD '99* [CD-ROM]. A collaborative project of the IDEA Partnership Projects (through project ASPIIRE at The Council for Exceptional Children) and the Western Regional Resource Center at the University of Oregon.

Liang, B. A. (2000). *Health law & policy: A survival guide to medicolegal issues for practitioners.* Woburn, MA: Butterworth-Heinemann.

Office for Civil Rights, United States Department of Health and Human Services. (2002). *Standards for privacy of individually identifiable health information (Unofficial version) (45 CFR Parts 160 and 164).* Retrieved March 17, 2003, from *http://www.hhs.gov/ocr/combinedregtext.pdf*

United States Department of Health and Human Services. (2002). *Fact sheet: Administrative simplification under HIPAA: National standards for transactions, security and privacy.* Retrieved March 15, 2003 from *http://www.hhs.gov/news/press/2002pres/hipaa.html*

CHAPTER 6

Fraud

INTRODUCTION

Fraud is lying or intentionally deceiving the reader of your documentation, especially if it is used to obtain reimbursement for services (Bailey & Schwartzberg, 2003). Fraud can take many forms, but in this book we will only be talking about it in terms of documentation. Fraud can be obvious, as when a therapist documents that a client received services on a day that the client did not receive services. It can also be subtle, as when a therapist documents that a client is making slower progress than the client really is in order to keep the client on the caseload longer. Fraud charges can be filed against the practitioner and the facility if the codes used to bill for services do not match the written description of services in the progress notes and related documentation (e.g., log sheets).

▼ MEDICARE FRAUD ▼

According to Kornblau and Starling (2000, p. 27), there are six "acts prohibited by Medicare and Medicare fraud and abuse provisions:

- Making false claims for payment
- Making false statements for payment
- Billing for visits never made
- Billing for nonface-to-face therapy services
- Paying or receiving kickbacks for goods and services
- Soliciting for, making an offer for payment, paying or receiving payment for patient referrals."

Medicare has strict penalties for fraud. It can cost the practitioner money, jail time, and one's license to practice occupational therapy. There are both civil and criminal penalties (Bailey & Schwartzberg, 2003; Kornblau & Startling, 2000; Liang, 2000). Filing false claims, that is, for services not rendered, can be punishable by fines up to $25,000 and 5 years in jail (criminal sanctions) and an additional $2,000–$10,000 in civil fines for each false claim, as well as an additional $10,000 and payback of triple damages under two additional parts of the law (Kornblau & Starling, 2000; Liang, 2000). Besides these costly consequences, a person participating in fraud can be excluded from ever participating in any federal reimbursement program such as Medicare, Medicaid, Veteran's Affairs, Public Health Service Programs, and other government-funded programs (AOTA, 2000a; Kornblau & Starling, 2000; Liang, 2000). Obviously, the occupational therapist is best advised to be truthful and accurate in all documentation in order to avoid claims of fraud.

▼ OTHER FORMS OF FRAUD ▼

To avoid allegations of fraud, the therapist must be knowledgeable of the regulations, must follow those regulations, and document with sufficient accuracy and honesty. There have been numerous cases where occupational therapists and others have been accused of fraud because they documented that they provided intervention to a client on a specific date when in fact they did not. Making an honest error on the date of service is one thing; creating fictional progress notes is another. Fraud investigators are trained to know the difference. Over the last several years, Medicare has stepped up efforts to catch occupational therapists who attempt to obtain Medicare reimbursement through fraud. If you know that someone else has committed fraud, and you do not report it, you can be charged with conspiracy to commit fraud (Kornblau & Starling, 2000).

Fraud can be more subtle. It can be any documentation that is meant to deceive the reader, especially if payment is sought for that service (Fremgen, 2002). For example, under Medicare, only the time the client spends in contact with the therapist is considered billable time. That means the time an aide spends taking a client to and from the clinic, time spent resting in the therapy room, and time the therapist spends documenting care or on the phone talking to other caregivers are not billable time. It also means that documenting slower progress than is accurate in order to justify keeping a client on one's caseload longer, or faster progress than is accurate to look more effective, are considered fraudulent (Bailey & Schwartzberg, 2003).

The AOTA Code of Ethics (2000b) specifically states in Principle 6.C: "Occupational therapy personnel shall refrain from using or participating in the use of any form of communication that contains false, fraudulent, deceptive, or unfair statements or claims." This applies to occupational therapy documentation, advertising and promotional materials, speeches and in-services, or any other form of communication that an occupational therapist might engage in regardless of the setting. This is further elaborated in the AOTA *Guidelines to the Code of Ethics:* "Occupational therapy personnel do not fabricate data, falsify information, or plagiarize" (AOTA, 1998, 2.9) and, even more explicitly, "Occupational therapy personnel do not make deceptive, fraudulent, or misleading statements about the nature of the services they provide or the outcomes that can be expected" (AOTA, 1998, 2.1).

For example, an occupational therapist in private practice was accused of adding one billed unit of time (usually 15 minutes of direct service) for every visit that the occupational therapists working for her submitted to her for billing. If the therapists documented in a progress note that the client was seen for a 30-minute session, and marked 30 minutes (two units) on the billing record, the owner of the company would submit the bill for 45 minutes (three units). She did this without the knowledge of the therapists. The therapists found out that this was happening because the family of the client brought a copy of the bill in to the occupational therapist to see why they were being billed for 45-minute visits when they were scheduled for 30-minute visits. The therapists started asking questions and the owner said that she was simply adding a unit to account for the time the therapists spent in documenting services, time on the phone with the client's doctor, cleaning up after sessions, and other miscellaneous clinic expenses. The therapists did some more digging and found that the owner was destroying the progress notes when they were 1 month old, or as soon as the next intervention plan was written. The family reported the fraud to the HMO that was paying for services, and the therapists resigned and then reported the fraud to the state regulatory board. If the allegations proved to be true, the owner could face major penalties and will probably lose her license. Insurance fraud is a federal crime. The Federal False Claims Act, 31 U.S.C.A. §3729-3733, allows whistleblowers, those who report fraud and who help in the prosecution of the case, to receive 15–25% of the monies recovered (damages, civil penalties, and treble damages) from a false claim (Kornblau & Starling, 2000).

Exercise 6.1

Which of the following scenarios constitutes fraud, and which is just carelessness?

1. A therapist dates her notes "Jan. 3, 2003" when in fact the date is January 3, 2004.

2. A therapist writes in her note on Monday that the client was weaker on her right side than on her left. On Wednesday she writes that the client was weaker on her left than on her right. On Friday she writes that although the client is showing improvement in function on her right side, it remains weaker than her left.

3. A therapist bills for hot packs when in fact the client soaked her hand in a bowl of warm water.

4. A therapist bills for a 45 minute session when in fact the client was in the room for 45 minutes, although for 20 of those minutes the client rested while the therapist worked with another client.

5. A therapist realizes that she wrote a progress note in the wrong chart, so she uses white-out to cover up her error.

SUMMARY

Fraud is a form of lying that is absolutely illegal. Fraud happens when an occupational therapist documents in such a way as to create a false perception by the reader about what has actually transpired. Examples of fraud include documenting that you spent more time with a client than you really did, describing progress that is faster or slower than reality, or billing for services not rendered. There can be severe criminal and civil penalties for fraud. AOTA, in the *Code of Ethics* (2000), explicitly prohibits occupational therapists from making false statements. The best advice is to document accurately and be truthful in everything you do.

REFERENCES

American Occupational Therapy Association. (1998). *Guidelines to the code of ethics.* Retrieved January 5, 2001, from *http://www.aota.org/members/area2/links/link04. asp?PLACE=/members/area2/links/link04.asp*

American Occupational Therapy Association. (2000a). *Final civil fraud and abuse penalties rule.* Retrieved May 12, 2002, from *http://www.aota.org/members/area5/links/link56. asp*

American Occupational Therapy Association. (2000b). Occupational therapy code of ethics. *American Journal of Occupational Therapy, 54,* 614–616.

Bailey, D. M., & Schwartzberg, S. L. (2003). *Ethical and legal dilemmas in occupational therapy.* Philadelphia: F. A. Davis.

Fremgen, B. F. (2002). *Medical law and ethics.* Upper Saddle River, NJ: Prentice Hall.

Kornblau, B. L. & Starling, S. P. (2000). *Ethics in rehabilitation.* Thorofare, NJ: Slack.

Liang, B. A. (2000). *Health law and policy: A survival guide to medicolegal issues for practitioners.* Woburn, MA: Butterworth-Heinemann.

CHAPTER 7

Plagiarism

INTRODUCTION

Plagiarism is a form of cheating and theft that has become very pervasive across the country. Plagiarism is defined as "using another's work without giving credit" (*http://sja .ucdavis.edu/avoid.htm,* 5/23/02, ¶ 2). It includes using someone else's exact words or using someone else's ideas, even if the wording is changed, without giving credit to the originator or the idea or words. Because of the availability of sample intervention plans, student papers, and research papers on the Internet, it is appropriate to discuss plagiarism in the context of a book about documentation. In occupational therapy practice, there are times when an occupational therapist has to put together a report, cite evidence to support practice, or present an in-service with handouts. Each of these situations presents an opportunity for plagiarism.

▼ AMERICAN PSYCHOLOGICAL ASSOCIATION STANDARDS ▼

Since the American Occupational Therapy Association (AOTA) uses the American Psychological Association (APA) standards for writing in the profession, all examples in this book are cited in APA style.

Here is a passage as it appears in the APA Publication Manual, Fifth Edition (2001).

Quotation marks should be used to indicate the exact words of another. *Each time* you paraphrase another author (i.e., summarize a passage or rearrange the order of a sentence and change some of the words), you will need to credit the source in the text. (p. 349)

Below is a paraphrase of that same passage in which proper credit is given to the author.

According to the American Psychological Association (2001), the exact words of another should be enclosed in quotation marks. Rearranging the order of a sentence, summarizing a passage, or changing a few of the words is paraphrasing (APA, 2001). A credit for the source needs to be included each time a source is paraphrased (APA).

▼ TYPES OF PLAGIARISM ▼

Here is an example of outright plagiarism:

Quotation marks must be used to indicate the exact words of another, along with a citation of the author, year, and page number. Paraphrasing is rearranging the order of a sentence and changing some of the words or summarizing a passage. Each time a source is paraphrased, you need to give credit to the original author.

In this case, the writer added a few original words, but one cannot tell where any of the ideas come from and whether any of the words are directly taken from a source. Here is the same paragraph with proper citation:

> "Quotation marks must be used to indicate the exact words of another" (APA, 2001, p. 349) along with a citation of the author, year, and page number. Paraphrasing is rearranging the order of a sentence, changing some of the words, or summarizing a passage (APA). Each time a source is paraphrased, you need to give credit to the original author (APA).

This paragraph demonstrates a common pitfall that people often fall into: They think that the author of the passage has said what needs to be said in the best possible way, so why paraphrase it? Isn't it safer to quote than to paraphrase? They proceed to write papers that are simply strings of quotes linked with a few transitional phrases in the person's own words. While this may feel like a safe way to go, papers that are strings of quotes are difficult to read; all those quote marks and citations get in the way of the flow of the paper. Also, some professors believe that when a student overuses quotes, the student is not taking proper responsibility for completing the assignment (Hashimoto, 1991).

Quotes can enhance a paper, but only when used to support the writer's idea (thesis of the paper) by adding a new take on it. If a writer uses a quote to show that someone else who knows better is thinking the same way as the writer, the quote becomes redundant (Hashimoto, 1991). For example, if I make a thesis statement in a paper that students use excessive quotes, then follow that with the quote "Too often, they use quotations just to restate their own positions" (Hashimoto, 1991, p. 170), I am being redundant and not really adding anything meaningful to my paper.

Another form of plagiarism that can occur happens when students share their work. If you have a friend who took a pediatric occupational therapy course last semester, and you are taking it this semester, your friend might offer you her intervention plans "to look at." If you use them to write your own intervention plans, you are stealing his or her work unless you give credit on your assignment (i.e., "Mary Smith contributed to this assignment"). Most of the time, instructors want you to do your own work, so even if you did give your classmate credit on your assignment, your instructor would probably either make you redo it without help or fail you on that assignment. Using a fellow student's work prevents you from learning and gaining skills needed for the real world. If this was a pattern of behavior, more serious consequences could occur, up to and including expulsion from the program or the school. Disciplinary action can also be taken against the student who did the work herself and then shared it with someone who copied it, because this contributes to the problem of cheating. Clinicians plagiarize when they copy someone else's intervention plan wording. This may be a breach of confidentiality as well.

Many people learn to cheat in middle and high school, and by the time they get to college or the workplace it is so commonplace that they do not see the problem with it. According to a survey administered by Who's Who Among American High School Students in 1998, of the 3,123 students responding, 80% said they had cheated on an exam (Bushweller, 1999, as cited in McMurtry, 2001). Of those who had admitted to cheating, half did not think there was anything wrong with it. Even more astonishing to me is that a poll by *U.S. News* found that 90% of college students believe that those who cheat never get penalized for cheating (Kleiner & Lord, 1999). Another study conducted by Duke University's Center for Academic Integrity showed that 75% of all college students admitted to cheating at least once (Kleiner & Lord). These are big numbers, and the trend is that they are getting bigger by the decade. Survey results like this have gotten the attention of college administrators everywhere, and faculty are examining their academic integrity policies.

I have heard occupational therapy students complain that occupational therapy instructors make too big a deal about plagiarism. Many try to argue that in other majors, instructors do not appear to care if a student plagiarizes. This is a lousy argument. It is not true that other disciplines do not care. However, in a profession where competence and integrity are essential, catching cheaters at an early stage in their careers can help keep the profession respectable. Plagiarizing in school and getting away with it could start one on a slippery slope toward falsifying documentation and engaging in fraud as a clinician.

Clinicians seem to want to share what they know with others in the hope that it helps some situation. Often, an occupational therapy department can only afford to send one practitioner to a workshop. When that person comes back from that workshop, he or she copies the handouts for the other members of the department and presents an in-service on it. Unless the practitioner has written permission to copy and distribute those handouts, he or she is committing plagiarism. If a clinician copies exercises out of a textbook to give to a client or client's caregiver to use in a home program, it could be considered plagiarism unless the textbook gives readers permission to copy and distribute material. Even copying journal articles for everyone in the department or on a committee is plagiarism unless you have written permission from the publisher.

By any professional standard, plagiarism is wrong; it is a form of stealing. The American Occupational Therapy Association Code of Ethics (2000) states "Occupational therapy personnel shall accurately represent the qualifications, views, contributions, and findings of colleagues" (principle 7.B). This is further elaborated in the AOTA *Guidelines to the Code of Ethics*: "Occupational therapy personnel do not fabricate data, falsify information, or plagiarize" (1998, 2.9). Whether you are a student or a clinician, representing anyone else's work as your own is a violation of professional ethics.

▼ PREVENTING PLAGIARISM ▼

How can you protect yourself against allegations of plagiarism? The first rule of thumb is that when in doubt, cite a source. If reading something someone else wrote puts a thought in your head and it comes out your fingertips onto the paper (or computer screen), then cite it. Things that are general knowledge, such as using sunscreen can prevent sunburn or that more falls happen to elderly people in the winter in Vermont than in the summer, do not need to be cited.

To make an allegation of plagiarism against a student, a teacher needs to be pretty sure the work was copied, or at least paraphrased from an identifiable source. New Internet search engines such as Google.com™ and Turnitin.com™ make it easy for instructors to find out if a student has copied someone else's work. The instructor can simply type in a phrase and search the Internet to see if it has been used by someone else on the Internet. If an instructor finds a student has used someone else's work, there can be serious consequences for the student. To find out what could happen if you got caught cheating or plagiarizing, check out your school's policy on academic integrity, honor code, or plagiarism policy. If you were to get caught using someone else's words when you are a clinician, you would be subject to disciplinary action from your employer, AOTA, the National Board for Certification of Occupational Therapists, and, depending on your state regulations for licensure or registration, disciplinary action from your state regulatory board as well.

This can be scary stuff. It almost makes one afraid to write anything. Chances are that all the good phrases have been taken, that is, "it's all been said before" (author of quote unknown). Bob Newhart had a comedy sketch in which he theorized that if you put a group of monkeys in a room with a typewriter apiece, sooner or later by random efforts they would reproduce all the world's great literature. There are common phrases that everyone uses so that it would be impossible to give credit to any one author. Sometimes two people who have never met can come up with similar word sequences. This cannot be helped.

According to the Georgetown University Honor Council Web page, one way to protect yourself is to allow yourself time to do it right. If you are writing a 12-page paper at 11:59 P.M. the night before it is due at 8:00 A.M., you could inadvertently leave out some quote marks or forget to cite a source. It might seem easier at that point to copy someone else's paper (or buy one off the Internet) than to stay up all night working hard on it. If you find yourself in this kind of situation, it is better to risk a lower grade on the paper (by not being thorough enough, making spelling errors, wandering off topic, etc.) than to risk the disciplinary consequences of an academic integrity violation (*http://www.georgetown.edu/honor/*

plagiarism.html, section 4). Of course, the best course of action is to not get yourself into this kind of situation in the first place.

Purdue University offers a printable handout on their Web page for avoiding plagiarism (*http://owl.English.purdue.edu/handouts/research/r_plagiar.html*). In it there are suggestions for what you can do during the writing process and how your finished product should look. They suggest coding your paper during early drafts with "Q" for quote, and then coding the rest with either an "S" when the material comes from any source, and "ME" when it is your own idea or insight. They also suggest summarizing or paraphrasing from memory, rather than while reading the material. One other suggestion is that you can call something common knowledge if you find the same information in five different sources, and each time the author did not document a source for it.

Exercise 7.1

Practice paraphrasing the following sentences.

1. "Client-centered therapy requires active participation of the client in the process of evaluation and intervention" (Schwartzberg, 2002, p. 62).

2. "Countersignature of a treatment plan, insurance form, prescription for medication, progress note, or similar document is usually tantamount to declaring oneself responsible, vicariously, for the treatment in question" (Gutheil, as cited in Bailey & Schwartzberg, 1995, p. 89).

3. "To protect confidentiality, medical records should not be released to third parties without the patient's written consent" (Fremgen, 2002, p. 160).

4. "The classical form of psychoanalysis is that originated by Freud at the beginning of the twentieth century" (Hagedorn, 1997, p. 85).

5. "Wordiness is every bit as irritating and uneconomical as jargon and can impede the ready grasp of ideas" (APA, 2001, p. 35).

6. "Occupational therapy is the art and science of helping people do the day-to-day activities that are important to them despite impairment, disability or handicap" (Neistadt & Crepeau, 1998, p. 5).

SUMMARY

When you plagiarize, you not only cheat the originator of the material out of his or her proper credit, you cheat yourself by not really learning the material. Occasional honest mistakes can usually be tolerated, but repeated instances of the same type of error in citing sources could be used to show a pattern of carelessness that amounts to plagiarism. A student who plagiarizes can expect to fail the assignment or the course, or be expelled from the program. Blatant and repeated plagiarism can lead to expulsion from a school. Plagiarism done by a professional can result in loss of a job or even a career in occupational therapy. There are ways to prevent plagiarism. Allowing plenty of time to complete written work, learning how to properly cite sources, and summarizing or paraphrasing from memory are a few of the ways that plagiarism can be prevented.

REFERENCES

American Occupational Therapy Association. (1998). *Guidelines to the code of ethics.* Retrieved January 5, 2001, from *http://www.aota.org/members/area2/links/link04 .asp?PLACE=/members/area2/links/link04.asp*

American Occupational Therapy Association. (2000). *Occupational therapy code of ethics. American Journal of Occupational Therapy, 54,* 614–616.

American Psychological Association. (2001). *Publication manual of the American Psychological Association* (5th ed.). Washington, DC: Author.

Avoiding plagiarism. Retrieved May 23, 2002 from *http://sja.ucdavis.edu/avoid.htm*

Bailey, D. M. & Schwartzberg, S. L. (2003). *Ethical and legal dilemmas in occupational therapy* (2nd Ed.). Philadelphia: F.A. Davis.

Fremgen, B. F. (2002). *Medical law & ethics.* Upper Saddle River, NJ: Prentice Hall.

Georgetown University Honor Council. (2002). Retrieved May 5, 2002 from *http://www .georgetown.edu/honor/plagiarism.html*

Hagedorn, R. (1997). *Foundations for practice in occupational therapy* (2nd ed.). Edinburgh, Scotland: Churchill Livingstone.

Hashimoto, I. Y. (1991). *Thirteen weeks: A guide to teaching college writing.* Portsmouth, NH: Boynton/Cook.

Kleiner, C., & Lord, M. (1999, November 29). The cheating game. *U.S. New and World Report.* Retrieved May 10, 2002, from *http://www.usnews.com/usnews/edu/college/ articles/cosheata.htm*

McMurtry, K. (2001). e-cheating: Combating a 21st century challenge. *T.H.E. Journal Online.* Retrieved June 13, 2002, from *http://www.thejournal.com/magazine/vault/ articleprintversion.cfm?aid=3724*

Neistadt, M. S., & Crepeau, E. B. (1998). *Willard & Spackman's occupational therapy* (9th ed.). Philadelphia: Lippencott-Raven.

Purdue University Online Writing Laboratory. (1995–2002). *Avoiding plagiarism.* Retrieved June 16, 2002, from *http://owl.English.purdue.edu/handouts/research/r_plagiar.html*

Schwartzberg, S. (2002) *Interactive reasoning in the practice of occupational therapy.* Upper Saddle River, NJ: Prentice Hall.

Clinical Documentation

▼ INTRODUCTION ▼

Now that we have some of the basics out of the way, we can get to the actual writing of occupational therapy documentation. This section explores the different types of documentation that occupational therapy practitioners write when working with clients whose ability to participate fully in life is diminished or at risk due to physical, psychological, or developmental issues. Typically, in clinical settings, payment for services is sought from third-party payers such as insurance companies, managed care organizations, government programs, or from the clients themselves. Occupational therapy services may be provided in medical or psychiatric hospitals, clinics, or long-term care settings as well as in the clients' homes, sheltered workshops, group homes, or other facilities.

▼ CLINICAL DOCUMENTATION ▼

Clinical documentation typically consists of documentation of the client's referral for services, a summary of the evaluation results, intervention plans, documentation of progress, attendance records, discontinuation summaries, and follow-up documentation (if any). Table III.1 shows each step of the occupational therapy process and the corresponding documentation for each step. In essence, for each step of the occupational therapy process there is documentation to go with it. Each of these types of documentation is discussed in the chapters in this section.

Regardless of the type of clinical documentation, certain conventions for good documentation must be followed. While there may be differences between the documentation written by an occupational therapist in a hospital in Los Angeles and an occupational therapy assistant in a sheltered workshop in Bangor, Maine, all documentation must be well written, accurate, and clear.

▼ AOTA STANDARDS FOR DOCUMENTATION ▼

The American Occupational Therapy Association (AOTA) has standards for documentation. The AOTA document *Guidelines for Documentation of Occupational Therapy* (2003) lists 13 elements that must be present in any clinical documentation:

1. *Client identification:* The client's full name should be on every page, along with the client's case number, if there is one (see also Fremgen, 2002). The case number may be a medical records number or room/bed number, whichever is used at a particular facility or program.

TABLE III.1 Occupational Therapy Process and Clinical Documentation

Steps in the Occupational Therapy Process	Types of Documentation
Client identification	Referral or physician's order Contact note
Screening	Screening report Contact note
Initial evaluation (occupational profile and analysis of occupational performance)	Evaluation report or evaluation summary
Intervention planning	Intervention plan (treatment plan, plan of care)
Intervention	Attendance logs Progress flow sheets Progress notes (SOAP, DAP, or narrative notes) Contact notes
Reevaluation (intervention review)	Revised intervention plans
Discontinuation (discharge)	Discontinuation (discharge) summary
Follow-up	Follow-up note Contact note

Source: AOTA (2003)

2. *Date and type of contact:* Each document should be dated with the day, month, and year (see also Fremgen, 2002; Ranke, 1998). Documentation of occupational therapy sessions (evaluation or intervention) often includes the time of day and sometimes the length of the session (see also Ranke). Dates and times are used to show the chronological order of events. The type of contact (i.e., screening, evaluation, intervention plan, etc.) should be specified.

3. *Type:* The type of documentation should be clearly stated, as should the name of the facility/agency and department. For example, the type of document may appear at the top of the page, and the name of the department may be under the signature line.

4. *Signature:* The writer should sign the document using at least his or her first initial and full last name followed by the appropriate professional designation (e.g., OTR, COTA, OT/L, OTA/L, etc.) (see also Fremgen, 2002; Ranke, 1998). Using initials only is usually not sufficient. In some cases, such as on an attendance log, the occupational therapist might simply place his or her initials in the space for each day. At the bottom of the page there should be multiple signature lines so that for each set of initials appearing on the page, there is a full name and credentials written out to clearly identify the person who worked with the client.

5. *Placement of signature:* Notes should be signed directly at the end of the note; there should be no space between what is written and the signature (see also Ranke, 1998). This can help prevent someone else from tampering with your documentation. Some facilities have the staff draw a wavy line where there is blank space between the end of a note and the signature.

6. *Countersignature:* As required by state or facility regulations, occupational therapists must countersign the signatures of occupational therapy assistants and students. This countersignature signifies that the occupational therapist has read the document and is in agreement with the conclusions drawn by the writer. This also provides documentation of supervision, which is required by law.

7. *Terminology:* All terminology used, including abbreviations, must be recognized by the facility as acceptable (see also Fremgen, 2002; Ranke, 1998). Official documents of the profession may be used to define terms, or the facility may specify terminology to be used by all professionals at the facility.

8. *Abbreviations:* Use only abbreviations approved by the facility/agency (see also Borcherding, 2000; Fremgen, 2002; Ranke, 1998). There is usually a list that is used by all disciplines. Some common abbreviations are listed in Chapter 1 of this book. However, just because an abbreviation is listed in this book does not mean that it will be recognized at your facility or in your program.

9. *Corrections:* Follow facility rules for correcting errors. Correct errors by drawing one line through the word(s) in error and initialing your error (see also Borcherding, 2000; Fremgen, 2002; Ranke, 1998). No erasures or correction fluid should be used. Do not scribble out a word or cross out a single letter or part of a word. Some facilities want errors dated. For example:

KMS 8/21/03

Client completed 15 ~~repititions~~ *repetitions of bicep curls.*

10. *Technology:* Follow professional standards and agency/facility policies and procedures for use of technology in documentation.

11. *Record Disposal:* Follow federal and state laws as well as agency/facility policies and procedures for proper disposal of records. (See Section II of this book.)

12. *Confidentiality:* All federal, state, and agency/facility rules and regulations for confidentiality must be obeyed. (See Section II of this book.)

13. *Record Storage:* All federal, state, and agency/facility rules and regulations for storage of records must be obeyed. (See Section II of this book.)

In addition to these standards, there are other common considerations. For example, most documentation is done in blue or black ink because often the documents must be copied and other colors of ink do not photocopy well (Borcherding, 2000; Fremgen, 2002). Never document in a permanent medical record using a pencil (it is erasable). Some facilities do not allow practitioners to document using erasable pens. Other facilities require the ink to be waterproof (Borcherding, 2000). Of course, when documentation is done on computer, the default color of ink used by most printers is black.

Another common consideration is that all handwritten documentation needs to be legible (Fremgen, 2002; Kuntavanich, 1987; Ranke, 1998). For some people, this means printing rather than writing in script (Fremgen). Again, if documentation is done on the computer, usually legibility is not a problem unless the printer is running low on ink, as long as the font size is large enough that people with varying visual acuity can read it (10- or 12-point size font).

Finally, all of the considerations in Chapter 4 about documenting with CARE and Section II (ethical and legal considerations) apply. All documentation must be clear, accurate, and relevant, and exceptions must be documented.

▼ STRUCTURE OF THIS SECTION OF THE BOOK ▼

Chapter 8 focuses on documentation of the initial contact a clinician has with a client. This includes referrals for intervention, physician's orders, and screenings.

Chapter 9 discusses the ways in which evaluation reports are written. As part of that discussion, the purposes and focus of evaluations, methods of recording evaluation data, interpreting the data, and summarizing the data are presented.

Chapter 10 centers on goal setting. Clinicians may set goals as part of an evaluation report or as part of an intervention plan. Several methods for writing goal statements are offered.

Chapter 11 presents methods for documenting intervention plans. Specific information about documenting progress summaries and intervention methods/strategies are set forth.

Chapter 12 addresses various forms of progress notes. The two most common kinds of progress notes are SOAP and narrative formats. This chapter looks at these and other formats in detail, with practice opportunities for the readers of this text.

Finally, Chapter 13 presents discontinuation (discharge) summaries. It offers information on documenting the plan for discontinuation and for follow-up if needed.

REFERENCES

American Occupational Therapy Association. (2003). *Guidelines for documentation of occupational therapy.* Retrieved June 27, 2003, from *http://www.aota.org/members/area2/docs/ra2.pdf*

Borcherding, S. (2000). *Documentation manual for writing SOAP notes in occupational therapy.* Thorofare, NJ: Slack.

Fremgen, B. F. (2002). *Medical law and ethics.* Upper Saddle River, NJ: Prentice Hall.

Kuntavanich, A. (1987). *Occupational therapy documentation: A system to capture outcome data for quality assurance and program promotion.* Rockville, MD: American Occupational Therapy Association.

Ranke, B. A. E. (1998). Documentation in the age of litigation. *OT Practice, 3*(3), 20–24.

CHAPTER 8

Client Identification (Referral and Screening)

INTRODUCTION

There are several different ways in which an occupational therapy practitioner can discover that she or he has a new client. Depending on the setting in which the occupational therapist works, she or he can find out by phone, fax, a conversation in a hallway, a written note (a prescription-like form or a handwritten order in a chart), or by a computer alert system. This notification usually comes in the form of a referral or an order.

▼ REFERRALS ▼

A referral is a suggestion from someone that a particular client would benefit from occupational therapy services. Occupational therapists can receive referrals from almost anyone. A parent can call up and refer a child for services. A nurse can refer a client who is struggling to stay in his or her home despite failing health. A chiropractor can refer a client who needs work on body mechanics. A dentist can refer a client with severe jaw pain. There are no rules or regulations preventing an occupational therapist from receiving referrals from anyone. However, third-party payers, such as managed care organizations and governmental reimbursement systems, often will not pay for services provided to a client with only a referral, unless the referral comes from a physician.

▼ ROLE DELINEATION OF REFERRALS ▼

The AOTA has established standards for referrals. These can be found in the *Standards of Practice for Occupational Therapy* (1998) in Appendix C of this book. These standards require that registered occupational therapists are responsible for receiving and responding to referrals (and orders). *The Standards of Practice* (1998) also require occupational therapists to refer clients to other practitioners (other occupational therapists with specific expertise or other professionals) when a client needs a provider with expertise beyond that of his or her own. This is also a standard in the AOTA Code of Ethics. In order to ensure appropriate referrals, it is incumbent upon both the occupational therapist and the occupational therapy assistant to educate referral sources on the appropriateness of referrals for occupational therapy services (AOTA, 1998). The AOTA standards do not allow occupational therapy assistants to receive or respond to referrals (AOTA, 1998).

▼ ORDERS ▼

An order is a referral written by a physician. It is like a prescription. Just as a pharmacy must fill a prescription written by a licensed physician, an occupational therapist must comply with a physician's order. Many people use the phrase "physician referral" rather than "physician order." The AOTA (1998) prefers the term "physician referral." If a client is referred to occupational therapy, often an order from a physician (or nurse practitioner, chiropractor, optometrist, or other legally defined health care professional, depending on state and payer regulations) is required in order to get paid for providing services. There is no national requirement that says occupational therapists need a physician's order or referral before providing services. Some state licensure laws and some payers require a physician's order for an occupational therapist to see a client.

If an occupational therapist receives a referral for occupational therapy services, and talks to the referral source to find out why the referral was made, the occupational therapist can then contact the physician and ask for an order (or referral). When contacting a busy physician, the occupational therapist needs to have a pretty solid idea of why the client would benefit from occupational therapy evaluation and intervention. In fact, whether or not a busy physician is involved, the occupational therapist and occupational therapy assistant need to clearly understand and articulate why occupational therapy services would be beneficial for every client served by occupational therapy.

It is up to the occupational therapist, using his or her best clinical judgment, to determine if the referral or order for occupational therapy is appropriate. It is also up to the occupational therapist to determine if additional orders are needed. For example, I have seen orders come through to a rehabilitation department (occupational therapy, physical therapy, and speech-language pathology) for physical therapy for ADLs. The physical therapy staff hand the order to the occupational therapy department and have the occupational therapists call the doctor to explain that it is occupational therapy that works on ADLs and request that the doctor change the order. Conversely, I have seen orders come through for occupational therapy to provide diversional activities. Generally speaking, third-party payers do not pay for diversional activities, so it behooves the occupational therapist to discuss the situation with the physician and clarify appropriate terminology that would be acceptable to insurance companies. The occupational therapist should also consider whether a referral to recreation therapy might be more appropriate for the client than occupational therapy.

Physician orders (referrals) need to contain certain information. The order (referral) should specify the full name of the client, the date, and sometimes the time the order was written, the full name and credentials of the physician, the reason for the referral (order), and the frequency and the duration of occupational therapy services (AOTA, 1995). Frequency refers to how often the intervention sessions will occur. Duration refers to how long it is expected to take to meet the needs of the client. Some settings also require intensity of intervention to be included in the order. Intensity refers to the length of time for any one session. An order (referral) for occupational therapy services six times a week (frequency) for three weeks (duration) of 30-minute sessions twice a day (intensity) would satisfy this part of the requirements. If any of these factors are missing, and they often are, the occupational therapist is responsible for contacting the physician to clarify the orders. Sometimes, the occupational therapist completes the evaluation, then, based on the results of the evaluation, contacts the physician to clarify the frequency, intensity, and duration.

An ongoing order is often needed for continued payment for services, especially from Medicare. Having the client's physician sign the plan of care (intervention plan) serves as ongoing orders. Medicare identifies this process as certification and recertification (Prabst-Hunt, 2002). Medicare requires this recertification every 30 days for anyone receiving outpatient occupational therapy (Part B), and the physician has the right to make any changes to the care plan that the physician deems necessary.

Exercise 8.1

Identify the parts of these referrals:

1.

7-10-04	Gertrude Silverstein
8:03 a.m.	#399-76-8223
	room 408B

Occupational therapy to evaluate and treat for R hemisphere stroke bid for one week. Focus on ADL's and IADL's. Provide adaptive equipment as needed along with training in the use of the equipment. Anticipated discharge date 7/17/02.

Dr. Sara Bellar

_____ Date of referral   _____ Name of physician
_____ Name of client   _____ Frequency
_____ Duration   _____ Intensity

_____ Reason for referral
Is this an adequate referral?   yes   no
Why or why not?

2.

| Jonathan Apple |
| May 31, 2004 |

Occupational Therapy as needed for ADLs.

Dr. Don Touchme

_____ Date of referral   _____ Name of physician
_____ Name of client   _____ Frequency
_____ Duration   _____ Intensity

_____ Reason for referral
Is this an adequate referral?   yes   no
Why or why not?

After receiving a referral or order, the occupational therapist makes contact with the client. Often a screening occurs at the first meeting of occupational therapist and client. A screening is a brief check of a client to see if further evaluation or intervention is warranted. It often is based on observations of a client and chart review without the direct intervention of an occupational therapist. Screenings are generally not reimbursable, but can be a good way to identify potential clients for reimbursable services. In most situations, a screening can be done without a physician referral or order.

In some settings, the occupational therapist routinely screens potential clients. This is referred to as a type I screening (Collier, 1991). For example, an occupational therapist working in a nursing home might screen all new admissions to the facility, or an occupational therapist in private practice might screen visitors to a local health fair. In other settings or at other times, the occupational therapist may only screen after receiving a referral. This is referred to as a type II screening (Collier). Then, if the screening demonstrates a need for occupational therapy services, an order can be obtained.

A screening is not a substitute for an evaluation. Chapter 9 explores evaluations more thoroughly. Evaluations are more thorough and specific than screenings and are generally reimbursable. It may be tempting at times to use a screening as a substitute for a complete evaluation when time is of the essence. Do not do it. As mentioned in Chapter 2, the word "assessment" means screening in some settings, and is used as a synonym for evaluation in other settings. Be sure you know how the word is used at your facility/agency and for the reimbursement system used.

According to Collier (1991), there are several general guidelines for when to do screenings:

- Screenings are done only when you believe that the potential problems you will find in your screening can be positively affected by occupational therapy intervention. You do not want to conduct screenings for problems that are beyond occupational therapy's scope of practice. For example, you do not want to screen for problems with articulation of words, a speech-language pathologist would do that.
- Screenings are best done when they are timely, that is, they are done at a time when intervention would be effective. It sounds obvious, but you would not screen for developmental delays in high schoolers; you would screen for delays in preschoolers.
- There must be a reason to believe that the population you are screening will have some people who demonstrate the problem you are screening for. If you are screening a healthy population, you must expect that at least a small percentage of people will ultimately need your services.
- Occupational therapy intervention must be available to help alleviate the problems you identify. It makes no sense to provide screenings where or when there are no services available to work on the problems found.
- Finally, use screening methods that you believe are valid and reliable. This does not mean they need to be standardized, but that your methods will consistently find persons with the problems you are looking for.

There are four possible outcomes of screenings. The first is that the client may in fact need occupational therapy intervention. The second is that the client does not need intervention right now, but there is enough concern that it would be worth rescreening in a few months (or whatever time period you think is appropriate). Next is the possibility that the client needs a referral to some other professional. Finally, the client may not need any intervention at all.

▼ ROLE DELINEATION FOR SCREENINGS ▼

The AOTA has established standards for screenings, which can be found in the *Standards of Practice for Occupational Therapy* (AOTA, 1998) in Appendix C of this book. The occupational therapist is responsible for conducting the screening; however, an occupational therapy assistant, under the supervision of an occupational therapist, may contribute to the screening. The occupational therapist is responsible for selecting the proper tools and methods for screening. Either the occupational therapist or an occupational therapy assistant, under the supervision of an occupational therapist, communicates the results of the screening results and recommendations to other members of the care team, or other appropriate persons.

▼ CONTACT NOTE ▼

A brief note is usually entered into the medical record to acknowledge that the referral/order was received or that the screening took place. This note contains the date and time the referral was received, and when the client is scheduled to begin the evaluation. If you did a screening, the note should also contain the bottom-line results of the screening. Below are two examples of contact notes.

> 5/2/02. 10:35 A.M. Order received for occupational therapy evaluation and intervention. Introduced myself to the client and scheduled her to come to the clinic this afternoon to begin evaluation process. K. Sapp, OTR/L.

> 5/2/02. 10:35 A.M. Received referral for occupational therapy evaluation and intervention. Results of screening show that client would likely benefit from occupational therapy intervention to improve functional use of both arms and hands. Evaluation scheduled for this afternoon. K. Sapp, OTR/L

Contact notes are also used at other points during the occupational therapy process. The AOTA *Guidelines for Documentation of Occupational Therapy* (2003) recommend that all contacts between the occupational therapist or occupational therapy assistant and the client be documented, including telephone contacts and meetings with others. Missed sessions should be documented using a contact note (AOTA; Fremgen, 2002). AOTA guidelines further recommend that client or caregiver training be documented in a contact note, being sure to include the names of those present for the training and the client's response (if present).

In some settings, a contact note is written for each contact with a client, including each intervention session. These notes include specific intervention participation (type of intervention and client response to the intervention), significant communication to or from a client, modifications made to the environment or tasks, and/or any equipment (assistive or adaptive devices) fabricated or modified (AOTA, 2003). Some settings prefer a more complete progress note (SOAP, DAP or narrative format) (see Chapter 12). Some settings use a combination of the two, writing a contact note for every client contact, and a SOAP, DAP, or narrative note on a weekly or biweekly basis to summarize the client's progress.

Exercise 8.2

In which of the following situations would it be appropriate to do a screening?

1. A doctor's order comes to the occupational therapy department in an acute care hospital to evaluate a client.

2. You work in a hand therapy clinic. Your caseload has fallen off recently. There is a health fair coming to the strip mall across the street from your clinic. The health fair coordinator suggests that you offer free grip and pinch strength testing.

3. You have a friend who is a building supervisor for a new assisted living facility. She would like you to come once a month to screen all new residents for things like fall prevention and other safety concerns. The facility does not have occupational therapy staff on site. You work in a preschool nearby and have never worked with the elderly before.

4. A nurse asks you to look at a resident of the nursing home at which you work. The resident has been taking longer and longer to eat, and is now the last one to finish even though they serve him first. She asks you to observe the client while he eats lunch and tell her whether you think she should ask the doctor for orders for occupational therapy.

SUMMARY

The occupational therapist usually makes contact with a client after an order or referral is received for services. The referral can come from any source including the client or the client's family, other health, social service, or education professionals or physicians. Most payers require either a referral or an order from a physician.

A screening is often the first contact an occupational therapy practitioner has with the client. Sometimes screenings are routinely done for all new admissions to a program or facility. Other times, screenings are conducted at the request of another health, social service, or education professional. Screenings are brief and are generally based on chart review, interview, and observations. A screening helps determine if a full-blown evaluation would be beneficial.

A contact note is usually written to verify that the occupational therapist has received the referral or order, a screening was done, and to indicate whether further evaluation and/or intervention will be necessary. In addition, a brief contact note may be written to document every subsequent contact the occupational therapist or occupational therapy assistant has with the client throughout the course of occupational therapy service delivery. The contact note documents communication with the client or client's caregiver as well as a description of the interventions implemented and the client's response to the intervention. Contact notes are also written to document reasons for missed sessions and the content of telephone conversations with the client.

REFERENCES

American Occupational Therapy Association. (1995). Elements of clinical documentation. *American Journal of Occupational Therapy, 49,* 1032–1035.

American Occupational Therapy Association. (1998). Standards of practice for occupational therapy. *American Journal of Occupational Therapy, 52,* 866–869.

American Occupation Therapy Association. (2000). Occupational therapy code of ethics—2000. *American Journal of Occupational Therapy, 54,* 614–616.

American Occupational Therapy Association. (2003). *Guidelines for documentation of occupational therapy.* Retrieved June, 27, 2003, from *http://www.aota.org/members/area2/docs/ra2.pdf*

Collier, T. (1991). The screening process. In W. Dunn (Ed.), *Pediatric occupational therapy: Facilitating effective service provision* (pp. 10–33). Thorofare, NJ: Slack.

Fremgen, B. F. (2002). *Medical law and ethics.* Upper Saddle River, NJ: Prentice Hall.

Prabst-Hunt, W. (2002). *Occupational therapy administration manual.* Albany, NY: Delmar.

CHAPTER 9

Evaluation Reports

INTRODUCTION

The initial evaluation report is the single most important document that you will write. All of the other documents (progress notes, intervention plans, discontinuation summaries) are dependent on a clear and valid initial evaluation report. Evaluation reports demonstrate the need for occupational therapy services. If a need for your services is not documented, why should anyone pay for them? Without documentation of an evaluation, it is difficult to identify the client's level of function prior to intervention. In other words, a baseline is needed from which you, other team members, and payers can see progress (Moyers, 1999).

This chapter focuses on the components of a well-written evaluation report. The evaluation report is dependent on the skills of the occupational therapist in collecting and interpreting data. This book does not cover specific instructions for conducting evaluations, nor will it recommend specific assessment tools. There are many resources available to occupational therapists that describe selecting and administering the proper assessment tool and interpreting data. This chapter assumes you have the data and now need to write about it.

▼ CORE CONCEPTS OF EVALUATIONS ▼

Polgar (1998) identifies three main purposes for doing an evaluation: Evaluations are done to (1) describe a client's current level of performance, (2) to predict future function of that client, and (3) to measure the outcomes of occupational therapy intervention. While there may be times when you conduct an evaluation without providing intervention afterward, often you will need to write your evaluation report with all three purposes in mind. As a result, you will need to describe the unique circumstances of your client's situation, predict future function through goal setting, and establish a baseline from which future performance can be measured and compared.

Occasionally, an evaluation is completed and no intervention is needed. In this case, the evaluation serves as documentation of a client's function at the point in time of the evaluation. If another evaluation is completed at a later date, it can be used to compare to the initial evaluation, to see if functional skills have been gained or lost. If the occupational therapist is functioning in a consultant role, the evaluation may be written with the expectation that others will carry out the intervention. In this case, careful attention to the language of the evaluation report will be needed so that those charged with implementation will understand exactly what needs to be done.

Moyers (1999) identifies the focus of the evaluation process as centering "on roles and performances in occupations (Fisher & Short-DeGraff, 1993) rather than beginning with evaluation of impairments (Trombly, 1993)" (p. 264). It would follow, then, that the focus of your evaluation report would be on engagement in occupations rather than on client factors that influence performance. The *Occupational Therapy Practice Framework* (AOTA, 2002) suggests "the evaluation process is focused on finding what the client wants and needs to do and on identifying those factors that act as supports or barriers to performance" (p. 616).

Both of these perspectives suggest a "top-down" approach to conducting the evaluation. A top-down approach considers occupational performance first and then discerns the factors that contribute to the occupational performance (Stewart, 2001). Some models and frames of reference also support the top-down approach; however, others support a "bottom-up" approach. In a bottom-up approach, client factors are evaluated first, then occupational performance is addressed. This is why it is so important to base one's evaluation process on a particular model or frame of reference. It gives you a starting point and direction in which to proceed. The model or frame of reference will guide the critical thinking of the occupational therapist in the selection of evaluation methods and assessment tools, as well as the language by which the occupational therapist will describe occupational performance strengths and deficits. Refer to Chapter 3 of this book for further discussion on the influence of models and frames of reference.

Two of the most prominent concepts driving occupational therapy practice today are evidence-based practice and client-centered practice (Law, Baum, & Dunn, 2001). Evidence-based practice means that to the extent possible, you must be prepared to show that your interpretation of the data collected is supported in the literature. This demonstrates to those reading your evaluation reports that you are current in your knowledge of occupational practice and that you know what is effective.

Being client-centered means that the client is a full partner in the evaluation process (Law et al., 2001). As a partner, the client's subjective experiences, as well as the occupational therapist's objective observations, are both critical to the evaluation process. The establishment of occupational therapy outcomes (goals) is a collaborative effort between the client and occupational therapist.

▼ COMPONENTS OF AN EVALUATION REPORT ▼

Evaluations vary on many factors. Some are comprehensive; some are problem specific. Some are standardized, formal assessments; some are nonstandardized, informal, activity-based evaluations; most use observation. There are checklists and self-reporting tools. Remember, evaluation is the process and assessments are the tools (AOTA, 1998). Documentation of evaluation results may be referred to using different terms: assessment summary report, evaluation summary, evaluation report, evaluation note, or assessment report and plan. In this book, the term "evaluation reports" is used.

Hinojosa and Kramer (1998) state that an occupational therapist must consider several factors when conducting an evaluation:

- The development (biological and personal) of the person
- Contexts
- The client's relationship with others
- The client's engagement in occupations
- The quality of occupational performance
- The relationship between the client's development (physical and psychosocial) and engagement in occupations.

They go on further to identify beliefs that occupational therapists hold about evaluation (Hinojosa & Kramer, 1998). The first is that the evaluation process is ongoing throughout the service delivery continuum and it is a dynamic and interactive process. Second, we know that assessment tools can have biases, and so can the people who administer them. Assessment tools can have biases in terms of gender, culture, geographic region, educational level or socioeconomic status of the test taker. Test administrators, including occupational therapists, can carry expectations, personal prejudices, and preconceived notions into the testing situation. Of course, it is hoped that assessment tools that are selected are as free of bias as possible, and that occupational therapists try to not let biases influence the way they administer the test or interpret it. The third belief is that the client's perspective, as well as that of the client's family and caregivers, is incorporated into the evaluation process. Finally, the evaluation report should provide the reader with a comprehensive picture of the client. The report reflects the person's occupational roles, occupational performance, performance skills and patterns, contexts, activity demands, and client factors (AOTA, 2002).

As with all clinical documentation, certain elements must be present in an evaluation report. Besides the usual identification information (client name, date of birth, gender, and diagnoses), the reason for the referral, when the referral was made and who made the referral, and the type/amount of service requested are also included (AOTA, 2003). Assessment tools used in the evaluation process are listed and references are made to other reports, such as the physician's history and physical examination used by the occupational therapist. Precautions and contraindications that could interfere with or cause problems during occupational therapy evaluation and intervention are clearly stated. Examples of precautions and contraindications are that the client could not find his or her own way out of the building in case of a fire, that the client's blood pressure drops dangerously low when seated at a 90° angle, or that the client is combative. Each of these is something any occupational therapy staff member who works with or transports the client to the clinic needs to know.

Listing the appropriate diagnoses is not as easy as it sounds. You need to identify which condition (there usually is more than one diagnosis, often identified by the referral source) the occupational therapy interventions are being designed to address. If a client has an upper respiratory infection, diabetes, chemical dependency, and a broken hip, which one is the primary condition you are addressing? The term "diagnosis" is used primarily to satisfy third-party payers. In nonmedical settings, a primary concern or occupational deficit may be used instead of a medical diagnosis.

A critical section of the evaluation report is the occupational profile. In this section of the evaluation report, the occupational therapist "describes the client's occupational history and experiences, patterns of daily living, interests, values, and needs" (AOTA, 2002, p. 616). The occupational therapist is trying to understand, from the client's perspective, what the client wants and needs. This requires using a client-centered approach. The occupational therapist needs a solid understanding of the client's past experiences and contexts, current occupational strengths and areas that are problematic, and priorities/desired outcomes (AOTA, 2002, 2003).

Next, the results of the evaluation are documented. The client factors, contexts, and activity demands (AOTA, 2002) that affect occupational performance are identified and prioritized. AOTA (2003) suggests expressing one's confidence in the test results. This can be accomplished by stating whether test scores are consistent with observed behavior. For example, a test may show that a client has poor muscle strength, yet the client is observed using that muscle against gravity during dressing. Or a test could show that a client is not able to follow three-step directions, but during an activity in the occupational therapy room, the client complied perfectly when you asked him to "Pick that up, put it on the shelf over there, and then come back and sit in that chair." The results need to be summarized and relate clearly to the occupational profile (AOTA, 2003).

Some evaluation reports will also include the initial Intervention Plan in the form of long-and short-term goals; intervention approaches and methodology; the anticipated frequency, duration, and intensity of occupational therapy services; and recommendations for other services. Goal writing is addressed in Chapter 10 and intervention planning is covered in Chapter 11.

▼ ROLE DELINEATION IN THE OCCUPATIONAL THERAPY EVALUATION PROCESS ▼

The occupational therapist is responsible for the occupational therapy evaluation process (AOTA, 1998). An occupational therapy assistant, under the supervision of an occupational therapist, may contribute to the process. Either an occupational therapist or an occupational therapy assistant may educate the client and others (as appropriate) about evaluation procedures and the reasons for the evaluation.

The occupational therapist determines the most appropriate assessment tools to use (AOTA, 1998). The occupational therapy practitioner administering the assessment is responsible for following established protocols for administration of standardized tests.

The occupational therapist is responsible for summarizing, analyzing, and interpreting the data (AOTA, 1998). He or she also uses that information to develop an appropriate intervention plan based on the client's current functional status. The occupational therapist follows established guidelines for documentation of evaluation results in a time frame and format accepted by the facility/agency, payer requirements, applicable accreditation agency standards, and state and federal laws and regulations. The occupational therapist also follows confidentiality standards in communicating the results of the evaluation process to others involved in the care of the client. An occupational therapy assistant, under the supervision of an occupational therapist, may contribute to these processes.

Finally, AOTA (1998) standards state that it is the occupational therapist that makes recommendations for evaluation or intervention by other professionals, based on the occupational therapy evaluation results. In practical terms, this means that the occupational therapist has ultimate responsibility for every stage of the evaluation process. However, an occupational therapy assistant can be a very valuable contributor to the evaluation process. As appropriate to the skill of the occupational therapy assistant and the condition of the client, the occupational therapist can delegate parts of the evaluation process to the occupational therapy assistant. State licensure laws may contain specific language describing criteria for delegation of duties to an occupational therapy assistant as well as the type and amount of supervision required. It is always prudent to check with your state's licensing (or registration or other form of regulation as appropriate) authority for specific requirements.

To illustrate this process, let's pick a client to evaluate.

Case: Jacob Olsen

Jacob "Jake" Olsen is a 20-year-old college basketball star. He is a junior at a major Big Ten school. He has been a starting forward since his freshman year. Since this school has a large athletic department, there are university employees whose only job is to see that the student athletes pass all their courses. Jake loves playing basketball, but not studying for classes, so he appreciates these "tutors." One of the tutors will even write his papers for him since she is paid to type them anyway; she just recycles papers she has typed for other athletes. Jake's other love is computer games. When he is not sleeping, eating, or on the basketball court, he is leaning over his laptop computer (he is a tall man, the desks are at heights for normal people), playing galactic battle–type games with his joystick. Over time the hours and hours he spent bent over and pressing the button on the top of the joystick have taken their toll on his neck, shoulders, wrist, and thumb. He has pain from his neck to his fingers on his shooting arm. The pain in his thumb has gotten so bad that the trainer advised him to see the team physician. He was diagnosed with "game playing thumb," a combination of tendonitis and osteoarthritis. The physician gives him a thumb support splint to rest the thumb, with strict instructions not to use the thumb for the next couple weeks.

Without basketball or computer games, he is bored. The coach and his fellow teammates are angry with him. He is in constant pain. The pain pills help, but he feels drained of all energy and motivation. His appetite has decreased. The doctor referred him to occupational therapy to use heat/cold to reduce the inflammation, electrical stimulation to assist in pain relief, and to "cheer him up," in other words, to keep him motivated.

Using the model of human occupation, the occupational therapist begins collecting data as part of the occupational profile by talking with him. Although she was tempted to give him a lecture on ethics, personal responsibility, and the good of the team, she restrained herself. Instead she finds out that the areas of occupation that currently concern Jake are that he has nothing to do with his time, no games to play, and writing is impossible (he can't take notes in class now that he has time to go to class and the tutors won't go for him). He wants to get back to his games as soon as possible; he is just itching to do some-

TABLE 9.1   Descriptive, Interpretive, and Evaluative Statements

Type of Statement	Examples
Descriptive	She wore a red dress.
	He sat down on the edge of the bed and took off his shoes.
	He ate everything on the right side of his plate, leaving the food on the left side untouched.
	She looked over her left shoulder and mumbled, "Get away" six times in the half hour she was in the room. No one was standing behind her.
	She said "please" and "thank you" consistently throughout the session.
Interpretive	She usually wears red dresses.
	He had to sit down on the edge of the bed to take off his shoes.
	He did not appear to notice the food on the left side of his plate.
	She seemed to be hallucinating about someone standing too close behind her.
	She demonstrated awareness of her manners.
Evaluative	She wore a beautiful red dress.
	He was too lazy to bend over and take his shoes off.
	He is careless.
	She acted like a crazy person.
	She is a pleasant person.

thing beside watching TV or going to classes. He wears sweats so dressing is not a problem, and all his meals are prepared for him, so these are not areas of concern.

Based on this information, the occupational therapist can select appropriate assessment tools to measure his motor deficits, his play/leisure choices, collect subjective data on his level of pain, and evaluate the ergonomics of his desk and chair. She delegates some of the testing to the occupational therapy assistant. Based on the data she and the occupational therapy assistant collected, the occupational therapist concludes that the factors affecting his occupational performance are motor skills (poor posture at the computer, repetitive stress on the joints of his thumb), energy (lack of it), dominating habits (computer games dominate his leisure time), and adaptation (anticipating problems, and modifying the environment or his task to accommodate for problems). These factors form the basis of her occupational analysis.

After she collects and synthesizes this data, she identifies the supports and barriers to his full engagement in the occupations he loves. She identifies his strengths and areas in need of improvement in the analysis of occupational performance. She and Jake then sit down together to write goals and identify a targeted outcome.

▼ WRITING THE REPORT ▼

Evaluation reports must contain objective information (Cook, 1991). When reporting your findings, record what you saw or heard (occasionally taste, smell, or touch is reported). Findings could be test scores, quotes from the client, observations, or measurements. It is important to keep the findings separate from your interpretation of those findings.

Descriptive, Interpretive, and Evaluative Statements

In writing, there are descriptive, interpretive, and evaluative statements. Descriptive statements are objective; they describe what you can see, hear, taste, touch, or smell. Interpretive statements are based on observations or data, but draw some inference or conclusion about the observation or data. Evaluative statements pass judgment on something, you can feel whether the person making the statement feels good or bad about it, satisfied or dissatisfied, angry or accepting. Table 9.1 gives examples of the different kinds of statements.

Exercise 9.1

Determine whether each statement is a *description* of an event or person, an *interpretation* of an event or person, or an *evaluation* about an event or person?

1. _____ She ate corn flakes for breakfast.
2. _____ She eats corn flakes for breakfast.
3. _____ She could care less what she eats for breakfast.
4. _____ The client's breath smelled like alcohol.
5. _____ Bobby likes to play with blocks.
6. _____ Jake abuses the system of tutors for scholar-athletes.
7. _____ Jake got a high score of 3,203,485 in Galactoids.
8. _____ Jake usually plays computer games 8–10 hours per day.
9. _____ Jake sat with his body forward at 60°, his elbows resting on his knees.
10. _____ Jake's poor posture contributes to his neck, back, and shoulder pain.

Reporting Data and Interpreting It

Interpreting data can be tricky. Often people use phrases like "appears" or "seems to." If that is the preferred wording at your facility or program, then use it. Otherwise, stay away from these phrases because they make you sound unsure of yourself. When you are interpreting data/findings, stay away from evaluative statements.

When you record test scores on a test blank, you are reporting raw data. In the evaluation report findings section, you can report a summary of the data collected, or name specific tasks that the client completed. For example, you could state that the child caught a 10-inch ball on five out of seven attempts. Or you could say that the child completed all test items at the 2-year level, and completed two of the five items at the 2-year, 6-month level. In the interpretation section, you could report the age level of the child's performance, a percentile rank compared to a normal population, or describe client factors that interfere with optimal occupational performance. When you identify a client's needs, you are making an interpretation of the data. For example, when you say that a child needs to work on fine-motor coordination to bring skills up to age level, or needs to improve gross-motor skills to enable him to explore and interact with her environment, you are making an interpretive statement. Recording data is recording facts; interpreting data gives the data meaning and context.

Exercise 9.2

Using "R" for report and "I" for interpretation, identify which of the following statements are a report of information and which are an interpretation of information.

1. _____ The client completed her meal in 26 minutes.
2. _____ The client did not complete the task of looking up the phone number for "time and temperature" and making the call.
3. _____ The child is functioning at an age equivalent of 3 years, 6 months.
4. _____ Annette completed all tasks at the 3-year, 6-month level.
5. _____ The client has severely limited range of motion in her left arm.
6. _____ Toby has an attention span of about 3 minutes.

When you are interpreting the data and paving the way for your plan, it is important to keep the principles of efficiency and effectiveness in mind (Law, et al., 2001). Since the evaluation report may be used by payers to determine if the services will be paid for, you need to make convincing arguments that occupational therapy intervention is necessary to improve the quality of life for your client. Using Jake as an example, one argument could be that poor posture will contribute to life-long recurring joint injuries and pain. Teaching him ways to arrange his furniture and computer could prevent future injuries. In clinical settings, you often have to show that your services are medically necessary, which may be defined differently by different payers. You can make your arguments more convincing by demonstrating that there is support in the literature for your conclusions (interpretations) and your plan for intervention. You also have to demonstrate that what you plan to do with the client is uniquely based on occupational therapy principles, and not something that could be done through the use of other disciplines in place of occupational therapy.

Exercise 9.3

Given the data provided, write a brief interpretation of that data.

1. *Findings:* Client drooled throughout the meal. He coughed and gagged with water and juice, but not with applesauce, mashed potatoes, or Jell-O. When he chewed, he frequently opened his mouth and protruded his tongue with food on it. Sometimes food fell off his tongue back onto his plate. He was provided with eating utensils, but he did not use them. Client scooped food with both hands, putting large quantities into his mouth at one time. He swallowed five times during the entire meal.
   Interpretation:

2. *Findings:* Active range of motion is within normal limits on the right side, but the left shoulder moves 80° in flexion and 70° in abduction (normal is 180° in both directions). Client moved her elbow between 80° flexion and 40° extension (normal is 0–150°). She had no active movement of the forearm, wrist, or fingers. Passive range of motion is within normal limits in all joints and directions.
   Interpretation:

Suggested Evaluation Report Format

Figure 9.1 contains a sample evaluation report format. Notice that there are four sections; background information, findings, interpretation, and plan. You can remember these parts with the mnemonic "BiFIP." The first section is for background information. It provides the context for the rest of the report. In the format presented here, the *OT Practice Framework* (AOTA, 2002) provides the structure for the next two sections. The second section is for reporting the findings. This is where objective data is reported, using descriptive language. In as few words as possible, explain the client's current level of performance. It is not necessary to list the client's level of function for every possible activity of daily living (ADL) if only a few areas are affected by his or her current condition. Refer back to Chapter 2 for explanations of each item listed on the format. Next is the interpretation section, sometimes referred to as the analysis portion. You want to use interpretive statements in this section to help the reader make sense of your findings. Finally, there is the plan section. This is where you set goals in collaboration with your client, and determine the methodology you will employ to help your client meet those goals. The ultimate goal, according to AOTA (2002), is the client's "engagement in occupation to support participation in life" (p. 609). In writing goals, you will need to specifically state which area or areas of occupation the client will participate in. In collaboration with your client, establish concrete, measurable, timely goals. Goal writing will be covered in Chapter 10. Intervention planning will be discussed in Chapter 11.

The BiFIP format is one of several possible formats for writing evaluation reports. A format simply provides a structure for presenting information in an organized fashion. Sec-

```
┌─────────────────────────────────────────────────────────────────────────┐
│          OCCUPATIONAL THERAPY EVALUATION REPORT and INITIAL INTERVENTION PLAN │
│                                                                           │
│  BACKGROUND INFORMATION                                                   │
│  Date of report:                          Client's name or initials:     │
│  Date of birth &/or age:                  Date of referral:              │
│  Primary intervention diagnosis/concern:                                 │
│  Secondary diagnosis/concern:                                            │
│  Precautions/contraindications:                                          │
│  Reason for referral to OT: (or questions to be answered)                │
│  Therapist: (Print or type your name, sign and date the report at the end.) │
│                                                                           │
│  Assessments performed: (Give a brief description of the method(s) used to gather evaluation │
│  data; i.e., interview, informal observation, name of formal assessments, etc.) │
│                                                                           │
│  FINDINGS                                                                 │
│  Occupational Profile: (Describe the client's occupational history and experience, patterns of │
│  living, interests, values, and needs that are relevant to the current situation.) │
│                                                                           │
│  OCCUPATIONAL ANALYSIS:                                                   │
│         Areas of occupation:                                             │
│         Performance skills:                                              │
│         Performance patterns:                                            │
│         Client factors:                                                  │
│         Activity demands:                                                │
│         Contexts:                                                        │
│                                                                           │
│  INTERPRETATION                                                           │
│  Supports and Hindrances to Occupational Performance:                    │
│                                                                           │
│  Prioritization of Need Areas:                                           │
│                                                                           │
│  PLAN                                                                     │
│         Mutually agreed-on long-term goals:                              │
│         Mutually agreed-on short-term goals:                             │
│         Recommended intervention methods and approaches:                 │
│         Expected frequency, duration, and intensity:                     │
│         Location of intervention:                                        │
│         Anticipated D/C environment:                                     │
│                                                                           │
│                                                                           │
│  _____                                        │
│  Signature                    Date                                       │
└─────────────────────────────────────────────────────────────────────────┘
```

FIGURE 9.1   Occupational Therapy Evaluation Report and Initial Intervention Plan

tions will vary in length based on the amount of information you have to present. Sometimes the structure is invisible; the report is written in a narrative format with a different paragraph for each section.

There are also forms, such as the HCFA 700 (used for Medicare Part B clients), for reporting evaluation results and the initial plan of care (see Appendix G). The trick with using a form such as the Medicare form is to fit all your information in the space provided and still be legible. The Medicare forms are available from electronic sources and can be done on the computer, eliminating the legibility issue. There are also numerous electronic evaluation report formats for writing evaluation reports on a computer. These usually come as part of a documentation system purchased by a facility or agency for use by all members of the intervention team. In facilities/agencies using electronic data entry and reporting, training is provided to all staff that use the system.

Complete the evaluation report below on Jake Olsen. You may invent test results and other information for this exercise, knowing you would never do such a thing in "real life." The results and additional information you create must be consistent with the case.

OCCUPATIONAL THERAPY EVALUATION REPORT and INITIAL INTERVENTION PLAN

BACKGROUND INFORMATION
Date of report: 1-15-04   **Client's name or initials:** Jacob Olsen
Date of birth &/or age: 6-25-84   **Date of referral:** 1-14-04
Primary intervention diagnosis/concern: Tendonitis of (R) thumb; neck, back, and (R) arm pain
Secondary diagnosis/concern: Depression
Precautions/contraindications: Thumb immobilized until 1-28-04
Reason for referral to OT: Immobilization of thumb interferes with daily life tasks
Therapist: *(use your name with OTS or OTAS as your credential if you are a student)*

Assessments performed: Observation and interview, UMOT interest inventory, ergonomic assessment of dorm room chair and desk, and the Multiple Dimension Hand Assessment.

FINDINGS
Occupational Profile:

Occupational Analysis:
    Areas of occupation:
    Performance skills:
    Performance patterns:
    Client factors:
    Activity demands:
    Contexts:

INTERPRETATION
Supports and Hindrances to Occupational Performance:
Prioritization of Need Areas:

PLAN
    Mutually agreed-on long-term goals:
    Mutually agreed-on short-term goals:
    Recommended intervention methods and approaches:
    Expected frequency, duration, and intensity: 3x/wk for 2 weeks, 45-min. sessions
    Location of intervention:
    Anticipated D/C environment:

Signature   **Date**

▼ RE-EVALUATION ▼

Evaluation is an ongoing process. While the focus of this chapter has been on documenting an initial evaluation, there is an element of evaluation that occurs throughout the intervention process. At every intervention session, the occupational therapy practitioner makes observations, collects information about changes in the client's circumstances and performance, and sometimes makes adjustments in the intervention methodology. If the intervention is going to occur over several weeks or more, periodic re-evaluations are conducted.

Re-evaluation may be formal or informal. Informal re-evaluation occurs every time the occupational therapist revises the intervention plan (see Chapter 11). A formal re-evaluation may involve repeating previous testing so that changes in performance can be measured and documented. Often this occurs when a client is close to being discontinued.

Nielson (1998) suggests that re-evaluation is a three-step process: data collection, reflection, and decision making. Data collection involves gathering subjective and objective information relative to the targeted outcomes identified by the client and clinician. Reflection is a thought process centered on the client's current status, changes in status since the last evaluation, and a judgment on the effectiveness of the current intervention plan. In the decision-making step, the occupational therapist decides whether the current intervention plan is sufficient, whether it should be changed in some way, or whether the client is ready to be discontinued from occupational therapy services.

SUMMARY

The evaluation report is a critically important document. When another team member or a payer reads your evaluation report, he or she should have a clear picture of how the client is functioning and what the hope is for change. The report will justify the need for occupational therapy involvement in this case. All the rest of the work you do with that client hinges on an evaluation report that shows a strong need for your services, clearly states where the client is starting from, and establishes a doable plan.

In the evaluation report, describe your findings/data and then interpret them. Without findings, an interpretation is meaningless. The interpretation cannot stand alone; there must be data/findings to back it up. There is a difference between descriptive, interpretive, and evaluative statements. In the findings section, only descriptive statements should be used. In the interpretation sections, interpretive statements are used. Evaluative statements have no place in evaluation reports. Be absolutely sure you distinguish between reporting information and interpreting it. Follow all the guidelines for general documentation as well as professional standards for evaluation reports.

The occupational therapist is responsible for conducting and documenting the evaluation process. An occupational therapy assistant may contribute to the process. The occupational therapist is also responsible for making referrals to other professionals if the client has needs that are better met by another professional.

There are many formats for reporting evaluation results. Medicare has a form that is available in both electronic and paper formats. Other vendors sell documentation systems that include evaluation formats. The format presented in this chapter is a paper-based format called "BiFIP," which stands for background information, findings, interpretation, and plan. The AOTA describes the evaluation process in *The Occupational Therapy Practice Framework* (2002). The evaluation process is client-centered.

Re-evaluation occurs periodically throughout the course of occupational therapy service delivery. It may be formal or informal. It should contain subjective input from the client and client's caregivers as well as objective data gathered through observation and testing. The re-evaluation helps the occupational therapist determine whether the current intervention plan is sufficient, needs adjustment, or if the client is ready to be discontinued from occupational therapy services.

REFERENCES

American Occupational Therapy Association. (1998). Standards of practice for occupational therapy. *American Journal of Occupational Therapy, 52,* 866–869.

American Occupational Therapy Association. (2002). Occupational therapy practice framework: Domain and process. *American Journal of Occupational Therapy, 56,* 609–639.

American Occupational Therapy Association. (2003). *Guidelines for documentation of occupational therapy.* Retrieved June 27, 2003, from *http://aota.org/members/area2/docs/ra2.pdf*

Cook, D. G. (1991). The assessment process. In W. Dunn (Ed.), *Pediatric occupational therapy: Facilitating effective service provision* (pp. 35–72). Thorofare, NJ: Slack.

Hinojosa, J., & Kramer, P. (1998). Theoretical basis of evaluation. In J. Hinojosa & Kramer (Eds.), *Evaluation: Obtaining and interpreting data.* Bethesda, MD: American Occupational Therapy Association.

Law, M., Baum, C., & Dunn, W. (2001). *Measuring occupational performance: Supporting best practice in occupational therapy.* Thorofare, NJ: Slack.

Moyers, P. A. (1999). The guide to occupational therapy practice. *American Journal of Occupational Therapy, 53,* 247–322.

Nielson, C. (1998). Reevaluation. In J. Hinojosa & P. Kramer (Eds.), *Evaluation: Obtaining and interpreting data.* Bethesda, MD: American Occupational Therapy Association.

Polgar, J. M. (1998). Critiquing assessments. In M. E. Neistadt & E. B. Crepeau (Eds.), *Willard & Spackman's occupational therapy* (9th ed., pp. 169–184). Philadelphia: Lippincott.

Stewart, K. B. (2001). Purposes, processes, and methods of evaluation. In J. Case-Smith, (Ed.), *Occupational therapy for children* (4th ed., pp. 190–213). St. Louis, MO: Mosby.

CHAPTER 10

Goal Writing

INTRODUCTION

Setting appropriate goals, ones that can be measured and are realistic, can help you demonstrate that you did indeed help your client. The trick is to set the goals so that the client can meet them. The goals cannot be so easy that they are not meaningful, yet not so hard that they cannot be accomplished in the time you have to work together. In other words, they have to represent a just-right challenge.

Goal writing is an essential step in both the evaluation and intervention process. Goals are often first established as part of the evaluation process, and then revised as part of the intervention process. Goals guide the direction of interventions. They help occupational therapists and occupational therapy assistants determine the effectiveness of their interventions. If a client is meeting goals, the intervention is likely to be appropriate. If a client is not meeting established goals, perhaps a different approach or intervention method should be tried.

▼ ROLE DELINEATION IN GOAL WRITING ▼

Goals are established in collaboration with the client, or if the client is unable to collaborate, the client's caregiver or guardian (AOTA, 2002). Primary responsibility for the development of intervention plans and goal setting rests with the occupational therapist, however, occupational therapy assistants may contribute to the process (AOTA, 1998). The *AOTA Occupational Therapy Standards of Practice* (1998) further states that the occupational therapist establishes "client-centered goals that are clear, measurable, behavioral, functional, contextually relevant and appropriate to the client's needs, desires, and expected outcomes" (AOTA, 1998, Standard V).

▼ GOAL DIRECTIONS ▼

The frame(s) of reference you used in determining your evaluation strategies is used to help you frame your goals (see Chapters 3 and 9). The type of setting in which you are working will impact the wording of the goals you write. In writing goal statements, there are a limited number of directions the goals can go. AOTA (2002), in *The Framework,* suggests the types of outcomes (goals) of occupational therapy intervention are that you can work with your client to enhance or improve occupational performance, improve client satisfaction with functional skills and abilities, improve role performance, adapt responses to challenges, promote health and wellness, prevent dysfunction, or improve the client's perception of his or her quality of life. *The Framework* further presents the following intervention approaches: create or promote, establish or restore, maintain, modify, or prevent. These intervention approaches can be used to help determine the direction a goal will take. Moyers (1999), in *The Guide to Occupational Therapy Practice,* describes five kinds of outcomes: occupational performance, prevention, general health, satisfaction, and quality of life.

Based on a synthesis of these two documents, goal directions can be summarized as restorative, habilitative, maintenance, modification, preventive, and health promotion.

Restorative Goals

Restorative goals (rehabilitative or remediative) are used when you have a client who used to be able to do something, but now cannot (AOTA, 2002). This usually happens when there has been an illness or injury. Occupational therapy practitioners working in hospitals, rehabilitation facilities, nursing homes, outpatient clinics, home health, or psychiatric facilities typically write restorative goals. These goals are written to reflect a desired change in function. Examples of restorative goals include:

- By discharge, client will feed herself three meals a day independently.
- By July 15, 2005, with one prompt, client will state three strengths about herself.
- The client will return to work as a carpenter, consistently using good body mechanics, by August 1, 2005.

Habilitative Goals

Goals that teach new skills are often called habilitative goals. Habilitation refers to teaching skills that the client never had, typically because of delayed development. This is different from rehabilitation, which seeks to restore a lost function, to help a client relearn a lost skill. Habilitative goals are often used with children whose development is delayed, or when teaching new skills to adults with developmental disabilities. Examples of habilitative goals include:

- Eric will write his name legibly on all his school papers by June 10, 2004.
- Pahoa will consistently package the correct number of products, using adaptive jigs if needed, in the sheltered workshop by September 1, 2004.
- Emmalee will demonstrate increased mobility by independently moving from prone on the floor to standing by November 3, 2004.

Maintenance Goals

Maintenance goals seek to keep a client at his or her current level of function despite disease processes that normally would cause deterioration of function (AOTA, 2002). These goals would be written in long-term care or outpatient settings. One concern about maintenance goals is that many third-party payers will not pay for them. The payers often only want to pay as long as progress is being made. A maintenance goal is seen as an indication that progress is no longer being made. Examples of maintenance goals include:

- Client will maintain independence in dressing for the next 3 months.
- Client will actively participate in a current events group eight times in the next 30 days.
- For the next 6 months, client will continue to live in her own home with minimal assistance of home health aide.

Modification Goals

Modification goals (also called compensation or adaptation goals) seek to change the contexts around the activity rather than change the skills and abilities of the client (AOTA, 2002). In other words, instead of increasing the strength and range of motion of an elderly client, address adapting the environment or tools used to complete the task. These goals are difficult to write in the sense that they can sound prescriptive and limiting. The trick is to be general enough to allow you to experiment and see what products work best, yet specific enough that you have some direction. Examples of modification goals include:

- By August 12, 2004, Pyter will open boxes, cans, and bags with the use of adaptive equipment as needed so that he can independently prepare meals at home.
- By discharge, client's home will be modified to allow wheelchair access both inside and outside the house.
- In 3 months, the client will return to work with workplace modifications as needed to allow completion of essential functions of the job.

Preventive Goals

Preventive goals are written to assist persons who are at risk of developing occupational performance problems (AOTA, 2002). The person may or may not be completely healthy at the time the goal is written. Examples of preventive goals include:

- By discharge, client will demonstrate proper body mechanics while lifting.
- By next session, Reed will list five strategies for removing himself from situations that tempt him to engage in the use of cocaine.
- By next week, Chenyse will identify three friends she can call for help when she begins to feel depressed or overwhelmed.

Health Promotion

Goals that relate to health promotion are more often seen in emerging areas of practice rather than in traditional occupational therapy practice (AOTA, 2002). Health promotion goals may apply to an individual, group, community, or organization. In these settings, there is usually no attempt to correct a performance deficit; rather, the emphasis is on enhancing the contexts and activities to enable maximum participation in life (AOTA, 2002). Examples of health promotion goals include:

- By the end of this class, parents will demonstrate minimal competency in infant massage.
- Playground surfaces will be replaced to provide a safer play environment for children by May 25, 2005.
- Within the next 3 months, create raised gardens at the community center so that wheelchair-bound gardeners can access their own garden plot.

▼ GOAL SPECIFICS ▼

Goals are also written for varying amounts of time. Long-term goals are overarching goals that guide the intervention to a definite conclusion. Often, long-term goals are the goals that, when met, will determine the time to discontinue therapy. Some facilities call them discharge goals. If a client is expected to receive services for more than one year, then the long-term goal might reflect the progress expected by the end of a year.

Short-term goals are written for specific periods of time, and change from time to time, leading up to the achievement of the long-term goal. In some settings, short-term goals are called objectives (Richardson & Shultz-Krohn, 2001). For example, if the long-term goal is to become independent in dressing, the first short-term goal might address dressing in clothes that have no fasteners, such as sweats. The next short-term goal might include zippers or Velcro. The next might include buttons, snaps, hooks, or ties. The last one might include outerwear (especially in cold climates) such as parkas, mittens, boots, hats, and scarves.

The way in which you refer to your client in the goal statement will vary by facility or program. In some facilities, the preferred phrase is "the client." In others, it is "the patient," "the resident," or "the participant." Some programs prefer you use the client's first or last name. The best advice is to either ask your supervisor what his or her preference is, or read the goals written by others in the department.

There are several formats for writing goals, but all of them require the use of action words (verbs). Figure 10.1 is a list of some verbs (there are more than those on this list, but these give you an idea) that can be used in goal writing.

Of course, a lot depends on how you use the word. For example, when you use the verb *focus* in reference to vision rehab, you can see if the client is focusing on an object. If you use *focus* in reference to thought processes, can you see that?

Verbs that are not action-oriented would rarely, if ever, be used in occupational therapy goals. These are listed in Figure 10.2.

Except for maintenance goals, most goals need to describe change, and how that change will be measured. Figure 10.3 shows examples of ways to measure change. However, depending on the unique wants, needs, and circumstances of each client, there are many other ways to document change as well. For example, attainment of health status, level of prevention of dysfunction, and client perception of life satisfaction, role performance, or quality of life may be measured qualitatively rather than quantitatively.

accesses	calculates	digs	generalizes
accomplishes	calls	diminishes	gets
accommodates	changes	discriminates	gives
achieves	chooses	discusses	grips
acquires	chops	displays	grooms
acts	clasps	distributes	goes
adapts	cleans	does	handles
adheres	clears	doffs	has
adjusts	closes	dons	heeds
agrees	collaborates	draws	identifies
aligns	collects	dresses	improves
allows	comes	drinks	initiates
applies	communicates	drives	inquires
approaches	completes	dries	irons
arranges	complies	eats	interacts
asks	conforms	employs	is
asserts	confronts	endures	jumps
assists	connects	engages	keeps
attempts	contacts	establishes	knits
attends	continues	explores	knots
avoids	contributes	expresses	labels
bakes	converses	extends	leads
balances	cooperates	facilitates	leaves
bathes	coordinates	fastens	lies
becomes	corrects	feeds	lifts
behaves	creates	finishes	lists
bends	crochets	focuses	listens
breathes	crushes	folds	locates
brushes	cuts	follows	locks
builds	dances	gains	loosens
buttons	demonstrates	gathers	maintains
buys	develops	gazes	makes

FIGURE 10.1 Action Verbs. *Source: Dictionaire Jeans Anglais Français, Français Anglais. © Langenscheidt, KG, Berlin and Munich.*

manages	pursues	says	strengthens
masters	pushes	scrubs	stretches
meets	puts	secures	succeeds
modulates	questions	seeks	sucks
spreads	quits	selects	supports
moves	raises	sends	sustains
obeys	reaches	sequences	takes
obtains	reads	serves	talks
opens	rebuilds	sets	taps
organizes	records	sews	tastes
navigates	reduces	shares	tends
notices	reestablishes	shaves	terminates
paces	regards	shops	throws
paints	rehearses	shows	tightens
participates	rejoins	showers	toilets
pauses	relates	shuts	touches
pays	remarks	signs	tracks
pedals	reminds	simulates	transfers
performs	removes	sings	transports
picks	repairs	sits	tries
places	repeats	skis	types
plans	requests	sleeps	unwraps
plays	researches	slides	uses
positions	responds	snaps	utilizes
posts	rests	socializes	verifies
practices	restores	solves	vocalizes
prepares	resumes	sorts	volunteers
presses	returns	speaks	walks
prevents	reverses	specifies	washes
prints	reviews	stabilizes	watches
prioritizes	revises	stands	wears
procures	rinses	starts	wipes
promotes	rises	states	withdraws
propels	rolls	stays	works
provides	rotates	stirs	wraps
pulls	rows	stitches	writes
punches	rubs	stops	zips
purchases	runs	straightens	

FIGURE 10.1   (Continued).

commits	feels	loves	resolves
considers	forgives	perceives	respects
contemplates	hears	prefers	sees
decides	imagines	processes	senses
desires	infers	realizes	smells
determines	interprets	recognizes	sympathizes
empathizes	knows	reflects	thinks
enjoys	learns	remembers	wants
expects	likes	represses	

FIGURE 10.2   Verbs to Avoid. *Source: Dictionaire Jeans Anglais Français, Français Anglais. © Langenscheidt, KG, Berlin and Munich.*

Frequency or Consistency

- Percentage (number of successes divided by the number of opportunities for success)
- "A" out of "B" trials
- Consistently

Duration

- Time, such as number of seconds or minutes of sustained activity
- Number of repetitions

Assistance

- Maximum (75% or more of task)
- Moderate (50–74% of task)
- Minimum (25–49% of task)
- Standby
- Set-up
- Adaptive equipment
- Verbal cuing/prompts
- Physical cuing
- Independently

Quality of Performance

- Number of errors
- Accuracy
- Amount of aberrant task behavior (i.e., tremors, off-task behavior)
- Amount of pain perceived by client
- Adherence to safety precautions

Level of Complexity

- Amount of instruction
- Number of steps in the process
- Cognitive level
- Multitasking

Participation

- Attend
- Engage
- Initiate
- Transition
- Interaction
- Adapts to environmental signals or social cues
- Obtain needed tools and equipment

Other

- Express feelings
- Specific task completion
- Variety of environments in which desired behavior will occur
- Level of cooperation
- Complete steps of a task

FIGURE 10.3 Ways to Measure Change. *From Moyers (1999).*

There are many systems for formulating goals. In this chapter, I share four of these with you. I do not propose that any one system is better than the others; they are all just different. It is good to be familiar with more than one system, as one never knows which system one's supervisor will prefer.

ABCD

Ginge Kettenbach (1990) proposed the "ABCD" method: **A**udience, **B**ehavior, **C**ondition, and **D**egree. The **audience** represents the person who will do the behavior. The *behavior* is what the audience will do. The *condition* describes the circumstances around the behavior. The *degree* describes how well the behavior must be done to meet the goal.

Usually, the **audience** is the client (Kettenbach, 1990). Since occupational therapy practice is client centered, this makes sense. Occasionally you might write a goal for a caregiver, but you should never write a goal for what you, the occupational therapist, will do (Kettenbach). What you plan to do belongs in the plan, not in the goal.

A **behavior** is usually something you can see or hear the person doing or saying. Examples of behaviors include reaching, dressing, carrying, demonstrating, expressing, eating, or crocheting. Behaviors represent an action and thus are stated as verbs (Kettenbach, 1990). However, not all verbs represent action. Refer to the word lists earlier in this chapter.

Conditions, circumstances that support the behavior, help to clarify the goal (Kettenbach, 1990). Conditions can represent something in the environment that is necessary for the behavior to occur (Richardson & Schultz-Krohn, 2001). For example, in the goal "The client will independently dress herself in clothes that have no fasteners," *clothes that have no fasteners* is the condition. The client needs access to clothes that do not have fasteners (elastic-waist pants, pull-over tops) in order to meet the goal. Conditions can also be the amount of cuing or assistance needed.

The **degree** is the measurable part of the goal (Kettenbach, 1990). It tells the reader how many, what percent, what degree, or other distinguishing characteristic of the behavior. The degree has to be realistic, functional, and identify a specific time frame. Realistic means that you can reasonably expect the client to achieve the goal in the time frame you establish. Functional means the goal describes an area of occupational performance. The time frame is when you realistically expect the goal to be met. This is dependent on the condition of the client, the frequency and duration of occupational therapy, and your professional knowledge and experience with similar types of clients.

Exercise 10.1

Identify the parts of the goal that correspond to the letters ABCD:

1. The client will prepare a complete meal (meat, vegetable, starch, beverage) independently on three consecutive days by Nov. 1, 2004. *(Client has osteoarthritis and diabetic neuropathy in her upper extremities.)*

    A:

    B:

    C:

    D:

---

2. The patient will bathe herself using adaptive equipment, if needed, in less than 15 minutes by next month. *(Client has a right hemiparesis.)*

   A:

   B:

   C:

   D:

3. Bobby will independently retrieve the tools necessary to complete his project in three of the next five sessions. *(Client has chronic schizophrenia and is seen in a day program.)*

   A:

   B:

   C:

   D:

FEAST

Another system for writing goals is FEAST by Sherry Borcherding (2000; see also Borcherding & Kappel, 2002). As with the ABCD method, each letter of the word *FEAST* represents a component of the goal.

F stands for **function**. Functions are the areas of occupational performance that the client hopes to improve or maintain, the focus of the goal. Examples of functions include dressing, eating, shopping, knitting, or navigating the neighborhood.

E stands for **expectation**. In conjunction with the client, you establish what the client will do. Phrases like "the client will" make the expectation clear.

A is for **action**. Actions are expressed as verbs and are often part of the function being addressed, so they may not be a separate part of the goal statement. Examples of action words (verbs) include make, do, reach, carry, write, lift, transfer, and demonstrate.

S stands for **specific conditions**. These are essentially the same as the "C" in the "ABCD" model. They identify the level of assistance or other conditions that are necessary for the client to meet the goal. For example, whether the client engages in the activity while sitting or standing, whether the client does it with help or independently, or which body parts will be involved. There may be more than one specific condition listed in the goal.

Finally, the T stands for **timeline**. Good goals give some indication of when you think the goal will be accomplished. This could be stated in terms of the number of intervention sessions, number of weeks, or a specific date.

Exercise 10.2

Identify the parts of the goal that correspond to the letters FEAST:

1. Client will demonstrate safe use of a sharp knife without cuing on three consecutive occupational therapy sessions by June 1, 2004. *(Client had a traumatic brain injury.)*

F:

E:

A:

S:

T:

2. Student will consistently write his name with each letter correctly formed by June 15, 2004. *(Client is in 8-year-old child with mental retardation.)*

F:

E:

A:

S:

T:

3. Client will retrieve her mail from the mailbox at the end of her driveway on three consecutive days by 4-17-04. *(Client is a middle-aged woman with agoraphobia.)*

F:

E:

A:

S:

T:

RHUMBA (Rumba)

A third method for writing goals is RHUMBA (College of St. Catherine [CSC], 2001) or RUMBA (McClain, 1991; Perinchief, 1998). According to Perinchief (1998), the American Occupational Therapy Association (AOTA) developed RUMBA in the 1970s. A rhumba (also spelled rumba) is an Afro-Cuban folk dance that is especially rhythmic (*The New Encyclopedia Britannica*, 1985). In goal setting, the client represents the music, the goals must "dance" to the client's tune, and each of the parts of the goal must "rhumba" with each other (CSC, 2001). As with the other systems for goal writing, each letter in the word "rhumba" stands for something.

Relevant/**R**elates: *The goal/outcome must relate to something, be relevant.*
How Long: *Specify when the goal/outcome will be met.*
Understandable: *Anyone reading it must know what it means.*
Measurable: *There must be a way to know when the goal is met.*
Behavioral: *The goal/outcome must be something that is seen or heard.*
Achievable: *It must be realistic and doable.* (CSC, 2001, p. 1).

Let's examine each of these in more detail.

The "R" can stand for **relevant** (McClain, 1991; Perinchief, 1998). If a goal is relevant, it answers the question "So what?" Does achieving this goal really matter? Will it make a difference in the client's life? Think about what matters more, that the client can bend her elbow 40° farther or that she can now feed herself? Here are some examples of meaningless goals adapted from CSC's *Goal Writing: Documenting Outcomes* (2001):

1. I will take 94E to 90S, averaging 70 mph and 30 mpg, on Saturday, driving for approximately 7 hours, in my red '02 MX6, by myself, taking enough luggage for 3 days and food for the trip, stopping no more than 3 times.

   So what? What is the point of all of this? Where are you going? Is how you do it more important than getting there? What needs to be stated is the expected outcome, not the method for getting there.

2. Patient will count coins of varying denominations and combinations of up to $.77 with 65% accuracy on 3 of 5 tries each day for 7 of 10 days within 30 days.

   So what? How will this make a significant difference in a client's life? What happens if the patient counts $.77 with 60% accuracy on 4 of 5 tries for 6 of the next 10 days? Is the goal met? Will the next goal be $.78? How will you keep track of all this data? I do not understand this goal, it is too complicated.

The "R" can also mean **relates** (CSC, 2001). The long- and short-term goals must relate to an area of occupation (keep it functional), they must relate to each other, and they must relate to identified wants and needs of the client (the client's music) (CSC, 2001). In other words there must be a clear relationship between the areas of occupation identified during the evaluation process as being in need of intervention, the goal statements themselves, and the intervention strategies used to help meet the goals. For example, if in your evaluation you determine that the client needs to learn to hold a crayon using a three-point grasp, then the goals need to say something about holding a crayon, and the intervention needs to involve crayons. It would be inappropriate to identify the need to hold a crayon, set a goal to improve hand use (too vague), and then suggest intervention strategies using jungle gyms, large balls, and finger painting.

How long is a realistic estimate of the time you expect it will take to reach the goal (CSC, 2001). For long-term goals, that usually means when the client will be discontinued, which may be a specific date or an estimate such as 6 months or a year. For short-term goals, it could be a number of visits, a specific date, or, if you write a new intervention plan every 30 days, you can assume the short-term goals are meant to be met in 30 days. Since how you state the time frame will vary by the setting in which you are working, always check with your supervisor to see what the standard is in that setting. I have seen some goals that simply state that a client will do something on 3 consecutive days, and then the goal will be met. Well, that is not really putting a time limit on a goal. The client could do the task on 3 consecutive days next week, or 6 months from now. If I am paying for occupational therapy services, I want to know whether to expect the client to meet the goal in 2 weeks or 2 months. If a client needs to do something 3 days in a row, that may be OK as a measurement, but it does not tell me when to expect the goal to be met.

Understandable involves several dimensions. In order for the reader to understand the goal, it first has to be legible (McClain, 1991; Perinchief, 1998). Then it has to make sense to the reader, which means using easily understood, grammatically correct, accurately spelled language free from jargon and using only acceptable abbreviations. Use an active voice rather than a passive voice. This means you say that the client will do something rather than say that something will be done, that is, "The client will change her socks," rather than "The socks will be changed by the client." Again, check a grammar guide for more information on active voice. Finally, consider avoiding noncommittal language. Examples of noncommittal language include phrases like "will appear" or "will be able to."

You want the client to do something, not just look like she can do it. There is a difference between actually doing something and being able to do something. If you say the client will be able to feed himself, it does not necessarily mean he will do it. Maybe the nurse does it for him, even though he could do it if they let him. If you say the client will feed himself, it means he will do it himself. The goal has to be so clearly stated that anyone stepping in for you if you are sick will know, beyond a shadow of a doubt, what your plan was for providing services to a client.

If you look at the two goals mentioned under the relevant section of RHUMBA, you will see that in addition to not being relevant, they are also not understandable. The goals contain so many clauses and conditions that it is impossible to know what the focus of the goal really is. I can't even tell how to measure the second example.

Measurable is usually expressed as a quantitative statement that identifies how you will know when the goal is met (CSC, 2001). A goal is not met just because the time frame has elapsed. There has to be a measurement of function. You can measure progress as well as maintenance of function. Examples of measurements include frequency, accuracy, level of efficiency, consistency, grade, degree, speed, level of independence, or duration (CSC; McClain, 1991; Perinchief, 1998).

The **behavioral** component is the same as it was in the ABCD system. The behavior has to be observed, not inferred. It can be reflected as an action verb (see lists earlier in the chapter). By observed, I mean something you can see the client do or hear the client say (Perinchief, 1998). Since you cannot see or hear how a client feels or knows something, these would not be behaviors you would include in goal statements. You can hear a client express his feelings, but you can never be completely sure that because someone says he feels something that he actually feels it. You can see if a client can demonstrate a behavior, but that may or may not mean she understands it.

Achievable means that the goal is reasonable and likely to be met in the time frame established (CSC, 2001; McClain, 1999; Perinchief, 1998). It is reasonable given the condition of the client, the frequency and duration of projected occupational therapy sessions, and the contexts of the client and the environment. It is not overly ambitious or too easy.

Exercise 10.3

Identify the parts of the goal that correspond to the letters RHUMBA:

1. By January 2, 2005, the client will accurately cut and paste eight individual letters using the mouse with his left hand in 5 minutes or less. *(Client had a stroke affecting his dominant (right) hand and wants to become proficient at using a mouse with his non-dominant (left) hand.)*

   R:

   H:

   U:

   M:

   B:

   A: *You do not have enough information to answer this, but I assure you it is achievable.*

2. By June 26, 2004, the client will consistently catch himself each time he begins to make self-defeating/self-derogatory statements. *(Client is experiencing major depression and has committed himself to an inpatient psychiatric program following a failed suicide attempt.)*

   R:

   H:

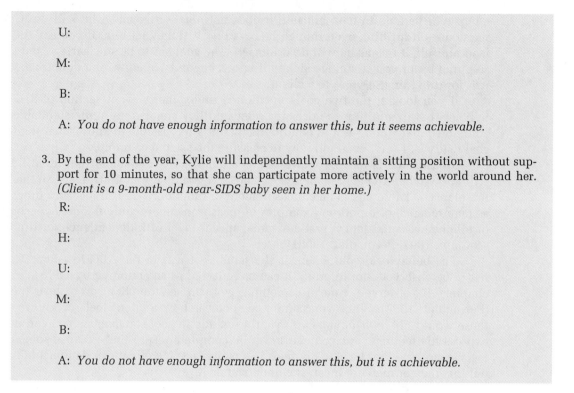

U:

M:

B:

A: *You do not have enough information to answer this, but it seems achievable.*

3. By the end of the year, Kylie will independently maintain a sitting position without support for 10 minutes, so that she can participate more actively in the world around her. *(Client is a 9-month-old near-SIDS baby seen in her home.)*

   R:

   H:

   U:

   M:

   B:

   A: *You do not have enough information to answer this, but it is achievable.*

SMART

The last system for goal writing is writing SMART goals. There are many versions of SMART goals as well. Angier (1995) says SMART goals mean goals that are specific, measurable, action-oriented, realistic, and timely. The University of Victoria Counseling Services (1996) uses SMART as an acronym for specific, measurable, acceptable, realistic time frame. Paul J. Meyer (2002) describes SMART as standing for specific, measurable, attainable, realistic, and tangible. In this book, SMART stands for significant (and simple), measurable, achievable, related, and time-limited.

Significant means that achieving this goal will make a significant difference in this person's life. This implies that you know your client's strengths and need areas so well that you know what will matter most to her (or him); in fact, your goals would ideally be developed in collaboration with her (or him), ensuring significance. By remembering to keep it simple you are more likely to achieve the goal and it will be easier to understand.

Measurable, as in RHUMBA, means that you have a clear target to aim for, and that you will know when the client gets there (CSC, 2001). The client will dress herself with no more than one verbal cue. The client will feed himself a whole meal in less than 30 minutes. Timothy will check his daily schedule every hour. These are incomplete goals, but I mention them here to emphasize the measurement component of goal writing. One common error I have seen in goal writing is goals that say the client will improve at something without stating how big the improvement must be. For example, the client will improve her accuracy at measuring dry ingredients. How much improvement is enough to say that goal was met?

Achievable also has the same meaning as it does in RHUMBA. It must be reasonable that the client could achieve this goal in the time allotted for it (CSC, 2001). Realistically, not every client will achieve every goal. When you first start out writing goals, you may have to guess a little at how much the client can achieve in your time frame. As you gain experience, your guesses will become more accurate.

Relates, in SMART as in RHUMBA, means that the goal clearly has a connection to the client's occupational needs as stated in the evaluation report (CSC, 2001). Long- and short-term goals relate to each other.

Finally, **time-limited** means the goal has a chronological end point (CSC, 2001). You know when to evaluate whether the goal is met. If the long-term goal is met, then it is time to discontinue services. If the short-term goal is met, then it is time to set a new short-term goal that gets the client closer to the long-term goal. If the short-term goal is not met at the designated time, then perhaps that goal needs to be either modified or continued.

Exercise 10.4

Identify the parts of the goal that correspond to the letters SMART:

1. By next week, client will demonstrate proper lifting techniques on 80% of opportunities for lifting boxes weighing 10 lbs. or more. *(Client had a back injury and is now being seen in a work hardening program.)*

   S:

   M:

   A: *Seems achievable given what we know.*

   R:

   T:

2. By April 22, 2004, Nellie will feed herself with a fork or spoon, spilling two or fewer times per meal. *(Nellie is in a long-term care facility with diagnoses of rheumatoid arthritis, COPD, and macular degeneration.)*

   S:

   M:

   A: *I think it is achievable in the time frame given.*

   R:

   T:

3. Mandy will cut out basic shapes with scissors within 1/4" of the line consistently by the end of the school year. *(Mandy is in first grade and has fine motor deficits that make her stand out from her classmates.)*

   S:

   M:

   A: *It is achievable.*

   R:

   T:

Exercise 10.5

Write a goal statement for the following cases using the format listed.

1. **ABCD:** This client has recently had tendon transfer surgery on his dominant hand. The surgeon wants you to make a splint and teach the client how to don and doff the splint. The hand will be immobilized for a week.

2. **FEAST:** This client was admitted yesterday after an episode of mania in which she got little sleep, shopped till she dropped, and then engaged in wild parties involving sex, drugs, and rock 'n roll. She is loud, often saying and doing things that embarrass other clients, and is in constant motion. Her husband admitted her to get her back on an appropriate medication routine.

3. **RHUMBA:** This client is 6 years old. She has cerebral palsy. She is in occupational therapy to learn to use a new electric wheelchair.

4. **SMART:** This client was badly burned in a terrorist attack. She has had numerous skin grafts. She is past the extreme pain phase, and now rates her pain level as very bad. In occupational therapy, she is working on increasing her reach and grasp with both arms while wearing compression garments.

SUMMARY

Goal writing is tricky business. You have to think about what the client wants or needs, what is a reasonable amount of time needed to meet the goal, how you will measure it, and assorted other conditions depending on the format you use for goal writing. Four separate formats for goal writing were presented: ABCD, FEAST, RHUMBA, and SMART. While there are subtle differences between them, they all result in well-written goals.

Goal writing is a collaborative process involving the occupational therapist and the client or client's surrogate (i.e., parent or guardian). An occupational therapy assistant contributes to this process.

Goals are written to help a client improve occupational performance, learn to do a new task, maintain function, modify or adapt contexts to enable performance, prevent occupational performance problems, or promote health (AOTA, 2002). The verbs used to show the action of the goal will vary by the direction of the goal, but all verbs used should be active rather than passive in nature. Word selection is also important in describing change and the measurement of change.

The ultimate goal in occupational therapy is "engaging in occupations that support participation in life" (AOTA, 2002, p. 609). For each client, the occupations the client wants or needs to engage in will be different. Long-term goals are written to describe the final outcome of occupational therapy intervention and are sometimes called discharge or discontinuation goals. Short-term goals are usually written for a specific period of time, often monthly, but may be written for a week, biweekly, or bimonthly. Long-term goals generally stay the same throughout occupational therapy service delivery, unless the client's life circumstances change. Short-term goals change or are revised often.

Goal writing is an essential part of both the evaluation and intervention processes. Goals give you a yardstick by which you can measure the effectiveness of the intervention approaches and methods used with a given client.

REFERENCES

American Occupational Therapy Association. (1998). Occupational therapy standards of practice. *American Journal of Occupational Therapy, 52,* 866–869.

American Occupational Therapy Association. (2002). Occupational therapy practice framework: Domain and process. *American Journal of Occupational Therapy, 56,* 609–639.

Angier, M. (1995). *Setting S-M-A-R-T goals.* Retrieved December 20, 2002, from *http://www.positiveath.net/ideasMA20_p.htm*

Borcherding, S. (2000). *Documentation manual for writing SOAP notes in occupational therapy.* Thorofare, NJ: Slack.

Borcherding, S. & Kappel C. (2002). The OTA's guide is writing SOAP notes. Thorofare, NJ: Slack.

College of St. Catherine. (2001). *Goal writing: Documenting outcomes* [Handout]. St. Paul, MN: Author.

Kettenbach, G. (1990). *Writing S.O.A.P. notes.* Philadelphia: F. A. Davis.

McClain, L. H. (1991). Documentation. In W. Dunn (Ed.), *Pediatric occupational therapy* (pp. 213–244). Thorofare, NJ: Slack.

Meyer, P. J. (2002). *Creating S.M.A.R.T goals.* Retrieved December 20, 2002, from *http:/achievement.com/smart.html*

Moyers, P. (1999). The guide to occupational therapy practice. *American Journal of Occupational Therapy, 53,* 247–322.

The new encyclopedia Britannica (14th ed., Vol. 10). (1985). Chicago: Encyclopedia Britannica.

Perinchief, J. M. (1998). Management of occupational therapy services. In M. E. Neistadt & E. B. Crepeau (Ed.), *Willard and Spackman's occupational therapy* (9th ed., pp. 772–790). Philadelphia: Lippincott.

Richardson, P. K., & Schultz-Krohn, W. (2001). Planning and implementing services. In J. Case-Smith (Ed.), *Occupational therapy for children* (4th ed., pp. 246–264). St. Louis, MO: Mosby.

University of Victoria Counseling Services. (1996). *Learning skills program: Smart goals.* Retrieved December 20, 2002, from *http://www.coun.uvic.ca/learn/program/hndouts/smartgoals.html*

CHAPTER 11

Intervention Plans

INTRODUCTION

The intervention plan is where the occupational therapist articulates what is going to happen in the course of occupational therapy intervention. It is based on the results of the evaluation and the wants and needs of the client or surrogate (i.e., parent or guardian) (AOTA, 1998b). The development and revision of the intervention plan are a collaborative effort between the occupational therapist, the occupational therapy assistant, and the client (AOTA, 1998b).

Establishing goals and determining intervention strategies that will be effective, and that third-party payers will pay for, is critical to the ongoing viability of your practice in occupational therapy. If you do not get paid for what you do, you will not be able to make a living at being an occupational therapy practitioner. To be paid for your services, you have to show that the intervention made a difference in your client's life. That is what motivates us to become occupational therapy professionals in the first place—we want to help make people's lives better.

As an example of what a payer considers as justifiable and reimbursable occupational therapy, read what Medicare uses as coverage criteria:

> Occupational therapy designed to improve function is considered reasonable and necessary for the treatment of the individual's illness or injury only where an expectation exists that the therapy will result in a significant practical improvement in the individual's level of functioning within a reasonable period of time. Where an individual's improvement potential is insignificant in relation to the extent and duration of occupational therapy services required to achieve improvement, such services would not be considered reasonable and necessary and would thus be excluded from coverage by Sec. 1862(a)(1) of the Social Security Act. Where a valid expectation of improvement exists at the time the occupational therapy program is instituted, the services would be covered even though the expectation may not be realized. . . . Once a patient has reached the point where no further significant practical improvement can be expected, the skills of an occupational therapist or occupational therapy assistant will not be required in the carrying out of any activity and/or exercise program to maintain function at the level to which it has been restored. . . . Generally speaking, occupational therapy is not required to effect improvement or restoration of function where a patient suffers a temporary loss or reduction of function (e.g., temporary weakness which may follow a prolonged bed rest following major abdominal surgery) which could reasonably be expected to spontaneously improve as the patient gradually resumes normal activities. . . . (AOTA, 2000a, section B, ¶2)

The key here is "significant practical improvement in the individual's level of functioning within a reasonable period of time" (AOTA, 2000a, section B, ¶2). This is where the professional expertise and judgment of the occupational therapist comes into play. The occupational therapist has to identify the frequency and duration of intervention so that it maximizes improvement in what payers say is a reasonable period of time.

▼ ROLE DELINEATION IN INTERVENTION PLANNING ▼

The occupational therapist is responsible for developing and documenting the intervention plan and complying with the time frames, formats, and standards required by the facility/agency, accrediting bodies, and payers (AOTA, 1998). An occupational therapy assistant under the supervision of an occupational therapist may contribute to the intervention plan. The intervention plan includes the frequency, scope, and duration of occupational therapy services. The occupational therapist or occupational therapy assistant under the supervision of the occupational therapist "reviews the intervention plan with the client and appropriate others" (AOTA, 1998, standard V.5).

You can see that the intervention planning process makes the client an active partner in the process. As in the evaluation process, it is client-centered. It also requires close interaction between the occupational therapist and the occupational therapy assistant. In some settings, the occupational therapy assistant is the professional who is at the facility day in and day out, while the occupational therapist makes periodic supervision visits to the facility to conduct evaluations, develop and revise intervention plans, and prepare discontinuation (discharge) plans and summaries. This is most likely to occur in settings where the clients are fairly stable, and the occupational therapy assistant is experienced and has demonstrated service competence in a wide variety of clinical skills. In situations like this, the occupational therapy assistant has more regular contact with the clients and can provide extremely valuable input to the occupational therapist regarding the skills and abilities of the client as they relate to occupational performance.

▼ CONCEPTS FOR INTERVENTION PLANNING ▼

To help your client make "significant practical improvement in the individual's level of functioning within a reasonable period of time" (AOTA, 2000a, section B, ¶2) you must select intervention strategies that will lead your client in the same direction as the mutually agreed-upon goal(s). This requires knowledge of both the skills and abilities of your client, and the qualities of the activities (occupations) so that there is a match between what the activity has to offer and what the client needs. For example, if a client has difficulty with problem solving, you need an activity that requires some problem solving, but at a level that is just a bit above where the client is currently functioning. In this case, perhaps problems that require abstract thought, such as story problems in math or "2-minute mysteries" type exercises, would be too hard. Instead, an activity that involves real-life situations with rules to follow, such as getting from one place to another within the building or using a substitutions list at the back of a cookbook, would be a better place to start.

An intervention plan is not engraved in stone; it is subject to change as the client's condition and contexts change. If the occupational therapist believes that a change in the goals or intervention strategies, including the frequency, intensity, or duration of intervention sessions, is needed, he or she writes up a new intervention plan. If the client is a Medicare recipient, the Medicare forms require a physician signature every 30 days so changing the frequency or duration on that form carries the weight of a doctor's order. Factors to consider when changing the frequency or duration include the client's potential to benefit from services, the degree of dysfunction, outcomes research on clients with similar conditions and interventions, potential for caregiver follow-through, and possible complications that could change the client's rate of progress (Moyers, 1999).

Intervention plans are established as soon as the occupational therapist determines that the client needs intervention. These are reviewed every 30 days (monthly) in most settings and with certain payers such as Medicare Part B and some managed care organizations. In some settings, the intervention plans may be reviewed every 60 days, quarterly, or semi-annually (twice a year).

▼ PARTS OF AN INTERVENTION PLAN ▼

The BiFIP format that was used in Chapter 9 can also be used to format an intervention plan. The background information, findings, interpretation, and plan sections may contain similar, yet different, content from an evaluation report.

The first intervention plan you write for any one client might be part of the evaluation report, or it may be a stand-alone document, depending on the policies of the facility at which you work. If it is part of the evaluation report, then there is no need to repeat identification/background information. However, if it is a stand-alone document, then you will need to include the same kind of identification information that you included on your evaluation report (AOTA, 2003):

- Client name, gender, and date of birth
- Date of the document (may be part of the signature) and the type of document; name of agency/facility and department
- Intervention diagnosis/condition and other diagnoses/conditions
- Precautions and contraindications
- Pertinent history (if there is new information since the evaluation was written)
- Reason for referral or physician's order

The next section of an ongoing intervention plan is findings. On an intervention plan the findings section is for reporting a brief summary of progress since the last intervention plan was written, within the client's current context. Then describe progress or lack thereof using the language of the *Occupational Therapy Practice Framework* (AOTA, 2002), addressing the client's performance in areas of occupation, and the performance patterns and skills, contexts, client factors, and activity demands that impact the client's occupational performance. Remember that in this section, you are reporting data, not interpreting it.

There is a difference between reporting on the current status of a client and reporting the progress made by that client (McQuire, 1997). According to McQuire, a status report tells what a person can do now with no comparison to prior performance, while a progress report contains some comparative statements. If you want to convince a payer or a referral source that you have provided a worthwhile service, you must choose your words carefully so they show progress. (There will be more information on this in the next section of this chapter.)

The third section of an intervention plan is for recording your interpretation of the findings. This is where you record any barriers or challenges to attaining the short- and long-term goals, and identify the client's current strengths and supports.

The fourth section of the intervention plan is for spelling out what you hope to accomplish in the next review period, adjustments to the short-term goals, intervention strategies, or the duration, frequency, and intensity of intervention sessions can be made. AOTA (2003) specifically states that the short-term goals must be "directly related to the client's ability to engage in desired occupations" (Standard II.A.2.b.).

Along with revising goals, you must determine appropriate intervention strategies and methods given the client's current condition and contexts (AOTA, 2003). For example, you will determine if a particular client is a good candidate for using adaptive equipment, or whether teaching the client an adaptive technique would be better. In the course of your occupational therapy education, you will learn many strategies for interventions. The persons reading your intervention plans (other facility staff, physicians, third-party payers, quality management personnel, lawyers, etc.) must be able to see the logical thinking that went into your plan. They have to see that if you set a long-term goal to improve someone's dressing skills, then the short-term goals and methods of intervention must also directly relate to dressing. Not everyone who reads your intervention plan will understand the link between improving dexterity and improving dressing, so if your intervention plan calls for stringing ¼-inch beads, it will not make logical sense. If, however, your intervention plan calls for learning to don and doff certain articles of clothing with certain types of fasteners, it will make logical sense. (More about this later in this chapter.)

AOTA (2003) also requires that the service delivery mechanisms and plan for discharge be included in this section. Service delivery mechanisms include such details as who will provide the services, where the services will be provided, and the frequency and duration of services. The plan for discharge includes criteria for discontinuing occupational therapy services, discharge disposition (where the client will be discharged to), and the need for follow-up care.

The last part of the intervention plan is for signatures. Every intervention plan needs to be signed by an occupational therapist. According to the *AOTA Occupational Therapy Standards of Practice*, "A registered occupational therapist develops and documents an intervention plan . . . a certified occupational therapy assistant may contribute to the intervention plan under the supervision of a registered occupational therapist" (1998b, Standard V.1). The *AOTA Guidelines for Documentation of Occupational Therapy Practice* (2003) suggests including the name and position of each person responsible for overseeing the implementation of the plan.

▼ SUMMARIZING PROGRESS ▼

Generally, you will write an intervention plan for a client every 30 days. Between intervention plan revisions, you will write progress notes (see Chapter 12). On your initial intervention plan, you will not be able to summarize progress, but on subsequent intervention plans you will. It is helpful to go back over the progress notes written over the last month (or whatever the interval between plans is in your setting) while you summarize changes since the last intervention plan was written.

You can either give the reader an accurate picture of progress, or you can choose your words so that progress appears faster or slower than it really is. However, if you describe faster or slower progress than reality, it is fraud (see Chapter 6). Do not do it. As stated in the AOTA *Code of Ethics*, "Occupational therapy personnel shall refrain from using or participating in the use of any form of communication that contains false, fraudulent, deceptive, or unfair statements or claims" (2000b, Principle 6.C). Further elaborated in the AOTA *Guidelines to the Code of Ethics*, "Occupational therapy personnel do not fabricate data, falsify information, or plagiarize" (1998a, 2.9) and, even more explicitly, "Occupational therapy personnel do not make deceptive, fraudulent, or misleading statements about the nature of the services they provide or the outcomes that can be expected" (1998a, 2.1).

So how do you describe progress accurately? Choose your words carefully. Understand how others interpret words. Some words are "loaded," that is, some readers will twist them in ways you never intended (see Chapter 1). When you write, "Continues to have difficulty with _____," a payer might read it as "not making progress." In reality, the client has made progress, but not as fast as you had hoped. Think about the difference between these words:

Attends	Participates
Understands	Complies or demonstrates
Approachable	Sociable

In each of these pairs, the word on the right is more active. If you write that a client attended occupational therapy sessions, a reader could interpret that as the client came into the room, but did not do anything. If you write that the client participated in the occupational therapy session, it does imply that the client engaged in the process. Someone can nod and say she understands, but unless you see them do it, are you sure she can do it? Approachable implies that one can go up to this person and initiate conversation. Sociable implies that this person is equally comfortable approaching others as he or others are approaching her. Figure 11.1 contains a list of words that convey progress or change.

Describing Physical Behavior

Adapts
Against gravity
Assistance
Athetoid
Awkward
Barely
Bouncy
Careful
Clumsy
Compensate
Complains
Completely
Consistent
Coordinated
Crooked
Creates
Crepitus
Delayed
Deliberately
Dependent
Difficulty
Easily
Effort
Effortless
Endurance
Energetically
Even
Exertion
Gently
Gracefully
Guarded
Haphazardly
Heavily
Hesitantly
Holds
Imitates
Inconsistent
Independent
Jerky/jerkily
Less
Limits
Maintains
Minimum
Mildly
Moderate
Modifies
More
Precise
Rapid
Regressed
Rigid
Roughly
Shaky
Slow
Smoothly
Softly
Spastic
Steady
Stimulating
Strength
Swiftly
Tentative
Thoroughly
Tires
Uneven
Violently
Withdraws
With ease
Writhe

Describing Social Behavior

Acceptable
Adapts
Aggressive
Agitated
Alert
Angry
Antagonistic
Anxious
Apathetic
Approachable
Appropriate
Argumentative
Argues
Asks
Attentive
Aware
Behaves
Boisterous
Bored
Careful
Changeable
Cheerful
Childish
Complacent
Complains
Complies
Confident
Confused
Consistent
Contributes
Consults
Converses
Cooperative
Curious
Decides
Demanding
Demands
Demonstrates
Dependable
Destructive
Diligent
Distractible
Drowsy
Easily upset
Elated
Empathetic
Encouraging
Engaging
Enjoys
Enthusiastic
Establishes
Euphoric
Evasive
Even disposition
Excessive
Excitable
Explores
Explodes
Expresses
Fearful
Flat affect
Flexible
Flexibility
Follows
Friendly
Fussy
Gathers
Giddy
Guarded
Hostile
Hyperactive
Immature
Impolite
Impulsive
Inappropriate touching
Inappropriate laughter
Inattentive
Incessantly
Inconsistent
Initiates
Intrusive
Involved
Irritable
Lethargic
Limits
Listens
Manipulative
Moody
Narcissistic
Observes
Obsessive
Overdependent
Pacing
Passive–aggressive
Permissive
Pleasant
Polite
Preoccupied
Proud
Quarrelsome
Receptive
Reliable
Reserved
Respectful
Responsible
Responsible
Restless
Reticent
Rigid
Satisfied
Seductive
Self-confidence
Sensitive
Shallow
Shy
Sluggish
Sociable
Socialize
Suspicious
Tenacious
Tense
Terse
Tolerant
Trepidation
Unaffected
Unassuming
Uncomfortable
Unpopular
Unrealistic
Vacillates
Volunteers
Withdrawn

Describing Cognition

Adapts
Alert
Attentive
Aware
Clarifies
Concentrates
Conscious
Consults
Decisive
Demonstrates
Determines
Distinguishes

FIGURE 11.1 Descriptive Words for Progress Notes

Distractible
Explores
Fidgety
Follows
Follows routine
Follows rules
Forgetful
Formulates
Identifies
Impatient
Inattentive
Inquisitive
Intellectually
   curious
Interprets
Knowledgeable
Is Realistic
Learns from
   mistakes
Needs reminders
Obtains
Organizes
Perseverate
Prefectionistic
Prepares
Prioritizes
Problem-solves
Reads
Refuses
Relaxed
Reliable
Retains
Seclusive
Selects
Thoughtful
Thoughtless
Writes

**Describing
Participation**

Attends
Contributes
Conversation
Diligent
Engages
Expresses
Eye contact
Industrious
Initiates
Participates
Quiet
Reserved
Responds
Responsive
Sociable
Solitary
Talkative
Team player
Terminates

**Describing
Appearance
and Touch**

Appropriate
Ashen
Bewildered
Blush
Body odor
Bored
Clean
Clenches teeth
Colors clash
Concerned
Damp

Dirty
Disheveled
Disordered
Disrepair
Drooling
Ecstatic
Erect posture
Excessive layers
Eyes get big
Fastidious
Flushed
Furrowed brows
Fussy
Glared
Goosebumps
Grimaces
Hot
   (temperature)
Ill-fitting
Mannerism
Monotone
Neat
Pale
Poised
Presents
Puffy
Raises eyebrow
Scarred
Shiny
Shivered
Sloppy
Slouched
   posture
Smiles
Sneer
Sweaty
Teary

Tired
Torn clothes
Unaware
Uncombed
Unkempt
Worn out

**Describing
Speech**

Babbles
Clear
Disarticulates
Echolalia
Expresses
Expressive
Flat
Gibberish
Grunts
Lisps
Mispronounces
Monotonous
Mumbles
Pressured
Rambles
Rapid
Repetitive
Slow
Slurred
Word
   substitutions

FIGURE 11.1   (Continued)

When you summarize progress over time, the focus needs to be on function. Describe the new occupations the client does now that he or she could not do last month (or whatever your time frame is). The World Health Organization's ICF document (see Chapter 2) contains a comprehensive list of activities that might be helpful to you as you think about function (WHO, 2002). Focusing on function means making sure you address what the client does, not the underlying skills and abilities. For example, if a client is now able to reach to the top shelf in the kitchen and bring down what she needs from that shelf without assistance, that is focusing on function. If instead you report that the client has increased range of motion to 170° in shoulder flexion, that is not reporting on function. Reporting increased range of motion is nicely measurable, but just because someone can move his arm farther does not necessarily mean he uses it to do anything, that his functional performance has improved. Another example would be describing ways a client demonstrates improved self-esteem rather than stating the client scores 26% higher on a test of self-esteem. Perhaps the client is now checking her appearance in the mirror before leaving her room, or she is expressing confidence in her skills.

How do you demonstrate progress? By choosing words that show change as much as possible while still being honest. On an intervention plan, it is not necessary to describe everything the client did over the past month, hit only the highlights, only ones that directly relate to the goals you set last month. To do otherwise would result in a lengthier document than you want to write and than anyone wants to read. Evaluation reports can be long, but intervention plans usually have limited space for recording progress.

What do you write if there has not been the progress you had hoped for? Explain what barriers to progress were encountered. There is probably a reasonable explanation for the lack of expected progress; maybe there was a medical complication or change in life circumstance that got in the way. Whatever the explanation, keep it simple and short. Explain how you will modify your intervention plan to encourage greater progress.

In some places, the payers allow maintenance therapy. In maintenance therapy, a client has a condition that is likely to cause functional deterioration. Occupational therapy intervention can delay or prevent this deterioration. If this is the case, showing progress is not expected, maintaining function is good. Do not try to describe progress when maintenance is the goal.

▼ DOCUMENTING INTERVENTION STRATEGIES ▼

Once you and the client have reviewed progress to date and revised goals toward which to work, your thoughts can turn toward intervention strategies to use to help the client meet those goals. Establishing and documenting the intervention plan is the responsibility of the occupational therapist; an occupational therapy assistant can contribute to the process (AOTA, 1998b).

The section of the intervention plan where the intervention strategies are listed may be called "interventions," "strategies," "approaches," "methods, " or some combination of these words. This is the section where you have to tell the reader what you plan to do to help the client meet his or her goals. For simplicity, the term "strategies" will be used here.

Strategies can include specific techniques for intervention that are suggested by the frame of reference you are using (see Chapter 3), the manner in which you approach the client, general principles for intervention, types of adaptive aids/assistive technology, or task/environmental modifications that will be tried (AOTA, 2003). It also includes whether the client would be best served in an individual or group session (Moyers, 1999).

As you develop intervention plans, remember that problem identification (evaluation results), goal setting, and intervention strategies all have to relate directly to each other. One way to ensure this interrelationship is to use a frame of reference to guide your thinking. Specific intervention techniques are usually explained by the frame of reference you are using. If you refer back to Chapter 3, you can see how knowledge of a frame of reference can direct your thinking about how to approach the client and the problem. For example, if you were using a biomechanical approach with a client who has had a stroke, your strategies would reflect splinting and range of motion exercises. If instead you were using a contemporary task-oriented approach, you would have the client practice functional activities that are meaningful to the client. If you were using a cognitive disabilities or cognition and activity approach, you would focus on ways to adapt techniques or the environment to enable task performance.

The way you approach the client should be specified in your intervention strategies section. This can have several meanings. It could mean that you identify whether you approach the client at eye level, whether you approach the client like you are the expert or a partner in recovery, or whether you approach the client at bedside or in the clinic. Will you follow the client's suggestions or will you be making suggestions? Will you be firm or flexible? Some of this will depend not only on the frame of reference, but also on the age and condition of the client and the philosophy of the program that is serving the client. For example, the program philosophy may emphasize clients taking an active role in their recovery, and all staff need to actively listen to what the client is saying, letting the client direct the activities he or she tries. Another program may have rigid rules to follow, and the client must obey staff directions.

The strategies section of the intervention plan is where you specify what types of assistive technology, adaptive equipment, or task/environmental modifications the client will try (AOTA, 2003). You also need to specify what home programs or training will be provided to the client or client's caregivers. Since your strategies are simply descriptions of what you will try during the plan period, you can suggest many options. If you put the specific type of equipment in the goal statement, you get locked into using that equipment. If the goal says that the client will do something with or without adaptive equipment, you are freer to experiment. Then in the strategy section, you can list several possibilities for different types of equipment or different techniques.

In addition to establishing goals and intervention strategies, the plan section includes the occupational therapist's recommendations on the frequency, duration, and intensity of occupational therapy intervention sessions (AOTA, 2003). Along with this information, some intervention plans may specify the location of intervention sessions (e.g., bedside, clinic, client's home) and the anticipated environment to which the client will be discharged (AOTA, 2003). The latter is usually only required if the intervention plan is written while the client is in a facility that houses the client overnight (e.g., hospital, nursing home, transitional care facility).

When you first start out writing intervention plans and client goals, it is not uncommon for your professor or supervisor to ask that you specifically state your rationale for the goals you set and the intervention strategies you suggest. This is actually a good way to start out because it forces you to articulate why you made the choices you did. In most clinical settings, your rationale will be implied; there will not be time or space to spell out your rationale on every intervention plan. To help you think about your rationale, consider the following questions:

- Why did you choose the goals you wrote down?
- How do they relate to the client's needs?
- How do your intervention strategies relate to each goal?
- What frame of reference (or model of practice) guided your thinking?
- Were there goals or strategies that you considered, but chose not to record? If so, why?

Exercise 11.1

For the following goals, suggest three activities that the client could engage in to help him or her reach his or her goals, and then state your rationale for the suggested activities.

1. Client: 2-year-old female with Down syndrome whose lack of coordination and low muscle tone interfere with her ability to engage in age-appropriate play activities.

    Goal: The client will successfully participate in three age-appropriate play activities by 6 months from now.

    Three suggested activities:

    Rationale:

2. Client: 54-year-old man with a traumatic amputation of his right arm just below the elbow.

    Goal: In the next 30 days, Mr. Smith will spontaneously begin to use artificial arm with hook to pick up solid objects.

    Three suggested activities:

    Rationale:

3. Client: 72-year-old woman with a total hip replacement.

   Goal: Ellie will dress herself independently, with or without the use of adaptive equipment, by April 10, 2005.

   Three suggested activities:

   Rationale:

4. Client: 28-year-old woman with postpartum depression.

   Goal: Naomi will initiate conversations with three people outside her family in the next 2 weeks.

   Three suggested activities:

   Rationale:

▼ SAMPLE INTERVENTION PLANS ▼

Figure 11.2 shows a sample intervention plan format. Sample intervention forms are also in Appendix G. Figure 11.3 contains three sample intervention plans (based on plans developed by occupational therapy students at the College of St. Catherine). They have been modified and simplified, listing only one long-term goal and two short-term goals, where in reality, there may be more goals than that. However, I will caution you to avoid setting too many goals in one plan. I have seen plans with eight or more goals that the writer expected to accomplish in a month. While the client may have lots of areas that need work, it would be better to focus on a few and do well with them than try to work on too many goals and not do as well.

▼ REVISING INTERVENTION PLANS ▼

The longer you work with a particular client, the more likely it is that you will need to revise your intervention plan. This is not necessarily a sign that your plan is not working, it just means that it takes time to effect significant changes in a person. Intervention plans are usually revised on a regular schedule, such as every 30 or 60 days, often dependent on the requirements of the third-party payer and/or the condition of the client.

Revising the intervention plan allows you to step back from day-to-day intervention and really evaluate whether the plan is working or not. If it is working, then maybe the time is right to take things to the next level. If it is not working, then this is a good time to figure out what you could do differently. Maybe you were too ambitious in your goal setting and need to set smaller goals. Maybe you were not ambitious enough and you need to set higher goals. Maybe you need to consider taking the interventions in a whole new direction. It is up to the occupational therapist to evaluate the effectiveness of the intervention plan. Any changes in the plan should be made in consultation with the client and/or client's caregiver (AOTA, 1998b).

OCCUPATIONAL THERAPY INTERVENTION PLAN

Background Information:

Date of report:	**Client's name or initials:**
Date of birth &/or age:	**Date of referral:** M F

Primary intervention diagnosis/concern:
Secondary diagnoses/concerns:
Precautions/contraindications:
Reason for referral to OT: *(or questions to be answered)*
Therapist: *(Print or type your name and credential, you will sign and date the report at the end.)*

FINDINGS

Occupational profile: *(Describe the client's occupational history and experience, patterns of living, interests, values, and needs from the client's perspective that are relevant to the current situation.)*

Progress *(Progress toward goals so far; reasons for progress or lack thereof.)*
    Areas of occupation:
    Performance skills:
    Performance patterns:
    Activity demands:
    Client factors:
    Contexts:

Equipment/orthotics issued:

Home programs/training:

INTERPRETATION

Analysis of occupational performance: *(Describe the barriers and challenges, supports and strengths.)*

PLAN

Long-term Goal	Short-term Goal	Methods/Approaches

Expected frequency, duration, and intensity:
Location of intervention:
Anticipated discontinuation environment:

_____
Signature   **Date**

FIGURE 11.2   Occupational Therapy Intervention Plan

OT Intervention Plan
FUNctional Rehab, Inc

Name: _Jamie Shooter_   **DOB:** _May 18, 1980_   **Date of Report:** _Nov. 3, 2003_
Precautions/Contraindications: _Non-weight bearing for six weeks_
Reason for referral: _Increase mobility for independence in self-care_

Occupational Profile: _Jamie was working as a human cannonball for the circus when he was seriously injured in a freak accident three days ago. He has multiple fractures of his lower extremities, a dislocated Ⓡ shoulder, and numerous contusions, cuts, and scrapes all over his body. He had a severe concussion with loss of consciousness for ten minutes following the incident. Prior to the injury he was healthy and physically fit._

Analysis of Occupational Performance: _Client is in a great deal of pain and resists moving quickly or through his entire range. He is totally dependent in transfers and dressing. He requires moderate assist for grooming and hygiene and minimal assist for feeding. Jamie expressed frustration with his condition, saying he is not used to lying around, he has always been active. He thinks boredom will be one of his biggest challenges because he knows he can recover from the physical injuries, but the recovery will not come as quickly as he would like. He loves his job and hopes to return to circus work, although he thinks the doctor is unlikely to recommend a return to being shot out of a cannon. He says he loves the rush he feels flying through the air, so if he can't do that, then maybe he will consider the trapeze._

Problems prioritized: #1 _Needs to increase mobility for self-care skills_
                             #2 _Needs to decrease dependence on others for self-care skills_
                             #3 _Needs to stay occupied_

Long-term goal:
Client will transfer independently from bed to wheelchair by Dec 15, 2003.

Short-term goals for Problem #1	Intervention approaches/methods for #1
By November 20, client will transfer from the mat table to the wheelchair with moderate assist on three consecutive tries.	Strengthening activities Instruction in safe techniques Practice pushing up on arms to bear weight on his arms without moving to another surface
By Dec. 1, client will transfer from the mat table to the wheelchair with stand-by assist and verbal cues as needed on three consecutive tries.	Strengthening activities Activities involving weight bearing on arms

Frequency of OT sessions: _2x/day_
Duration of OT sessions: _30 min._
Expected length of OT services: _6 weeks_

_____**Date:**_____

Signature (s)

FIGURE 11.3   Sample Intervention Plans

OT Intervention Plan
FUNctional Rehab, Inc

Name: _Loretta Mojo_   **DOB:** _4-28-99_   **Date of Report:** _Nov. 3, 2003_
Precautions/Contraindications: _Strong aversion to any touch_
Reason for referral: _Aversion to touch is interfering with everyday life_

Occupational Profile: _Loretta is a four-year-old girl with autism. She developed normally until she was 18 months old when she seemed to regress to earlier developmental stages. She has strong aversive responses to any form of touch. General health has been good, with only a few ear infections._

Analysis of Occupational Performance: _According to Loretta's mom, Loretta has become increasing aversive to almost any touch. She is removing her clothes because they appear to irritate her, making it difficult for Loretta to go out in public. She screams when anyone touches her. She fights her bath, especially getting her hair washed. She walks on tiptoes so that her whole feet do not have to touch the floor. Loretta's mom reports that Loretta is a very picky eater and will not let them hug her. This last point seemed to be of the greatest concern to her mom as evidenced by her tears at this point in the interview. Results of sensory integration testing confirm aversion to touch, and deficits in processing both tactile and proprioceptive input._

Problems prioritized: #1 _Needs to tolerate touch so that she can be hugged and give hugs_
#2 _Needs to tolerate touch so that she can wear clothes of varying textures and get her hair washed calmly_
#3 _Needs to increase the variety of foods she will eat_

Long-term goal:
Loretta will share hugs with parents and loved ones within one year.

Short-term goals for Problem #1	Intervention approaches/methods for #1
Loretta will receive one hug without withdrawal during three consecutive OT sessions within three months.	_Sensory integrative techniques for tactile processing that will gradually increase in duration and intensity. Begin with her applying the stimuli and moving toward the OT applying them._
Loretta will initiate a hug with a parent following OT sessions on 4 out of 5 opportunities within 5 months.	_Progressive touching activities such as handshaking, putting her arm around an object or person, and then to a hug._

Frequency of OT sessions: _2x/week_
Duration of OT sessions: _45 min._
Expected length of OT services: _1 year_

_____**Date:**_____
Signature (s)

FIGURE 11.3   (Continued)

OT Intervention Plan
FUNctional Rehab, Inc

Name: _Yolanda Odor_   **DOB:** _Jan. 18, 1957_   **Date of Report:** _Nov. 3, 2003_
Precautions/Contraindications: _none_
Reason for referral: _Needs to improve personal hygiene_

Occupational Profile: _Yolanda is a 46-year-old woman with schizophrenia. She has been living in community housing, however recent complaints of poor hygiene resulting in strong body odor has resulted in increasingly angry exchanges with housemates. According to Yolanda, she would bathe if she needed to, but she sees no need to. She also does not think that her bathing habits are anyone's business but her own. She also says she had been faithful in taking her medications, but has stopped taking them because she feels she no longer needs them._

Analysis of Occupational Performance: _Client has a very strong body odor; stringy, greasy hair, and has not shaved her legs or armpits in quite some time (judging by the length of the hair). During observation, she did not wash her hands no matter how soiled they became. She did not wash her hands after going to the bathroom. Client reports not using toothpaste, soap, or deodorant in weeks. She also says she does not notice any particular odor about her. Her clothes had multiple spots where food had landed on them._

Problems prioritized: #1 _Needs to improve personal hygiene skills_
                                 #2 _Needs to improve personal grooming skills_

Long-term goal:
Within one month, Yolanda will independently complete all personal hygiene tasks.

Short-term goals for Problem #1	Intervention approaches/methods for #1
Within one week, Yolanda will wash her hands with soap and water after each time she uses the toilet.	_Visual reminders in the bathroom_ _Coaching and verbal reminders_
Within three weeks, Yolanda will independently initiate showering at least 4 days per week.	_Adaptive equipment and instruction in the safe use of this equipment as needed_ _Calendar to keep track of showers_ _Coaching and feedback_

Frequency of OT sessions: _3x/week_
Duration of OT sessions: _60 min._
Expected length of OT services: _6 weeks_

_____**Date:**_____
Signature (s)

FIGURE 11.3   (Continued)

Exercise 11.2

This exercise is called "Create-a-Client." In this exercise, you will create an imaginary client and develop an intervention plan for this client. I suggest that you create a memorable client, someone you think would be fun to work with. You can create a serious case that is simple or complex, or you can create a bizarre and unique client. Use the form below to write about your client.

First, establish background information on your client. Create a memorable name for your client. Determine the client's age, diagnoses, and occupational profile. Then summarize the occupational needs of the client. Determine what performance skills, performance patterns, contexts, activity demands, or client factors contribute to the problems. Next, prioritize occupational needs and establish goals for this client. Finally, suggest intervention strategies.

Create-a-Client
I. Background Information
Name: _____ **Age:** _____
Diagnoses: _____
Occupational Profile:

II. Summary of Occupational Needs:

III. Prioritize Occupational Needs:
    1.
    2.
    3.

IV. One long-term and two short-term goals for top priority:
    LTG:

    STG:

    STG:

VI. Possible treatment/interventions:

SUMMARY

In this chapter you have learned about writing intervention plans. The intervention plan is a vital document that is used by payers to determine whether continued intervention is needed, by coworkers to communicate the client's current status and progress, and by the occupational therapy personnel to evaluate the effectiveness of intervention programs.

Generally speaking, a client receiving ongoing intervention from occupational therapy will have an intervention plan developed immediately after the evaluation, and then periodically until services are discontinued. Except when the client is working on maintenance goals, each successive intervention plan should show progress in the client's areas of occupation. If progress is not made, an explanation for the lack of progress must be given.

The occupational therapist is responsible for writing, revising, and communicating the intervention plan. An occupational therapy assistant contributes to the intervention planning process. It is a client-centered process.

In addition to necessary client identification information, intervention plans usually contain a brief summary of progress, revised goals, and intervention strategies. Intervention strategies include frequency and duration of services, manner of service delivery, place of service delivery, types of adaptive equipment/environmental adaptations, task modifications, home programs, and training for the client and the client's caregivers. While intervention plans are written in ink, they are not engraved in stone. They are expected to change as the client's circumstances and condition changes.

REFERENCES

American Occupational Therapy Association. (1998a). *Guidelines to the code of ethics.* Retrieved January 5, 2001, from *http://www.aota.org/members/area2/links/link04. asp?PLACE=/members/area2/links/link04.asp*

American Occupational Therapy Association. (1998b). Occupational therapy standards of practice. *American Journal of Occupational Therapy, 52*, 866–869.

American Occupational Therapy Association. (2000a). *Coverage of occupational therapy services.* Retrieved January 5, 2001, from *http://www.aota.org/members/area5/links/ LINK18.asp?PLACE=/members/area5/links/link18.asp*

American Occupational Therapy Association. (2000b). Occupational therapy code of ethics–2000. *American Journal of Occupational Therapy, 54*, 641–616.

American Occupational Therapy Association. (2002). Occupational therapy practice framework: Domain and process. *American Journal of Occupational Therapy, 56*, 609–639.

American Occupational Therapy Association. (2003). *Guidelines for documentation of occupational therapy.* Retrieved June 27, 2003, from *http://aota.org/members/area2/ docs/ra2.pdf*

McQuire, M. J. (1997). Excellence and efficiency in documentation. *OT Practice, 2*(12), 36–41.

Moyers, P.A. (1999). The guide to occupational therapy practice. *American Journal of Occupational Therapy, 53*(3), 247–322.

World Health Organization. (2002). *International classification of function.* Geneva, Switzerland: author. Retrieved May 22, 2002, from *http://www3.who.int/icf*

CHAPTER 12

SOAP and Other Methods
of Documenting Ongoing Intervention

INTRODUCTION

Progress notes come in different sizes and formats, but they are all intended to provide a record of intervention sessions. In most cases, progress notes are written following each intervention session; however, in some cases, they may be written weekly or other time interval.

Progress notes should be more than simply a listing of the types of activities in which a client has engaged. They are called progress notes because they are supposed to show progress. Therefore, the notes need to include information about the client's response to interventions and how current performance is different from previous performance (AOTA, 2003). Any unusual or significant event, assistive or adaptive equipment issued or tried, and any client/caregiver instruction also need to be documented (AOTA, 2003).

There are three main kinds of progress notes: narrative, SOAP, and DAP (FIP). Narrative notes are notes that are written in paragraph form. SOAP and DAP (FIP) notes have specific labeled sections. All three types of notes are discussed in this chapter. In addition, ways to document progress in checklist or graphic forms, such as progress flow sheets and attendance logs, are discussed.

▼ ROLE DELINEATION FOR PROGRESS REPORTING▼

The occupational therapist, with contributions from the occupational therapy assistant, performs reevaluation during the ongoing intervention process (AOTA, 1998; AOTA, 2003). He or she documents changes in the client's occupational performance, short-term goals, and anticipated discharge environment (AOTA, 1998). The occupational therapist is responsible for modifying the interventions as the client's contexts, wants, needs, and responses to interventions change (AOTA, 1998). The occupational therapy assistant, under the supervision of an occupational therapist, offers suggestions for modifying intervention methods (AOTA, 1998). Progress notes may be written by either the occupational therapist or occupational therapy assistant (AOTA, 1998). Notes written by an occupational therapy assistant are usually reviewed and cosigned by the occupational therapist when required by statute, regulation, accrediting agency, payer, or facility/agency policy (AOTA, 1998).

Documentation of progress requires that the occupational therapist and occupational therapy assistant work closely together. As mentioned in Chapter 11, in some settings, the occupational therapy assistant works without onsite supervision by an occupational therapist. Depending on state licensure or registration laws, the stability of the clients, and the service competency of the occupational therapy assistant, an occupational therapist may provide onsite supervision a couple days a week, once a week, or once every couple weeks. When the occupational therapist does not see the client on a daily basis, he or she relies heavily on the occupational therapy assistant to report changes in the client's condition and client's performance in areas of occupation. The occupational therapist uses this information along with his or her own observations, interviews, and data gathering to recommend any modifications to the ongoing implementation of intervention. These modifications are documented in progress notes and revised intervention plans.

▼ SOAP NOTES ▼

SOAP notes are another of medicine's acronyms. SOAP stands for **S**ubjective, **O**bjective, **A**ssessment, **P**lan, which are the component parts of this type of progress note. One of the advantages of this type of note is that it is quite common and the reader knows just what kind of information to find in what part of the note. Professionals from all health care disciplines write them. The SOAP format can also be adapted for use as an evaluation report or discontinuation summary (Borcherding, 2000; Borcherding & Kappel, 2002).

Dr. Lawrence Weed is credited with developing SOAP notes in the 1960s as part of his efforts to make client charting more client-centered (Borcherding, 2000; Borcherding & Kappel, 2002; Kettenback, 1990). He reorganized a client's medical record so that there would be a master list of the client's problems from the perspective of all the disciplines working with the client, and then a section for progress notes that all disciplines could write in (as opposed to separate sections of the chart for each discipline). Weed named this system the Problem Oriented Medical Record (POMR). The SOAP note format has become so popular that today, even if facilities do not use POMR, the SOAP note is still the preferred format for note writing.

Here are some sample progress notes written in SOAP format.

Case 1: Helen, Alzheimer's client in day care setting

S: "Where do I go? What do I do?"

O: Upon entering the building, Helen waited for her daughter to tell her which way to turn. Once in the room, she helped herself to a cup of coffee. Then she sat down and sipped her coffee until she received further instructions. She imitated the exercises that the group leader demonstrated. Halfway through the exercise group, she stood up, put her coffee cup in the garbage, and thanked everyone for a pleasant experience. She started to leave the room. She blushed and hid her face when told that the group was not over yet.

A: Helen appears to be dependent on the verbal cues of others in her environment to direct her behavior. In the absence of verbal cues, she gets confused.

P: Pair verbal and visual cues for Helen, or use verbal cues alone. Continue to encourage participation in small-group activities. Provide a structured environment with a consistent, posted schedule. Continue monthly occupational therapy consultation.

Bobbi Babinski, OTR/L 11-1-03

Case 2: 27 y.o. with LCVA (Bob)

S: "I used to be able to do this without thinking about it. Now I have to concentrate so hard on it I wonder if it's worth it."

O: Client participated in a 30-minute occupational therapy session to work on functional activities with his unaffected (nondominant) hand. Bob attempted to use a computer mouse with his left hand by playing a game of solitaire. He moved quickly to the general area that he wants the mouse to be. He moved slowly and hesitantly to the precise spot he needed, however, he often overshot the mark. Bob

---

clicked the mouse with his index finger easily, however, he had minimal success holding the mouse button down while dragging the mouse. It took 20 minutes to complete one game of solitaire.

A: Bob has not yet achieved adequate coordination with either hand to allow him to perform mouse activities to his satisfaction.

P: Try a touchpad mouse. Encourage moving slowly and carefully. Practice using left hand for other activities during the day. Continue twice daily occupational therapy as per plan of care.

Carrie Ingwater, COTA/L 3-2-03

Bobbi Babinski, OTR/L 3-2-03

Subjective

The subjective part of the SOAP note usually refers to the client's subjective comments about problems, complaints, life circumstances, goals, current performance, limitations, or other pertinent comments (Borcherding, 2000; Borcherding & Kappel, 2002; Kettenbach, 1990; Kuntavanish, 1988). You may directly quote the client or paraphrase, but direct quotes must be marked as such with quotation marks. A direct quote can be very effective at illustrating the client's attitude, use of language, denial, or loss of memory. However, simply writing "I feel icky" does not really tell the reader much (Borcherding & Kappel, 2002; "Tips On Medical Progress Notes," 2002). If a client says that, ask him or her for clarification, then write down the client's description of his or her aches, pains and feelings. "I feel tired and my chest and shoulder hurt" conveys more specific information. A relative or caretaker may also say something that is significant, and these comments can also be recorded in the subjective section of the SOAP note. Sometimes a client is nonverbal. If that is the case, you can document nonverbal communication such as smiles, nods, and gestures as appropriate.

Some people advocate using statements like, "Client denies feeling suicidal" ("Sample Medical SOAP Notes," 2002). I think the word "denies" sounds like you do not believe the client; it sounds judgmental. I prefer wording such as "Client reports she is not having suicidal thoughts."

Pick your "S" carefully. Make sure it is relevant to the topic you will write the rest of your note about. For example, if you are writing a SOAP note about the client's functional skills in meal preparation, an "S" about how the weather is making the client's knee hurt is not really relevant. If there is nothing relevant to report in the "S" section, you can draw a circle with a line through it (Ø) to indicate that you thought about it but there was nothing relevant to write about. Leaving it blank might look like you forgot to write something there.

Exercise 12.1

Which of these statements belong in the subjective section of the SOAP note?

1. _____ Ndebe appeared tired and listless.
2. _____ Client said she is hearing voices telling her to cut her hair.
3. _____ Raësa got dressed by herself today.
4. _____ Cyndee's mother said that Cyndee has not been sleeping well the past 3 nights.
5. _____ "I am fat and ugly."
6. _____ Client is resistant to all suggestions.
7. _____ "Where am I?"
8. _____ Client made several lewd comments throughout the session, accompanied by sexually suggestive hand gestures.
9. _____ Saji's shirt was misbuttoned, untucked, and stained.

Objective

The objective section is the place for recording observations, data collected, and other facts (Borcherding, 2000; Borcherding & Kappel, 2002; Kettenbach, 1990; Kuntavanish, 1987). The information you record in this section should be the indisputable truth. It is harder than it looks to keep your interpretations out of this section. Remember the Description, Interpretation, Evaluation (DIE) discussion in Chapter 9? This would be a good time to review that material.

If the client made an attempt to open a carton of milk, but gave up before getting it open, would you say "The client was unsuccessful at opening a milk carton" or "The client is dependent in opening milk cartons"? Both sentences are probably true and accurate statements. The first sentence is descriptive of a particular event. The second is a generalization; it makes the claim that the client would be unlikely to open any milk carton. This makes the second sentence an interpretive statement that belongs in the "A" section rather than the "O" section.

Another consideration when writing the "O" section is that in some settings, the preference is to only document what the client can do, not what the client cannot do. In other settings, it is expected that both strengths and limitations will be documented. However, the "O" section should not read like a list of the client's failings.

The emphasis of this section should be on the client's performance, not simply a listing of activities the client engaged in. The actual intervention is not as important as how the client responded to the intervention (Borcherding & Kappel, 2002). Your powers of observation are essential in writing good progress notes. Record the client's reaction. Here are some possible "O" statements:

- Client pulled away from contact with the shaving cream.
- Client was dressed in plaid pants and a striped shirt.
- Jalele made fleeting eye contact with other members of the group.
- Client stacked the plates eight high on the bottom shelf of the overhead cabinet.
- Client instructed in use of stocking aid; she demonstrated proper use of it.
- Client dressed herself with minimal assist for shoes and socks.
- Selena entered the room and went straight to the coffee pot.
- Client spontaneously used his right hand to pick up his coffee cup.

Exercise 12.2

Which of the following statements belong in the "O" section of the SOAP note?

1. _____ The client's eyes were red and watery.
2. _____ Bob got angry.
3. _____ He pushed away from the table and left the room.
4. _____ She said she hated strawberries.
5. _____ Pevitra wants to be recognized for good behavior.
6. _____ Esai eats all of one food before eating the next food on his plate.
7. _____ The client appears bewildered when others get annoyed with him for invading their personal space.
8. _____ The client has a habit of twisting her ring around her finger during personal conversations.

Borcherding (2000) and Borcherding and Kappel (2002) suggest that the "O" section begin with a statement of where and why the client was seen. Some settings and payers also expect the note to contain the amount of time the client was in occupational therapy since the last progress note. For example, the section might start with this sentence: "Demitri participated in two 45-minute occupational therapy clinic sessions this week to develop age-appropriate social skills." Or "Etta received occupational therapy today for 60 minutes in her home to work on meal preparation and housekeeping skills."

The "O" section can be organized chronologically, that is, describing events in the order in which they happened (Borcherding, 2000; Borcherding & Kappel, 2002). This gives the reader a good idea of exactly what transpired during occupational therapy intervention sessions. If you are working with a client such as a child with sensory integration dysfunction where the sequence of interventions is important, then this is the best format.

Kettenbach (1990), Borcherding (2000), and Borcherding and Kappel (2002) suggest that objective data can be categorized to make the note appear more organized. Headings can be used to clearly identify separate topics such as test results, functional activities, or body parts. When reporting range of motion or strength data for multiple joints, a chart can be used to display the information. A chart is easier to read and refer back to than a long sentence with multiple measurements.

Exercise 12.3

Practice organizing the "O" section for the following case.

> You are working with a client who has severe rheumatoid arthritis, resulting in joint deformities of the fingers of both hands. He wants to be able to keyboard so he can email his son. On his right hand, the thumb IP joint can flex to 40°. Thumb abduction is 55°. The MCP joint can flex to 30°. The index finger has DIP, PIP, and MCP flexion of 45°, 85°, and 50°, respectively, with 35° of hyperextension at the DIP and 35° of MCP extension. There is ulnar drift of index, middle, ring, little fingers of 30°, 30°, 35°, and 40°, respectively. Both the middle and ring finger had 50° of DIP flexion. The little finger has no movement at the DIP joint. The PIP joint of the middle, ring, and little finger are 50°, 40°, and 30°, respectively. There is 30° of flexion and extension for the MCP joints. On his left hand, the thumb IP joint can flex to 40°. Thumb abduction is 55°. The MCP joint can flex to 70°. The index finger has DIP, PIP, and MCP flexion of 50°, 60°, and 50°, respectively. The index finger has 40° of hyperextension at the DIP joint and 40° of MCP extension. There is ulnar drift of index, middle, ring, little fingers of 20°, 30°, 30°, and 40°. Both the middle and ring finger had 30° of DIP flexion. The little finger has no movement at the DIP joint. The PIP joints of the middle, ring, and little finger flex to 60°, 50°, and 45°, respectively. There is 35° of flexion and 40° of extension for the MCP joints.

Fill in each of the tables below using the data in the paragraph above.

L	Thumb	R
_____	IP flexion	_____
_____	MCP flexion	_____
_____	Abduction	_____
	Index finger	
_____	DIP flexion	_____
_____	DIP extension	_____
_____	PIP flexion	_____
_____	MCP flexion	_____
_____	MCP extension	_____
	Middle finger	
_____	DIP flexion	_____
_____	PIP flexion	_____
_____	MCP flexion	_____
_____	MCP extension	_____
	Ring finger	
_____	DIP flexion	_____
_____	PIP flexion	_____
_____	MCP flexion	_____
_____	MCP extension	_____

Little finger

_____	DIP flexion	_____
_____	PIP flexion	_____
_____	MCP flexion	_____
_____	MCP extension	_____

Ulnar Drift

_____	Index	_____
_____	Middle	_____
_____	Ring	_____
_____	Little	

Finger	DIP flexion	DIP extension	PIP flexion	MCP flexion	MCP extension	Abduction	Ulnar drift
R Thumb			▓		▓		▓
L Thumb			▓		▓		▓
R Index						▓	
L Index						▓	
R Middle		▓				▓	
L Middle		▓				▓	
R Ring		▓				▓	
L Ring		▓				▓	
R Little		▓				▓	
L Little		▓			▓	▓	

Next, answer the following questions:

1. Of the three methods of presenting information (narrative, list, and table), which do you think is the easiest to read and understand?

2. Can you think of another way to organize this information?

Assessment

The assessment or "A" portion of the SOAP note is where you explain what all this data (the subjective and objective) means (Borcherding, 2000; Borcherding & Kappel, 2002; Kettenbach, 1990; Kuntavanish, 1987). This is where your professional judgment and skills come into play. Of all the parts of the SOAP note, this is the most important one, the part where you want to make the best impression on the reader.

In some facilities, the "A" section begins with a problem list (Ketttenbach, 1990). The data recorded in the "S" and "O" sections is analyzed, summarized, and prioritized. By listing the problems in order of importance to the client you let the readers (which often includes payers) know why occupational therapy is involved in this case. There is no need to use complete sentences in the problem list. Examples of problems could be:

- Impaired self-care skills
- Decreased hand function

- Decreased job skills
- Low self-esteem
- Limited access to services in his community
- Difficulty feeding herself
- Limited attention to tasks

Typically, in those facilities where the "A" section includes a problem list, the "A" section also includes both long- and short-term goals and a summary. The summary explains to readers the correlations between the "S," "O," and "P" sections, justifies your recommendations, clarifies progress made, explains any difficulties in obtaining information, and makes suggestions for further testing.

Here is an "A" section using this type of format:

A: Problem list: Limited ROM in Ⓡ shoulder, impaired dressing, grooming, and hygiene skills.

Long-term goal: By discharge, return to independence in dressing, grooming, and hygiene.

Short-term goals: In two sessions, pt. will grasp objects at shoulder height without moving his trunk.

In three sessions, pt. will use both hands to shampoo his hair.

In three sessions, pt. will use both hands to dry and style his hair.

Summary: Pt. is using trunk rotation to substitute for Ⓡ shoulder flexion. He has improved since last visit in that he now is using his Ⓡ arm for some tasks. Would benefit from continued occupational therapy.

In other facilities, the "A" will be presented in a more narrative way without listing problems or setting goals. In this method, the "A" would consist of wording similar to what one would write in the summary sections of the "A" part of the note above.

Examples of "A" statements would be:

- Client is independent in dressing.
- Laleh needs verbal cues to stay on task.
- She is ready to go on a home visit.
- He has difficulty with impulse control.
- Client is dependent in toilet transfers.
- Client is able to manage her own medication routine.

It might seem unnecessary to remind you that what you write in the "A" section must directly relate to what you write in the "S" and "O" sections, but this has consistently been one of the hardest things for students to learn to do. Often what happens is that students write great "A" statements, but when you look at the "O" section, there is nothing supporting the conclusions drawn in the "A" section. For example:

S: Client reported pain in his shoulder every time he moves in any direction

O: Client twisted his trunk and extended his Ⓡ elbow to reach objects in front of him rather than flexing his shoulder. Once positioned, he grasped various objects including a cup, a glass, a fork, a scissors, and a pen.

A: He writes legibly with his right hand.

P: Continue OT sessions 3x/wk to improve functional use of RUE.

While the "O" does mention that he grasped a pen, there are no observations related to actually using the pen. The "A" is a big leap of thinking and it is unsupported by anything in the "O" or "S" sections. A better "A" for the note above would be, "He is protecting his shoulder by substituting trunk and elbow movement for shoulder movement. However, this is an improvement over last session when he refused to use the hand/arm at all." The "A" section is not the place to bring in new information (Borcherding, 2000). Everything you write in "A" has to be supported with evidence in the "S" and "O" sections.

One technique that can be helpful in writing "A" sections that connect to "S" and "O" sections is to go through the first two sections sentence by sentence and ask yourself what it means for the client (Borcherding & Kappel, 2002). Ask yourself what it is about what the client said or did that is important enough to write down. What does it tell you about the client's performance in areas of occupation? What does it tell you about performance skills, patterns, or client factors? You may find a difference between what the client said and what the client did. You may notice whether or not there has been an improvement in function.

Exercise 12.4

Which of these statements make good "A" statements on SOAP notes?

1. _____ She has to be told to come out of her room.
2. _____ Client tried to use the TV remote control to call home.
3. _____ Client completed 75% of the task without assistance.
4. _____ Usha does not interact with peers.
5. _____ He can use public transportation independently.
6. _____ Ashton can tolerate a moderately noisy environment for up to 10 minutes.
7. _____ Client's statements are inappropriate to the situation.

In addition to the interpretation of data, justification of the goals, inconsistencies, progress, difficulty in obtaining information, and suggestions for further intervention (Borcherding, 2000; Borcherding & Kappel, 2002; Kettenbach, 1990), you can also include information on the client's strengths, deficits, and motivation (Kuntavanish, 1987). The keys are to not restate the "O" in "A," and be sure that every statement in "A" is supported by evidence in "O."

Exercise 12.5

1. Write an "A" for the data presented in Exercise 12.3.

2. Write an "A" for the following cases ("S" and "O" provided).

   Case 1: 3-year old boy with muscular incoordination and autism

   S: "Keep that away from me!" (response to presentation of plate of shaving cream)
   O: Deshaun received 45 minutes of occupational therapy intervention for sensory and motor skill development. He ran away when a plate of shaving cream was brought toward him. He tipped over his chair in his attempt to run away. As each new sensory activity was introduced, Deshaun started flapping his hands. At least five times during the 1-hour session, he bent over forward, placed his head on the floor, and rocked back and forth. He refused to go down a 3-foot long slide, or through a 5-foot long plastic tunnel. When held upside down by his ankles and swung gently, he repeatedly asked to do it again. He also asked to have the weighted blanket put on him three times during the session.
   A:

Case 2: 78-year-old man who had a stroke 1 month ago, resulting in left-sided hemiparesis and visual neglect (hemianopsia).

S: "I don't see why I can't drive myself to the golf course for a round of golf, I'm fine. They wouldn't have let me home from the hospital if there was anything really wrong. I can use the golf club for a cane on the course." Client says he has no problem with his left side and all this talk about "left side neglect" is just "garbage."

O: When client attempted to putt using a golf club, he put the club in his left hand and then grasped it with his right. His left hand consistently fell off the club during the back swing. When a plate with chips on the right side and dip on the left was placed in front of him, he ate only the chips, never the dip.

A:

Plan

The plan section is where you very clearly spell out what your plan is for helping the client achieve his or her goals. It often states the frequency, duration, and intensity of occupational therapy and suggestions for intervention. It can also include the location of the intervention sessions (i.e., bedside, clinic, or home) and equipment issued to the client (Kettenbach, 1990). The "P" section should be written with sufficient clarity that if you get sick and cannot come to work the next time the client is supposed to be seen, a substitute occupational therapy practitioner could step in and do what you would have done (Borcherding, 2000; Borcherding & Kappel, 2002).

Examples of the "P" statements include:

- Continue OT 3x/wk for self-care skills development. Try adaptive feeding equipment such as a plate guard and large-handled utensils.
- Continue OT bid, 5x/wk for brain injury retraining program. See in room in a.m. for dressing, grooming, and hygiene, and in clinic in the afternoon for meal prep, safety, and problem solving.
- As per plan of care, client will be seen 5x/wk for 30-minute sessions for the next 2 weeks. Will work on toilet transfers and manipulation of clothes necessary for toileting next visit. Caregiver instruction will be included.
- Client will participate in activity group and assertiveness group daily.

It is not uncommon to see the "P" section written with differing levels of specificity depending on the writer. Generally, the more specific the better.

Exercise 12.6

Which of these statements make good "P" statements?

1. _____ Practice writing his name three times per day.
2. _____ Engage client in conversations about child care.
3. _____ She should be more careful in the kitchen.
4. _____ Increase repetitions as tolerated.
5. _____ Instruct in splint care and maintenance.
6. _____ Client needs to spend more time on leisure occupations.
7. _____ Client will work on chewing food at least 10 times before swallowing.

The client, Susie, is a 4-year-old girl with cerebral palsy who is seen in an outpatient rehabilitation center. Although only a few notes are shown here, assume that the notes follow a similar pattern twice a week for several months.

Jan. 4, 2002
    S: No new complaints today
    O: Today we worked on fine motor skills using blocks and pegs.
    A: Susie tolerated everything fairly well today.
    P: Continue OT 2x/wk per plan of care.

Jan. 6, 2002
    S: No new complaints today
    O: Today we worked on functional activities for fine motor development including large and small pegs, using hand over hand assistance as needed.
    A: Susie tolerated everything fairly well today.
    P: Continue OT 2x/wk per plan of care.

Feb. 11, 2002
    S: No new complaints today
    O: Today we worked on:
        1) Grasp and release using small pegs and a pegboard
        2) Gross motor coordination using adaptive scissors
        3) Spatial relationships by stacking measuring cups
        4) Writing
    A: Susie tolerated everything fairly well today.
    P: Continue per POC 2x/wk.

March 17, 2002
    S: No new complaints today.
    O: Today we worked on PNF diagonal patterns by reaching for things while sitting on a large ball, weight-bearing by rocking back and forth while on all fours, throwing beanbags to work on grasp/release, and turning pages of a book.
    A: Susie tolerated everything fairly well today.
    P: Continue OT 2x/wk per plan of care.

FIGURE 12.1   Bad Example of SOAP Notes #1

Figures 12.1 and 12.2 show some sample progress notes. Read through them and see what you think about the quality of the notes. Consider how useful and informative the information is. Review the criteria for Documenting with CARE (Chapter 4).

All the SOAP notes in Figure 12.1 technically have subjective information in the subjective space, objective information in the objective space, and so on; however, the notes lack any really useful information. Figure 12.2 shows two SOAP notes where the objective and assessment sections contain information that belongs in the other section or have assessment statements that are not supported by objective information.

Exercise 12.7

Write the P section for each of the three cases in Exercise 12.5.

    Case 1: Client with severe arthritis
        P:

Case 2: Client with sensory defensiveness
    P:

Case 3: Client with left side neglect
    P:

The client, Susie, is a 4-year-old girl with cerebral palsy who is seen in an outpatient rehabilitation center. Although only a few notes are shown here, assume that the notes follow a similar pattern twice a week for several months.

Jan. 4, 2003
    S: "No"
    O: Today we worked on fine motor skills using blocks and pegs. She cannot seem to get a stack of more than three 1" cubes without knocking it down in the process of adding the fourth block. She lacks coordination to stack them higher. Using a whole hand grip on large pegs, she placed six in a row before she refused to do anymore.
    A: Susie did fairly well today. She was less resistive to fine motor tasks.
    P: Continue OT 2x/wk per plan of care.

Jan. 6, 2003
    S: "No"
    O: Today we worked on functional activities for fine motor development including large and small pegs. She needed hand over hand assistance with the small pegs. She could pick them up between her thumb and index finger, but could not get them to stand up in the holes.
    A: Susie needs to continue to work on fine motor tasks. She was unable to stack four or more 1" blocks.
    P: Continue OT 2x/wk per plan of care.

Feb. 11, 2003
    S: Ø
    O: Today we worked on:
        1) Grasp and release using small pegs and a pegboard to make a big square shape. She didn't seem to understand the concept of alternating colors to make a pattern.
        2) Fine motor coordination using adaptive scissors. She made a few snips on a piece of paper, but threw the scissors down when the OT tried to guide her to cut along a line.
        3) Spatial relationships by nesting measuring cups. She nested three cups (1/4 c., 1/2 c., 1 c.). She liked this activity, nesting and unnesting them repeatedly.
        4) Writing. She scribbled with a large crayon. She refused to make an S.
    A: Susie did fairly well today. She seems to be getting used to working with the occupational therapist.
    P: Continue per POC 2x/wk.

March 17, 2003
    S: "OK"
    O: Today we worked on PNF diagonal patterns by reaching for things while sitting on a large ball. She pulled plastic figures off a shelf and dropped them in a bucket. We worked on weight-bearing by rocking back and forth while on all fours. Once she got started rocking she didn't want to stop, she appeared overstimulated and excited. We worked on throwing beanbags to work on grasp/release, as well as turning the pages of a book. She is doing better at quickly releasing objects.
    A: Susie had a great day! She was happy throughout the session.
    P: Continue OT 2x/wk per plan of care.

FIGURE 12.2   Bad Example of SOAP Notes #2

Exercise 12.8

Label the statements below according to where they would best belong in a SOAP note. Use "S" for subjective, "O" for objective, "A" for assessment, and "P" for plan. Then use these statements to write one coherent SOAP note. You may add transitional phrases to make the note flow better.

1. _____ The client sat on the side of the bed waiting for dressing direction.
2. _____ The client is unable to initiate dressing.
3. _____ She walks to the kitchen when dressed carrying her purse, ready to go to day care.
4. _____ When told what clothes to put on she gets dressed.
5. _____ What am I supposed to wear?
6. _____ The buttons on her blouse are not lined up.
7. _____ While sitting there, she removes her nightclothes.
8. _____ Clothing will be carefully placed in proper sequence and laid out the night before so the client can see the clothes on the chair when she gets up.
9. _____ When given cues can dress herself with minor errors.
10. _____ She puts her anklets on under her TED stockings.

S:

O:

A:

P:

Exercise 12.9

Analyze the following SOAP notes. Tell what is good about them and what needs improvement.

Case 1: Client is a 78-year-old woman who had a stroke affecting her left side 3 months ago. Her left arm has been in a sling with only a little active range of motion in her elbow and shoulder. Then three days ago, she fell outside on the sidewalk, breaking her right arm. It is now in a cast. She is now attending an intensive program to facilitate movement in her left arm (constraint induced movement therapy [CIMT]).

S: "I felt so helpless with two useless arms. I can't believe I was able to feed myself with my left arm."

O: Client participated in 6 hours of outpatient occupational therapy today. Fitted with a universal cuff, she was able to feed herself using a spoon, with minimal spillage. It required her to use both elbow flexion and trunk movements to get the applesauce scooped up and into her mouth. It was the first time she had fed herself since breaking her arm.

A: Client is making progress in the functional use of her left arm. She was not able to get the spoon to her mouth yesterday.

P: Continue participation in CIMT program 6 days per week as established in plan of care. Provide adaptive equipment as needed.

Case 2: Client is a 19-year-old man who lost his left arm in a farm accident (he is right-handed) 3 weeks ago.

S: "I still can't believe my arm is gone. It's unreal. There are times I swear I can still feel it, like a fly crawling on it, but when I look there's nothing there. Nothing."

O: Withdraws from light touch within 1.5 inches of wound. He demonstrated proper stump wrapping technique. Instructed on how to massage area in preparation for artificial arm.

A: Stump is healing well and he is on track for getting an artificial arm. He is ready to be fitted with a temporary arm.

P: OT bid, 6 days per week, to reduce sensitivity of stump, prepare stump for artificial arm, and begin training in the use of an artificial arm.

▼ DAP NOTES ▼

DAP notes are very similar to SOAP notes in that each letter stands for one section of the note: **D**escription, **A**ssessment, and **P**lan. This format is less common than either the narrative or SOAP note. They can also be called FIP notes, as in **F**indings, **I**nterpretation, and **P**lan.

The description (findings) section is much like a combination of the "S" and "O" section of a SOAP note. In this section, you describe what you see and hear during the occupational therapy session. It can include quotes, paraphrases, observations, measurements, or test results. This is where you provide evidence that you are making progress. Be sure that everything in this section is fact based, and not a conclusion or inference on your part.

The "A" and "P" ("I" and "P" for FIP notes) sections are exactly like those in SOAP. Here are examples of DAP and FIP notes.

Case 1: Helen, Alzheimer's client in day care setting

D: Upon entering the building, Helen waited for her daughter to tell her which way to turn. "Where do I go? What do I do?" Once in the room, she helped herself to a cup of coffee. Then she sat down and sipped her coffee until she received further instructions. She imitated the exercises that the group leader demonstrated. Halfway through the exercise group, she stood up, put her coffee cup in the garbage, and thanked everyone for a pleasant experience. She started to leave the room. She blushed and hid her face when told that the group was not over yet.

A: Helen appears to be dependent on the verbal cues of others in her environment to direct her behavior. In the absence of verbal cues, she gets confused.

P: Pair verbal and visual cues for Helen, or use verbal cues alone. Continue to encourage participation in small-group activities. Provide a structured environment with a consistent, posted schedule.

Bobbi Babinski, OTR/L 11/2/2003

Case 2: 27 y.o. with LCVA (Bob)

F: "I used to be able to do this without thinking about it. Now I have to concentrate so hard on it I wonder if it's worth it." Client participated in a 30-minute occupational therapy session to work on functional activities with his unaffected (nondominant) hand. Bob attempted to use a computer mouse with his left hand by playing a game of solitaire. He moved quickly to the general area that he wants the mouse to be. He moved slowly and hesitantly to the precise spot he needed, however, he often overshot the mark. Bob clicked the mouse with his index finger easily, however, he had minimal success holding the mouse button down while dragging the mouse. It took 20 minutes to complete one game of solitaire.

I: Bob has not yet achieved adequate coordination with either hand to allow him to perform mouse activities to his satisfaction.

P: Try a touchpad mouse. Encourage moving slowly and carefully. Practice using left hand for other activities during the day. Continue twice daily occupational therapy as per plan of care.

Carrie Ingwater, COTA/L 3/2/03

Bobbi Babinski, OTR/L 3/2/2003

Exercise 12.10

Write concise SOAP notes and DAP notes for the following cases.

Case 1: Toddler boy with seizure disorder and sensory processing disorder (sensory hypersensitivity)

Tommy was brought to the therapy clinic today by his father. Although Tommy has been here twice a week for the last 3 months, and has always seen the same occupational therapist, he was resistant to separating from his father and coming with the OTR. He held on to his father and refused to let go. His father described breakfast this morning as very difficult. Tommy threw his sippy cup, refusing to drink from it. He spit out his oatmeal and pushed the spoon away. He asked for his bottle, and after a while dad gave up and gave Tommy his bottle. Tommy refused to sit in a chair in the clinic, so Tommy's dad held him in his lap at the table. Cheerios® and Chee-tos® were placed on the table. Tommy picked up a piece of the cereal and put it in his mouth. He held it in his mouth while putting two more pieces in. He gagged on them. Next he tried Chee-tos®. He smiled when he tasted it, but spit it out rather than swallow it once it softened in his mouth. He saw the orange residue on his hand and started flapping his hand and screaming. He allowed his father to wipe it off with a damp cloth. He took three sips of milk from a covered cup. He withdrew when his father tried to wipe his chin with the same cloth. His father then sat Tommy on the floor (carpeted), but Tommy immediately stood up and started bouncing up and down. The OTR tried to engage Tommy in playing with toy cars made of smooth plastic. He held on to one for 5 seconds, another for 3 seconds. He watched the whole minute the OTR played with the cars, but did not make any attempt to reach out and grab any cars. When presented with a toy tree that was bristly, Tommy refused to touch it. He kept two fingers (usually his left hand, but occasionally his right) in his mouth throughout most of the session. He cried and tried to jump off a low platform swing. Next Tommy was brought by his dad over to the water table. Tommy watched for a minute or two, but refused to put his own hands in, no matter how the OTR or his dad begged him to try it. Tommy rolled a ball between himself, the OTR, and his dad for a couple minutes. Although the OTR and his dad sat on the floor, Tommy remained standing. He did allow his dad to put him on the floor with his legs spread like the OTR and dad, but he only stayed like that for about 10 seconds. This is longer than he has ever stayed on the floor before in the clinic. At about halfway through the session, he left dad and held the OTR's hand as they walked over to the easel. Dad stayed by the door. After about 2 minutes, Tommy stopped scribbling and began to look for dad, dropped everything, and ran to hug dad around the knees. They sat back down at the table again and tried the Chee-tos® again. This time the OTR held one while Tommy licked the orange coating. He said it tasted good. The OTR asked Tommy to copy her while she demonstrated chewing without food in her mouth. Tommy moved his lower jaw up and down. Then she demonstrated taking a small bite of Chee-tos®, chewing and swallowing it. Tommy imitated her, and swallowed a small piece. He did this three times before starting to gag. OTR discussed with dad the possibility of trying the copying game at home at mealtime. Also discussed trying to engage Tommy in games where he sits on the floor. First try it with long pants on, then in shorts. Since some progress was observed today, I recommend continuing services twice a week.

S:

O:

A:

P:

D:

A:

P:

Case 2: 82-year-old woman who fractured the head of her left femur and then had a heart attack trying to crawl to a phone in her bedroom. She has been in the hospital for 10 days and is transferring to a transitional care facility in 2 days.

Mrs. Anderssen was seen today in her room for work on toilet transfers and dressing. She transfers from bed to wheelchair with minimal assist using a transfer belt and a pivot transfer. This is an improvement, since she was requiring moderate assist 2 days ago. She propelled herself to the bathroom and washed her face and upper body with a washcloth independently. The toilet seat is raised to same height as wheelchair seat. Toilet also has handrails. Client locked the wheelchair at a right angle to the toilet, put both hands on the arms of her wheelchair, and using both arms and her right leg, raised herself to standing. She moved her right hand to the toilet rail, pivoted on her right leg, and sat down on the toilet with stand-by assistance. She independently obtained and used toilet paper. She reached behind her and flushed the toilet while still sitting. Then she again used her arms and right leg to stand and then used a pivot transfer with minimal assist to get back to the wheelchair. She reports that except when OT is in her room, the nurses give her a lot of assist with toilet transfers. She has not yet tried toileting independently while wearing street clothes, which would require her to worry about adjusting her clothing. We will attempt to do it this afternoon.

She propelled herself into her room and in front of her closet. From her closet she used a long-handled reacher to get a hanger down from the hanging rod. She removed a sweat suit and replaced the hanger, again using the reacher. Then she got her bra and panties out of a drawer. She removed her gown and put on her bra (using the hook in front, then twisting it around and pulling up the straps) and sweatshirt without assistance. Next she used a sock aid to put on anklets. It took three tries and some verbal cues, but she did do it without physical assist. Then she used the dressing stick to put her panties and pants on and pull them just over her knees. This was a slow process and she expressed some frustration at how tired and slow she felt. Until she fell, she was a very active woman and participated in a local mall-walking club. It is probably because she was in good condition for her age that she has made the progress that she has. She slid her feet into Velcro sneakers with a long shoehorn. She pushed herself up to standing, pausing for a couple seconds to make sure her balance was good. She steadied herself with her left hand on the bed. Finally, she pulled her panties and pants the rest of the way up and then sat back down in her chair. The entire process of washing, toileting, and dressing took 35 minutes. She reports that it used to take her 10 minutes to do all that, although she didn't have to use all that extra equipment. She is progressing as planned. OTR left instructions for undressing with both Mrs. Anderssen and the nursing staff.

S:

O:

A:

P:

D:

A:

P:

▼ NARRATIVE NOTES ▼

If the narrative progress note is written directly in the client's medical record, it is usually done in a section of the medical record set aside for that purpose. Notes are entered as close to the time of intervention as possible since the notes are expected to be in chronological order. Therefore, narrative notes written directly in the medical record need to be dated, and often the time the note was written is also recorded (Fremgen, 2002; Ranke, 1998). Since the pages of the progress note section of a client's medical record are usually stamped with the client's identifying information, there is no need to repeat it in the note. The length of time of the intervention session is usually recorded.

If the progress notes are written on smaller forms (sometimes these forms come in duplicate or triplicate) and then taped into the chart, or written on a computer and sent to the client's record electronically, then you will need to provide identifying information about the client on your note. A computer may automatically record the date and time.

How do you show that your client is making progress? The easy way would be to write "The client is making progress." However, this would be woefully inadequate. Why should anyone reading the record take your word for it? You have to show that the client is doing something now that he or she could not do before; you have to show a change in the client's occupational performance.

Here are some sample narrative notes.

Case 1: Helen is an 84 y.o. female with Alzheimer's disease. She receives OT on a monthly consultative basis.

Helen attended her day program for people with Alzheimer's 5 days a week for the past month. She received social and recreational programming, one congregate meal, a short rest period each day, and occupational therapy consultation. In addition to Alzheimer's, the client has high blood pressure and circulatory problems in her left leg. She wears a TED stocking. Her medications are stable. She is a widow of 2 years.

Helen helped herself to coffee without asking for permission or directions. She stayed with the morning exercise group for about 20 minutes (it is a 45-minute group) each day. At about that time, she typically got up to throw her coffee cup away, and tried to continue on out of the room. Helen allowed the group leader to redirect her back to the group, and then she continued to participate in the exercises until she was told that the group is over. Then she asked what was next. When asked the name of the program, she said she was not sure she ever knew the name of it.

Helen has been consistent in her behavior for the last month. According to staff, she is less agitated since moving into small-group activities instead of the large group she was in 2 months ago. She is dependent on verbal cues for the completion of most activities. She expresses her confusion with frequent questions.

Helen will continue to attend the 5x/wk Alzheimer's program. Staff will provide her with a highly structured, small-group experience. The client will continue to ask many questions, and these will be responded to in short, simple sentences. Staff will post a daily schedule near the clock.

Bobbi Babinski, OTR/L Nov. 1, 2003

Case 2: 27 y.o. with LCVA (Bob)

Bob participated in a 30-minute session to work on functional activities with his unaffected (nondominant) hand. Bob attempted to use a computer mouse with his left hand by playing a game of solitaire. He moved quickly to the general area that he wants the mouse to be. He moved slowly and hesitantly to the precise spot he needed, however, he often overshot the mark. Bob clicked the mouse with his index finger easily, however, he had minimal success holding the mouse button down while dragging the mouse, such as when he wanted to move a card to a different pile. He expressed concern about how much more he had to concentrate on the movements than he had to when he used his right hand. It took 20 minutes to complete one game of solitaire.

Carrie Ingwater, COTA/L 3/2/03

Bobbi Babinski, OTR/L 3/2/2003

Case 3: 9-month-old infant who was found blue (not breathing) in her crib 2 weeks ago

Rina was seen today for a 30-minute session. She did not make eye contact with the occupational therapist, but she did respond to sound and to touch. She did not try to locate a toy by sight, but when a rattle was touched to her fingertips or the back of her hand, she turned her hand to grasp the rattle and shake it. From a prone position, she rolled to the right and to the left in response to noise. She rolled in a straight line to her right but was slower and less direct rolling to her left. Mild ATNR present, stronger when her head is turned to the left. Rina supported her weight on her right arm when prone on elbows with a toy in her left hand. After three attempts, she was not able to support her weight on her left arm when prone on elbows with a toy in her right hand. While she is able to use both arms to reach and grasp for toys, she is showing greater strength and endurance on her right side. Her vision continues to appear impaired. The plan is to continue to see Rina twice a day for the duration of her hospitalization to work on movement and play skills and to monitor for any sign of returning vision.

Stephanie Smith, OTR/L 7/02/03

Narrative format is also used to write a contact note. This is a note written to document contact with a client, but not necessarily during a therapy session. For example, when you instruct a caregiver in proper transfer techniques or splint care. A contact note could be written to document the reason for a missed intervention session. A contact note might also be used to document that you met the client and scheduled the client to come to the occupational therapy room to begin the evaluation (or for you to come to the client's room and begin the evaluation there if that is the plan). In a case like this, the contact note might look like this:

Saw Mrs. Smith in her room today. Explained what occupational therapy is and that she was referred to occupational therapy to work on her self-care skills. She said she understood her doctor's concern, but that she was sure that her left side was not affected by the stroke and that she really did not want to waste my time when I could be helping someone who really needs my help. She agreed to humor me and come to the occupational therapy clinic this afternoon at 1:30. I told her I would send an aide to come and bring her to the clinic. Britta Farver, OTR/L, 9-23-03

or

Went to client's room to bring her to the clinic. She said she felt really nauseous today, and a bit light-headed and would prefer to skip this afternoon's session. Checked with the nurse who was aware of the situation and concurred that she should not participate in occupational therapy this afternoon. Mika Vica, OTR/L, 9-23-03

Exercise 12.11

Write a narrative progress note based on the following cases:

Case 1: Kiki is a 6-year-old receiving occupational therapy following a car accident. She had a severe head injury. Last week she visually tracked a toy while supine over a 60° horizontal arc. She did not reach for the toy. During passive ROM to her upper extremities, she cried out with each movement. She was dependent in all her ADLs. This week, she tracked the toy while sitting over a 90° arc horizontally, and 40° vertically. She cried out during shoulder passive ROM, but not during elbow, wrist, or hand PROM. Showing about 10° active ROM in Ⓡ elbow spontaneously, but not on command. She remains dependent in all her ADLs. She received occupational therapy twice a day, 5 days this week, and once on Saturday.

Note:

Case 2: 88-year-old woman with osteoarthritis in her knees, COPD, and diabetic neuropathy who received home-based occupational therapy following hospitalization for pneumonia, resulting in diminished strength and endurance. She received occupational therapy twice a week and you write a note after each visit. Her goals are to prepare light meals for breakfast and dinner (Meals on Wheels for lunch), dress and undress herself without fatigue, and safe showers. In addition, the client wants to be able to take care of her houseplants and play solitaire, even though holding things in her hands is difficult. During this 45-minute visit, occupational therapy worked on using a kitchen stool to sit on while preparing a meal, shower transfers using the bath bench you brought for her to try, and trying adaptive equipment for dressing and card playing. (*Write the narrative note, using an educated guess on how much progress she has made since you saw her 3 days ago.*)

Note:

Flow sheets can show the progress a client is making on specific activities in a very concise way. Flow sheets are typically tables or graphs where measurements can be recorded at regular intervals, generally after each intervention session. It makes it easy for the reader to see at a glance whether progress is being made in a particular area of need for a client. For example, you could chart the length of time it takes for your client to complete a meal, the number of dishes the client unloaded from a dishwasher and put away in a cabinet, or the degrees of active range of motion of a client's wrist. When progress flow sheets are used, then the narrative, SOAP, or DAP note is often written weekly or biweekly rather than after every intervention session.

There are several advantages of using flow sheets to track progress. One is that they are easier to read than lengthy progress notes. The data recorded is kept to a minimum, and is organized in an easy-to-follow format. Second, instead of relying on someone saying a client has made progress, you have solid, objective data that shows the progress. Another advantage is a flow sheet contains a lot of data but uses minimal space, so it conserves paper. Using a flow chart keeps the clinician focused on interventions that are specific to the client's goals, and less chance to go off on tangents. It makes it easy for a substitute clinician to know what to expect a client to do in the next occupational therapy session. Third, flow charts provide reliable data that can be used to write progress summaries. In those settings where progress notes are written weekly or biweekly, a clinician who can reflect that data off the flow sheet will have written a more reliable note than one who writes from memory alone. This is particularly helpful if the client's medical record is ever called into court.

There are also disadvantages to using flow sheets. Often, there is space enough to record a number or other objective measurement, but not room for descriptions of performance. There is no place to record the client's reaction to the intervention. There may be a place to record new interventions, but there may not be, depending on the form used.

Figure 12.3 is a sample progress flow sheet for an adult with mental retardation being seen in a sheltered workshop. In this case, only brief objective data is recorded. Figure 12.4 is a sample of a progress flow sheet for a woman in a nursing home. The therapist records objective data in the appropriate box. It does allow for observations to be recorded as well as number of cues, number of repetitions, time to complete task, or whatever measure is included in the goal. Some forms use short-term goals rather than a problem statement.

Intervention \ Date	6-1-03	6-3-03	6-5-03	6-8-03	6-10-03	6-12-03	6-15-03	6-17-03	6-19-03	6-22-03	6-24-03
Number of correct packets assembled independently	6	6	7	6	7	7	7	8	7	8	
In 30-min. period, number of times client needed redirection	8	9	8	8	7	6	8	6	6	5	
Degree of assist needed in lunch line (dep = 5, max = 4, mod = 3, min = 2, indep = 1, P = physical, V = verbal)	3P 4V	3P 4V	3P 3V	3P 3V	2P 3V	3P 3V	3P 4V	2P 3V	2P 3V	2P 3V	
During lunch, number of times client engages in self-stimulatory behavior	6	7	6	6	6	6	5	6	5	5	

FIGURE 12.3 Sample Progress Flow Sheet A

In some settings, there may be a separate flow sheet for each goal area. If this is the case, you can graph progress. For example, if you were working on having a client with schizophrenia and ADD increase attention to task, you could graph the amount of time the client worked on a task before his first redirection, or the number of redirections in a 1-hour session. The graphs might look like Figure 12.5.

You can see at a glance that progress is being made, even before you read the data. Figure 12.6 shows a type of bar graph, but you could use a line graph where you connect the dots plotted like this as well.

Flow sheets must be signed at the bottom of the page, but each entry is usually simply initialed. There can be a key at the bottom that looks like the one on the bottom of Figure 12.5. This lets readers know who worked with the client on what day.

Progress flow sheets cannot entirely replace progress notes. They may decrease the frequency with which progress notes are written from daily to weekly or biweekly in some settings. Not every setting uses progress flow sheets.

▼ ATTENDANCE LOGS ▼

Attendance logs, at minimum, identify when the client had therapy. Many also identify which occupational therapy personnel worked with the client that day, and how long the therapy session was. Some also identify which type of intervention happened during which intervention session. An attendance log can be used for billing therapy services if it is designed to be compatible with the billing system used at that facility.

Most commonly, I have seen attendance logs on a clipboard in the department with a separate page for each client. When the client is discontinued, the attendance log may go in the client's permanent record, the department file, or the billing office, depending on facility policy.

Goal area	Date: 3-24-03	Date: 3-26-03	Date: 3-28-03	Date:
Dresss self in 15 minutes or less	21 minutes 2 verbal cues 1 physical prompt	21 minutes 1 verbal cue 1 physical prompt	19 minutes 1 verbal cue 1 physical prompt	
Feed self without spilling	Breakfast: Used fork; no spilling when stabbing meat, but did spill three times when scooping eggs.	Breakfast: Used fork for eggs, fingers for meat; eggs fell off twice.	Breakfast: Used spoon for oatmeal; no spilling.	
Actively participate in one group activity per day	Attended bingo game when aide escorted her, but did not play.	Attended current events group, made one comment in 30-min. session	Attended current events group, made two comments in 30-min. session	
Develop a repertoire of individual activities (6) in which to engage	Discussed former hobbies; used to enjoy crocheting, knitting, reading magazines and novels, cooking, walking, and dog grooming.	Showed her where magazines are kept for resident use and provided library cart schedule. Provided a large crochet hook and her choice of yarns.	Resident has 6 inches of a scarf crocheted. Reports that her hands hurt after a while. Told her about a program to crochet afghans for kids at homeless shelter.	

FIGURE 12.4   Sample Progress Flow Sheet B

min	9-3	9-4	9-5	9-6	9-9	9-10	9-11	9-12	9-13	9-14
15 min										
14 min										
13 min										
12 min										
11 min										
10 min										
9 min										
8 min									▓	
7 min									▓	▓
6 min							▓	▓	▓	▓
5 min				▓		▓	▓	▓	▓	▓
4 min		▓		▓	▓	▓	▓	▓	▓	▓
3 min	▓	▓	▓	▓	▓	▓	▓	▓	▓	▓
2 min	▓	▓	▓	▓	▓	▓	▓	▓	▓	▓
1 min	▓	▓	▓	▓	▓	▓	▓	▓	▓	▓
Date 2003	9-3	9-4	9-5	9-6	9-9	9-10	9-11	9-12	9-13	9-14
Initials:	KS	KS	KS	KS	CJ	KS	KS	KS	KS	KS

Signatures:

Initials	Names
KS	*Katerine Sanchez, OTR/L*
CJ	*Cecelia Jorgenson, COTA/L*
____	_____
____	_____

FIGURE 12.5   Sample Progress Graph

Attendance logs can be set up much like the first example of a flow chart, with dates across the top and interventions listed along one side. If the attendance log is used for billing, then the interventions are labeled so that they coincide with billing codes. In the box that correlates to the date and intervention, the clinician records the number of billable units of that intervention, or the number of minutes of that intervention. The biggest difference between the attendance log and the flow sheet is the attendance log does not include any data on the client's performance, only that a particular intervention was worked on.

▼ PHOTOGRAPHIC AND VIDEO DOCUMENTATION ▼

It is often said that a picture is worth a thousand words. If that is the case, then it would seem logical that visual evidence of a client's performance would strengthen the documentation. With the availability of digital cameras, visual documentation is getting easier and less cumbersome.

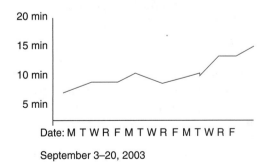

Date: M T W R F M T W R F M T W R F

September 3–20, 2003

FIGURE 12.6   Progress Graph

There are several ways in which visual evidence can be used. Still pictures of proper positioning of a client can be used both as an educational aid for clients and/or caregivers and as evidence of the caregiver/client education in the medical record. Before-and-after intervention pictures of resting hand position, posture, range of motion, sensory tolerance, or other intervention provide eloquent evidence of the effect of intervention.

SUMMARY

In this chapter we explored three types of progress notes. The narrative note is written in paragraph form, and often reads as if one is telling a story, which is in fact what one is doing. SOAP (subjective, objective, assessment, plan) and DAP (description, assessment, plan) perform the same function as narrative notes, but do it in a prescribed fashion. Progress notes do not simply list activities, they describe what progress has been made, how the client reacted to the interventions, and what functional skills the client has demonstrated.

SOAP notes are used by many health care disciplines in many settings. The "S" part of the note is where subjective information, such as the client's perspective on the problem, is recorded. The "O" is for objective data, the information about what the client did without judgment or interpretation. In the "A" section, you make sense out of the information in the "S" and "O" sections by interpreting it and assessing it. Finally, in the "P" section, you state what you plan to do with the client so that the client can achieve his or her goals.

DAP notes are also sometimes called FIP (findings, interpretation, plan) notes. They are very similar to SOAP notes. In the "D" section, you combine the subjective and objective information that would normally be recorded in separate sections in a SOAP note. In the "A" section you assess the meaning of the information in the "D" section, and in the "P" section you record the plan.

Narrative notes contain the same information as SOAP and DAP but the information is not labeled as such; rather, it is written in paragraph format. Narrative notes may be written in great detail, or may only hit the high points. A specific kind of narrative note, a contact note, may be written to document contact with a client or client's caregiver (as part of an occupational therapy session or outside of regular sessions), or to document the reason for a missed intervention session.

Progress flow sheets and attendance logs were also discussed in this chapter. These documents provide information on when a client received intervention, and to a limited extent, what was worked on. These documents can supplement, but not replace, writing progress summaries.

The occupational therapist is responsible for ensuring that progress reports get written in accordance with standards and regulations for timeliness and content and are communicated to the client or other involved party (in accordance with privacy regulations). Occupational therapy assistants, under the supervision of an occupational therapist, contribute to the process. Either the occupational therapist or the occupational therapy assistant may write the progress report. In most situations, as part of routine supervision, the occupational therapist will cosign notes written by the occupational therapy assistant.

REFERENCES

American Occupational Therapy Association. (1998). Occupational therapy standards of practice. *American Journal of Occupational Therapy, 52,* 866–869.

American Occupational Therapy Association. (2003). *Guidelines for documentation of occupational therapy.* Retrieved June 27, 2003, from *http://www.aota.org/members/area2/docs/ra2.pdf*

Borcherding, S. (2000). *Documentation manual for writing SOAP notes in occupational therapy.* Thorofare, NJ: Slack.

Borcherding, S., & Kappel, C. (2002). *The OTA's guide to writing SOAP notes.* Thorofare, NJ: Slack.

Fremgen, B. F. (2002). *Medical law and ethics.* Upper Saddle River, NJ: Prentice Hall.

Kettenbach, G. (1990). *Writing SOAP notes.* Philadelphia: F. A. Davis

Kuntavanish, A. A. (1988). *Occupational therapy documentation: A system to capture outcome data for quality assurance and program promotion.* Rockville, MD: American Occupational Therapy Association.

Ranke, B. A. E. (1998). Documentation in the age of litigation. *OT Practice, 3*(3), 20–24.

Sample Medical SOAP Note. (2002). Retrieved September 5, 2002, from *http://cpmcnet.Columbia.edu/dept/ps/2002/SOAPmed.html*

Tips on Medical Progress Notes. (2002). Retrieved September 5, 2002, from *http://cpmcnet.Columbia.edu/dept/ps/2002/SOAPmed.html*

CHAPTER 13

Discontinuation Summaries

INTRODUCTION

When the client achieves all of his or her goals, moves out of the facility, refuses to continue in the program, or achieves maximum benefit from occupational therapy, a discontinuation summary must be written (AOTA, 1998). This summary, also called a discharge summary, needs to show the client's progress from the beginning of occupational therapy services to the end. It is the final justification of your services.

The terms "discontinuation" and "discharge" are distinct but overlapping terms. Discontinuation occurs when a client stops, or discontinues, services from a particular provider. The term "discontinuation" is used in both *The Framework* (AOTA, 2002) and *The Standards of Practice for Occupational Therapy* (AOTA, 1998). The term "discharge" is often used to describe what happens when a client leaves a facility or clinic. *The Guidelines for Documentation of Occupational Therapy* (2003) uses the term discharge to describe the end of service delivery. Since services are often discontinued when a client is discharged, the words are often used interchangeably. In this book, the document that is written when a client stops receiving occupational therapy services is referred to as a discontinuation summary.

▼ ROLE DELINEATION IN DISCONTINUATION ▼

The occupational therapist determines when a client is ready to discontinue services (AOTA, 1998). The occupational therapy assistant may recommend discontinuing services to a client. The occupational therapist prepares, implements, and documents the discontinuation plan, including appropriate follow-up resources and reevaluation needs. The occupational therapy assistant contributes to the process of implementing the discontinuation plan and in documenting the changes in the client's engagement in occupations (AOTA, 1998, 2003).

▼ COMPONENTS OF A DISCONTINUATION SUMMARY ▼

In some facilities the discontinuation summary is an interdisciplinary effort. At a rehabilitation facility or rehabilitation unit of a hospital, members of the rehabilitation team may dictate their part of the summary, and have a secretary type up one report in a narrative format that includes information from occupational therapy, physical therapy, speech-language pathology, nursing, social work, psychology, and other represented disciplines. While dictation can save the clinical staff some time (you can talk faster than you can write), it requires a certain amount of skill. First, you have to speak clearly and spell out any terms that you think the secretary may not be familiar with. You have to identify the punctuation marks so the secretary knows when to include them. Be aware that every word or sound gets transcribed, so side conversations and "ums" and other "filler" words could show up in print. Long pauses waste time for the transcriber. You have to proofread the document for errors before you sign it. The advantage of the interdisciplinary format is that it gives a very complete picture of the client.

At other facilities there may be a form or format to follow for discontinuation summaries. Generally, no matter whether you dictate, fill out a form, or write the report electronically, the same basic information is provided. First, there is, as always, identifying information. Next is a summary of the occupational therapy services provided and the client's response to the intervention (AOTA, 2003). The *Guidelines for Documentation of Occupational Therapy* lists the following items that should be found in this part of the document (AOTA, 2003):

- Starting and ending dates of service
- Frequency/number of session
- Summary of the interventions provided
- Summary of the client's progress in occupational therapy goals
- Occupational therapy outcomes (engagement in occupations)
  - Initial status of client
  - Ending status of client
  - "Client's assessment of efficacy of occupational therapy" (AOTA, 2003, III.A.2.c.)

Finally, any follow-up plans, recommendations, or referrals to other professionals are documented. Of course, the occupational therapist signs and dates the document.

It is important to be comprehensive, yet concise when reporting on progress toward goals and occupational therapy outcomes. If a client has been receiving occupational therapy intervention for several months or more, you may want to focus more on the long-term goals than on each and every adjustment to short-term goals. However, if a client was seen for a few days to a few weeks, you may address each short-term goal.

When addressing the initial and ending status of the client in relation to engagement in occupations, the emphasis will clearly be on occupations rather than on changes in client factors, activity demands, or even contexts. However, contexts, especially those related to the client's discharge disposition, are very important. The client's discharge disposition is the place the client is being discharged to; it could be to the client's home, extended care facility, assisted living facility, home care, outpatient program, or other community-based service (Moyers, 1999). Your evaluation of the client's ending status is dependent on the discharge disposition.

In order to make appropriate recommendations for follow-up or referrals in the discontinuation summary, the discharge disposition is also essential (Moyers, 1999). If a client is being discharged to another facility, you need to know what services are available at that facility in order to make an appropriate referral. If the client will be receiving occupational therapy intervention at the new facility, it is helpful if the occupational therapists can talk with each other. However, in order to do that, permission to discuss the client's status must be obtained from the client or client's legal guardian in order to comply with confidentiality regulations (i.e., HIPAA; see Chapter 5). If a client is being discharged to his or her home, community-based services can be recommended, but the occupational therapist has to know what kinds of services are available in the area. This is where working as a team with a social worker can be a real help. For example, you might recommend that a client participate in a community-based 12-step program (i.e., Alcoholics Anonymous), join a health club or community-based exercise program, or seek further help from a vocational rehab program (Moyers, 1999).

You may recommend that the client come back in a few months for a recheck because you expect the client will progress or regress on his or her own and may need more occupational therapy at that time, or the client may have some medical interventions planned (e.g., surgery, botox injection) that will result in a change of functional status (Moyers,

1999). Orthotic devices or adaptive equipment may need to be checked periodically for wear and fit. For any of these reasons or others, recommending the client come back in three months for a recheck may be a good idea. However, if you make such a recommendation, be sure it is documented in the discharge summary.

Figure 13.1 shows a sample format for a discontinuation summary report. Figure 13.2 shows a sample completed discontinuation summary report.

▼ SOAP FORMAT ▼

Some facilities use the SOAP format for their discontinuation summaries (Borcherding, 2000; Borcherding & Kappel, 2002; Kettenbach, 1990). This would usually only happen in facilities that use the SOAP note format for reporting progress. In a discontinuation note, the "S" would describe something the client said about her progress, or the client's subjective description of current function. The "O" would report objective data regarding

---

Occupational Therapy Discontinuation Report

Date of report: Name:
Date of birth &/or age: Date of initial referral: M   F
Primary intervention diagnosis/concern:
Secondary diagnosis/concern:
Precautions/contraindications:
Reason for referral to OT:
Reason for OT discontinuation:

Therapist: *(Print or type your name and credential, you will sign and date the report at the end.)*

Description of OT intervention: *(Include service delivery model, duration/frequency of interventions, # of intervention sessions or beginning and end dates of interventions, location of interventions, and types of interventions provided.)*

Brief summary of progress toward goals: *(Statements of progress toward or achievement of long-term goals or reasons why goals were not met.)*

Occupational therapy outcomes:
   Initial performance in areas of occupation:
   (Concise summary of the client's initial performance in the areas of activities of daily living, instrumental activities of daily living, education, work, play, leisure, and social participation.)

   Current level of performance in areas of occupation:
   (Concise summary of current performance and expectations for performance within the contexts of the client's anticipated environments following discontinuation.)

Contextual aspects related to discontinuation:
(Concise summary of the cultural, physical, social, personal, spiritual, temporal, and/or virtual contexts.)

Discontinuation recommendations:
(Concise description of discontinuation plans, other referrals, follow-up, home program suggestions, support systems, and caregiver suggestions.)

_____   _____
Signature   Date

FIGURE 13.1   Sample Discontinuation Summary Report Format

Occupational Therapy Discontinuation Report

Date of report: Sept. 30, 2003   **Client's name:** Sadie Clapsaddle
Date of birth/age: March 26, 1974   **Date of initial referral:** Sept. 23, 2003   M   Ⓕ
Primary intervention diagnosis/concern: Depression with suicide attempt
Secondary intervention diagnoses/concerns: History of cutting
Precautions/contraindications: Do not allow to use sharp instruments without close supervision.
Count sharps at end of session.
Reason for referral to OT: Evaluate and treat for depression. Increase self-esteem.
Reason for discontinuation of OT: Completed 7-day inpatient program.

Therapist: Carla McShane, OTR/L

Description of OT intervention:
Sadie was seen in the occupational therapy clinic twice a day for 6 of the 7 days she was here.
Provided with unconditional support and encouragement. Participated in self-esteem and assertive-
ness group as well as task group.

Brief summary of progress toward goals:
Sadie's initial goal for herself was to begin to get involved in activities that interested her in the
past. She used to paint, but stopped painting when her children were little. Her children are now
teenagers. She also wanted to learn to say "no" to members of her family who demanded that she
do things for them, without feeling guilty and changing her mind because of it. She met both goals.

Occupational therapy outcomes:
Initial performance in areas of occupation:
Sadie initially sat with her head down; she did not initiate conversation or activities. She was
compliant with all therapist requests. She said nothing interested her anymore. Sadie did not
initiate any interactions with peers or staff. She did not comb her hair unless she was told to
do it. She reported that prior to her hospitalization, she just sat at home doing nothing. She
was not interested in painting, a hobby she gave up 14 years ago when she had her first
child.

Current level of performance in areas of occupation:
During her week here, she rehearsed saying "no" during role-playing exercises with the therapist. By the end of the week, when the therapist would ask Sadie for favors like "Could you
clean up the sink?" Sadie said "no" and stuck with that answer. If the therapist asked for volunteers to do something, Sadie literally sat on her hands to keep from volunteering. With the
help of the occupational therapist, Sadie signed up for a painting class through Sadie's local
community education program. Sadie reports that she is excited about taking a painting
class. She said she liked the paintings she made in occupational therapy. She met with her
husband and children and told them that they had to start doing some things for themselves
when she came home. They agreed to take on some of the work she usually does. Sadie
said she was amazed that her family was so unaware of her feelings. She made a commitment to express her feelings on a more regular basis, and they agreed not to "blow her off."
Sadie is returning to her home with twice a week outpatient visits with a counselor.

Contextual aspects related to discontinuation:
Home has been a stressful place for Sadie, but she and her family say they are committed to making things less stressful by sharing Sadie's load.

Discontinuation recommendations:
Sadie will participate in counseling sessions twice a week. She will attend a painting class through
community education.

Carla McShane, OTR/L   _Sept. 30, 2003_
Signature   Date

FIGURE 13.2   Sample Discontinuation Report

performance in areas of occupation. This can include both initial and ending data. The "A" would articulate your assessment or interpretation of the data in "O." You would summarize those areas where significant progress occurred, and identify areas where progress was not made. The "P" would be where you indicate home program instructions, follow-up recommendations, and referrals to other professionals. Figure 13.3 shows a sample format for a SOAP-based discontinuation summary. Figure 13.4 shows a SOAP-based discontinuation summary for the same client as in Figure 13.2.

Occupational Therapy Discontinuation Report

Date of report: **Name:**
Date of birth &/or age: **Date of initial referral:**   M   F
Primary intervention diagnosis/concern:
Secondary diagnosis/concern:
Precautions/contraindications:
Reason for referral to OT:
Reason for OT discontinuation:

Therapist: *(Print or type your name and credential, you will sign and date the report at the end.)*

S: *(Client's subjective description of progress or occupational performance)*

O: *(Description of occupational therapy services)*

Long-term goals	Initial performance	Ending performance

A: *(Your assessment [interpretation] of progress)*

P: *(Home programs, follow-up recommendations, and referrals to other professionals)*

_____   _____
Signature   Date

FIGURE 13.3   Sample Discontinuation Report, SOAP Format

Occupational Therapy Discontinuation Report

Date of report: Sept. 30, 2003   **Client's name:** Sadie Clapsaddle
Date of birth/age: March 26, 1974   **Date of initial referral:** Sept. 23, 2003   M   Ⓕ
Primary intervention diagnosis/concern: Depression with suicide attempt
Secondary intervention diagnoses/concerns: History of cutting
Precautions/contraindications: Do not allow to use sharp instruments without close supervision.
Count sharps at end of session.
Reason for referral to OT: Evaluate and treat for depression. Increase self-esteem.
Reason for discontinuation of OT: Completed 7-day inpatient program.

Therapist: Carla McShane, OTR/L

S: "I am looking forward to the painting class. It will be like taking a 'mini-vacation' twice a week."

O: Sadie was seen in the occupational therapy clinic twice a day for 6 of the 7 days she was here.
    Provided with unconditional support and encouragement. Participated in self-esteem and as-
    sertiveness group as well as task group.

Long-term goals	Initial performance	Ending performance
Sadie will say "no" and stick to that answer.	Client complied with all requests of the occupational therapist	Client said "no" to three requests on last 2 days of OT, did not change her answer.
Look people in the eye, maintain eye contact for 10 seconds	Client looked down, did not make eye contact	Maintained eye contact with therapist and peer for 10 seconds on six occasions in last 2 days of OT
Engage in painting with watercolors	Started painting after several prompts	Independently initiated painting upon entering OT clinic. Signed up to take painting class through community education.

A: Client made good progress. She achieved all of her goals. She is taking steps to take charge of
    her life, such as taking a painting class, talking with her family and negotiating shared work-
    loads, and not backing down once she says no.

P: Sadie will participate in counseling sessions twice a week. She will attend a painting class
    through community education.

_____Carla McShane, OTR/L_____   _____Sept. 30, 2003_____
Signature   Date

FIGURE 13.4   Sample SOAP Discontinuation Report

SUMMARY

The discontinuation brings closure to a case. It provides the final justification for the services that were provided. In this document, you provide an overview of the client's progress and plans for the future. Because it is a summary, it does not need to be a session-by-session recap of what happened. Rather, it hits the highlights and reflects progress toward occupational therapy outcomes.

A discontinuation summary may be written in narrative or SOAP format. Either way, the discontinuation summary must contain specific information about the client's change in status and recommendations for follow-up and referral to other services. Knowing the client's discharge disposition is essential for making accurate statements about the client's status at discharge and what services can be recommended after discontinuation of occupational therapy services.

REFERENCES

American Occupational Therapy Association. (1998). Occupational therapy standards of practice. *American Journal of Occupational Therapy, 52,* 866–869.

American Occupational Therapy Association. (2002). Occupational therapy practice framework: Domain and process. *American Journal of Occupational Therapy, 56,* 609–639.

American Occupational Therapy Association. (2003). *Guidelines for documentation of occupational therapy.* Retrieved June 27, 2003, from *http://www.aota.org/members/area2/docs/ra2.pdf*

Borcherding, S. (2000). *Documentation manual for writing SOAP notes in occupational therapy.* Thorofare, NJ: Slack.

Borcherding, S., & Kappel, C. (2002). *The OTA's guide to writing SOAP notes.* Thorofare, NJ: Slack.

Kettenbach, G. (1990). *Writing SOAP notes.* Philadelphia: F. A. Davis.

Moyers, P. (1999). The guide to occupational therapy practice. *American Journal of Occupational Therapy, 53,* 247–322.

School System Documentation

▼ INTRODUCTION ▼

In school systems the requirements for documentation are different than for occupational therapy services provided in clinical settings. There are clear federal guidelines about what to document and when. In this section of the book, we look at the documentation requirements for services provided to children through the school system. Minimal information about the actual delivery of services is covered.

▼ OVERVIEW OF SCHOOL SYSTEM DOCUMENTATION ▼

The Individuals with Disabilities Education Act (IDEA) dictates how educational services are provided to children with disabilities from birth to age 21. IDEA also provides guidelines about how to document those services. Under IDEA, there are three types of documents; notice and consent forms, the Individualized Family Service Plan (IFSP), and the Individualized Education Program (IEP). IDEA allows each state to develop guidelines for service delivery to children that further refine the federal law. In most states, services to these children are provided by local school districts. For children birth to age 2, some states provide services to children with special needs through the school district (coordinated by the state Department of Education), but in others, the primary provider of these services could be a home health agency or welfare agency (coordinated by the state Department of Health or Department of Human Services).

Throughout this section of the book, federal laws and regulations will be cited. However, examples of how these laws and regulations are implemented will come from individual states. This is because federal law requires states to offer certain services, document them, and inform families, but allows the states to determine the exact method of implementation and documentation of these services. States used as examples in this section of the book represent those in which information is more readily available on the Internet. It is not meant to imply that the states whose forms or regulations are cited have better systems than those who are not cited. I have tried to present information from different states representing a geographic cross-section of this country.

One of the biggest differences between school system documentation and clinical documentation is that school system documentation is intended to be shared with the child's family/guardian. When you document in a school system, you know that the parent or guardian will receive a copy of the document, and will read what you write. In a clinical setting, you know the physician and other team members will read the document, but only if a family asks for access to the documents will they be allowed to read what you wrote.

School systems may bill third-party payers (insurance companies, managed care organizations, or Medicaid), but not every district has elected to do so. Billing third-party payers may impact the type and frequency of documentation completed by occupational therapy personnel.

▼ ROLE DELINEATION IN SCHOOL SYSTEM DOCUMENTATION ▼

In school systems, most of the documentation is written through a team effort. The team may include teachers, special education teachers, school nurses, speech clinicians, school psychologists, and administrators, along with occupational and physical therapists. As a member of the team, the occupational therapist may write or verbally contribute to sections of the Notice and Consent Forms, IFSP, or IEP. Occupational therapy assistants may also contribute to development of the IEP and IFSP. If the occupational therapist is serving as the service coordinator for an infant or toddler, he or she will be responsible for ensuring that all required documentation is completed within established timelines. As described in the *Guidelines for Documentation of Occupational Therapy* (AOTA, 2003), the occupational therapist is responsible for completing the evaluation; an occupational therapy assistant may participate in the process. Specific rules for documentation written by the occupational therapist or occupational therapy assistant in school systems may vary from state to state. You can find these rules by checking with your state education agency (i.e., Department of Education). As always, the AOTA *Standards of Practice for Occupational Therapy* (1998) for role delineation in documentation apply (see Appendix C).

▼ STRUCTURE OF THIS SECTION OF THE BOOK ▼

Under IDEA, the contents of educational documentation including notice and consent forms, the IFSP, and the IEP are specified, however, the specific forms may be developed by the state education agency or the school district/local agency. Just as with documents in medical model settings, these documents are legal documents and can be called into court when there are lawsuits. It seems lately that there are more and more lawsuits involving the provision of special education and related services, especially issues around who will be responsible for paying for what services.

Notice and consent forms are designed to guarantee that the rights of the child and his or her family are respected. Some of these forms provide information or notice to the family, others seek parental consent to evaluate, provide, or change services (20 U.S.C. 1400 .615[b]). These are discussed in Chapter 14.

Documentation for children birth through age 2 are covered in Chapter 15. Each infant or toddler who qualifies for services under IDEA must have a written plan, called an Individualized Family Service Plan (IFSP), for the services he or she will receive. This chapter discusses the IFSP.

The last chapter of this section, Chapter 16, discusses the Individualized Education Program (IEP). This is generally written for children with special needs ages 3–21. For these children, occupational therapy is a related service rather than a special education service (AOTA, 1999; Office of Special Education Programs, 2000).

REFERENCES

American Occupational Therapy Association. (1998). Occupational therapy standards of practice. *American Journal of Occupational Therapy, 52,* 866–869.

American Occupational Therapy Association. (1999). *Occupational therapy services for children and youth under the Individuals with Disabilities Education Act* (2nd ed.). Bethesda, MD: Author.

American Occupational Therapy Association. (2003). *Guidelines for documentation of occupational therapy.* Retrieved June 27, 2003, from *http://aota.org/members/area2/docs/ra2.pdf*

Office of Special Education Programs. (2000). *Guide to the individualized education program.* Retrieved November 7, 2002, from *http://www.ed.gov/offices/OSERS/OSEP/Products/IEP_Guide*

CHAPTER 14

Notice and Consent Forms

INTRODUCTION

Whenever you work with children, you are working with a vulnerable population. As such, the federal government has developed regulations that protect the rights and interests of the child and his or her family. The forms that are used to protect the rights of recipients, inform families, and obtain consent are called notice and consent forms. Generally, the school system or agency will have these forms available for obtaining parent signatures and providing legally required notices.

Some states mandate that school districts use a prescribed set of forms; others allow each school district to develop its own set of forms. A survey by the Project Forum of the National Association of State Directors of Special Education (NASDSE) in 2002 showed that 17 states (34%) have mandated procedural safeguard forms and 10 (20%) states have forms for obtaining parental permission prior to initial evaluation of a student (Ahearn, 2002).

Figure 14.1 shows the language of the federal law (20 U.S.C. 1400 et seq.) relating to the types of notices and consent forms and their contents. No matter what type of form parents are asked to read or sign, they must be provided in the families' native language, including Braille or orally (34 C.F.R. § 300.503[c]; 34 C.F.R. § 303.403[c]).

▼ SERVICE COORDINATION ▼

Providing educational services to children is a team effort. It includes professionals from several disciplines as well as the parents, and when possible, the child. Because of the many people who could be involved in the team, there needs to be one person who takes responsibility for ensuring that everything that needs to be done gets done in a timely fashion. This person is referred to as the service coordinator (team leader). An occupational therapist can serve as the service coordinator for a child from birth through age 2 if designated as such by the Individualized Family Service Plan (IFSP) team (34 C.F.R. § 303.6). However, because occupational therapy is a related service (rather than a special education service) for children ages 3–21, an occupational therapist is usually not the service coordinator for preschool through school-age children. However, if designated by the Individualized Education Program (IEP) team, the occupational therapist can be the case manager (AOTA, 1999).

The service coordinator prepares the documents for parent notification and consent (AOTA, 1999; 20 U.S.C. 1400.615[b]). The service coordinator must provide parents with written information about procedural safeguards upon initial referral or evaluation, each notification of IFSP or IEP meetings, every reevaluation, and when the parents request it (34 CFR § 300.504[a]). This information accompanies notice and consent forms presented to families to ensure that families are fully informed about their rights.

Sec. 615. PROCEDURAL SAFEGUARDS

(a) ESTABLISHMENT OF PROCEDURES–Any State educational agency, State agency, or local educational agency that receives assistance under this part shall establish and maintain procedures in accordance with this section to ensure that children with disabilities and their parents are guaranteed procedural safeguards with respect to the provision of free appropriate public education by such agencies.

(b) TYPES OF PROCEDURES–The procedures required by this section shall include—

(1) an opportunity for the parents of a child with a disability to examine all records relating to such child and to participate in meetings with respect to the identification, evaluation, and educational placement of the child, and the provision of a free appropriate public education to such child, and to obtain an independent educational evaluation of the child;

(2) procedures to protect the rights of the child whenever the parents of the child are not known, the agency cannot, after reasonable efforts, locate the parents, or the child is a ward of the State, including the assignment of an individual (who shall not be an employee of the State educational agency, the local educational agency, or any other agency that is involved in the education or care of the child) to act as a surrogate for the parents;

(3) written prior notice to the parents of the child whenever such agency—

(A) proposes to initiate or change; or

(B) refuses to initiate or change; the identification, evaluation, or educational placement of the child, in accordance with subsection (c), or the provision of a free appropriate public education to the child;

(4) procedures designed to ensure that the notice required by paragraph (3) is in the native language of the parents, unless it clearly is not feasible to do so;

(5) an opportunity for mediation in accordance with subsection (e);

(6) an opportunity to present complaints with respect to any matter relating to the identification, evaluation, or educational placement of the child, or the provision of a free appropriate public education to such child;

(7) procedures that require the parent of a child with a disability, or the attorney representing the child, to provide notice (which shall remain confidential)—

(A) to the State educational agency or local educational agency, as the case may be, in the complaint filed under paragraph (6); and

(B) that shall include—

(i) the name of the child, the address of the residence of the child, and the name of the school the child is attending;

(ii) a description of the nature of the problem of the child relating to such proposed initiation or change, including facts relating to such problem; and

(iii) a proposed resolution of the problem to the extent known and available to the parents at the time; and

(8) procedures that require the State educational agency to develop a model form to assist parents in filing a complaint in accordance with paragraph (7).

(c) CONTENT OF PRIOR WRITTEN NOTICE–The notice required by subsection (b)(3) shall include—

(1) a description of the action proposed or refused by the agency;

(2) an explanation of why the agency proposes or refuses to take the action;

(3) a description of any other options that the agency considered and the reasons why those options were rejected;

(4) a description of each evaluation procedure, test, record, or report the agency used as a basis for the proposed or refused action;

(5) a description of any other factors that are relevant to the agency's proposal or refusal;

(6) a statement that the parents of a child with a disability have protection under the procedural safeguards of this part and, if this notice is not an initial referral for evaluation, the means by which a copy of a description of the procedural safeguards can be obtained; and

(7) sources for parents to contact to obtain assistance in understanding the provisions of this part.

FIGURE 14.1 Procedural Safeguards. (20 U.S.C. 1400.615)

▼ TYPES OF NOTICE AND CONSENT FORMS ▼

The Individuals with Disabilities Education Act (IDEA) requires that notice be given to parents (or guardians) whenever there is a proposal to initiate or change services, or when the agency refuses to initiate or change services (AOTA, 1999; 20 U.S.C. 1400.615[b]). The law requires that notices must be provided in the family's native language (AOTA; 34 C.F.R. § 300.503[c]; 34 C.F.R. § 303.403[c]) or "other way of communicating, such as sign language" (Families and Advocates Partnership for Education [FAPE], 2001, p. 1). Providing notice means that the agency has notified the parent or guardian; it does not mean that the parent has agreed to anything.

Evaluation (and Reevaluation) Notice and Consent

Parental consent is needed before an evaluation or reevaluation can be conducted (34 C.F.R. § 300.505[a][1]; 34 C.F.R. § 300.505[a][1]; 34 C.F.R. § 300.503[b]; 34 C.F.R. § 303.404). The notice has to include what action is being proposed, a rationale for that action, what procedural safeguards are available, and procedures for filing a complaint in that state (34 C.F.R. § 303.403[b]).

The service coordinator completes a form that details what areas are to be evaluated. Areas to be evaluated may vary from state to state in terms of wording, but usually include health, vision and hearing, social/emotional status, general intelligence, academic performance, communication status, and motor abilities (Illinois State Board of Education [ISBE], 2001). For each area to be assessed, the members of the team who will be involved in conducting the evaluation are listed. Finally, a reason for evaluating that area and a plan for doing so are documented. A copy of the form is presented to the child's family, and sometimes to the referral source. (An example of a consent for evaluation form can be found at *http://www.isbe.state.il.us/spec-ed/PDF/NoticeEnglishDataInput3-03.pdf.*)

Since the family or guardian will be reading this document, it is imperative that the writer use clear language, avoid abbreviations and jargon, and be especially careful to keep evaluative language out of any written document. The hardest part of the form to word appropriately is the explanation of the reason for assessing a particular area. You do not need to be very specific. You could say that you want to do a motor assessment to "determine student's ability to participate in preschool learning activities" (Minnesota Department of Children, Families, and Learning [MDCFL], 1997, Appendix A, p. 1). You could say that you want to do an assessment of functional skills to "determine the student's ability to perform self-care tasks & daily routines in the preschool environment" (p. 1). For an older child, you could say that you want to do an assessment of motor function to "determine the student's ability to participate in instructional activities/programs and complete class work requirements" (p. 2) or an assessment of transition skills to "determine post-secondary options" (p. 2).

Write a reason for doing the following assessments:

1. Peabody Developmental Motor Scales for a 5-year-old who has difficulty with both gross and fine motor skills, which cause her to stand out as "different" in her kindergarten class.

2. Test of Visual Perceptual Skills on a 6-year-old with attention deficits and mental retardation.

3. Clinical observations of neuromotor skills for a 7-year-old with cerebral palsy.

Meeting Notice

Since parents and guardians are so involved in this process, they need to be notified and invited to participate in all team meetings, especially meetings for developing the IEP or IFSP. Parents/guardians are vital to the success of school-based programs. The service coordinator must be sure that proper forms for notifying parents/guardians of team meetings are completed and delivered to the parents/guardians. At minimum, the notice of a team meeting must include the purpose, time, and place of the meeting, as well as identifying who will be at the meeting in addition to the parents (34 C.F.R. § 300.345[b][1]).

Other Notices

In addition to notifying parents when an evaluation is being conducted or a team meeting is being held, notices are required whenever services are initiated, changed, discontinued, or refused (34 C.F.R. § 300.503; Pennsylvania Department of Education [PDE], 2001). For example, if a school district proposes to make significant changes to the IEP or refuses to make changes requested by the family, or proposes to change a student's placement or refuses to change a placement (34 C.F.R. § 300.503; PDE, 2001), notice is required.

Here is a sample list of notice and consent forms used by school districts or state agencies (MDCFL, 1997; NASDSE, 2002):

- Referral for an initial evaluation
- Procedural safeguards notice
- Parental permission for initial evaluation/reevaluation
- Report of IEP/IFSP meeting
- Manifestation determination form
- Notice of a team meeting
- Consent to release private data
- Documentation of significant changes to Individual Education Program (IEP) plan
- Permission to start the program

Not every state agency or school district will require all of these forms. Complete information on which forms are required where you work can be found on the website for the Department of Education (or whatever agency is the lead agency for early intervention services) of your state.

SUMMARY

In school systems, there are several forms that are used to ensure that a child and his or her family's rights to notice and consent are protected. For children under age 3, an occupational therapist may be the service coordinator, thereby being the person responsible for the completion of notice and consent paperwork. For children over the age of 3, an occupational therapist may contribute to the notice and consent documents, but would not usually be the responsible person (case manager). As with all school system documentation, the writer needs to be sure that they are written so that parents of all educational levels can read them.

REFERENCES

Ahearn, E. M. (2002). *State special education forms.* Retrieved March 28, 2003, from *http://www.nasdse.org/FORUM/sped_forms.pdf*

American Occupational Therapy Association. (1999). *Occupational therapy services for children and youth under the Individuals with Disabilities Education act* (2nd ed.). Bethesda, MD: Author.

Families and Advocates Partnership for Education (FAPE). (2001). *Facts on hand: Informed parent consent for pre-school and school-aged children with disabilities.* Retrieved March 28, 2003, from *http://www.fape.org/pubs/FAPE-23%20Informed%20 Parent%20Consent.pdf*

Illinois State Board of Education. (2001). *Required special education notice and consent forms.* Retrieved March 28, 2003, from *http://www.isbe.state.il.us/spec-ed/PDF/ NoticeEnglishDataInput3-03.pdf*

Minnesota Department of Children, Families, and Learning. (1997). *Occupational therapy and physical therapy services in the schools: Minnesota state guidelines for practice.* St. Paul, MN: Author.

Minnesota Department of Children, Families, and Learning. (2000). *IFSP planning standards.* Retrieved October 24, 2002, from *http://www.cfl.mn.us*

Office of Special Education Programs. (2000). *Guide to the individualized education program.* Retrieved November 7, 2002, from *http://www.ed.gov/offices/OSERS/OSEP/ Products/IEP_Guide*

Pennsylvania Department of Education. (2001). *Special education: Revised forms and formats for special education: Procedural safeguards notice.* Retrieved March 28, 2003, from *http://www.patten.k12.pa.us/Fed_PA_Sp_Ed_Law/school_age_forms_and_ formats_IBM.htm*

CHAPTER 15

Individualized Family Service Plans

INTRODUCTION

The Individuals with Disabilities Education Act (IDEA), Part C (1997 revision, 20 U.S.C. 1400 et seq.), states that services provided to children with disabilities who are ages birth through age 2 are provided under an Individualized Family Service Plan (IFSP) (AOTA, 1999; Stephens & Tauber, 2001; 20 U.S.C. 1400 Part C Sect. 634). An IFSP is a written document that specifies the unique strengths and needs of a child and his or her family, the steps that will be taken to help the child achieve the outcomes desired by the child's family, and who is responsible for implementing and paying for services needed to meet those outcomes (AOTA, 1999; 20 U.S.C. 1400 Part C Sect. 636[d]).

▼ IFSP REQUIREMENTS ▼

Specifically, the IFSP must contain the following eight elements:

1. A statement of the infant or toddler's present level of performance of physical development, cognitive development, communication development, social or emotional development, and adaptive development, based on objective criteria;
2. A statement of the family's resources, priorities, and concerns relating to enhancing the development of the family's infant or toddler with a disability;
3. A statement of the major outcomes expected to be achieved for the infant or toddler and the family, and the criteria, procedures, and timelines used to determine the degree to which progress toward achieving the outcomes is being made and whether modifications or revisions of the outcomes or services are necessary;
4. A statement of specific early intervention services necessary to meet the unique needs of the infant or toddler and the family, including the frequency, intensity, and method of delivering services;
5. A statement of the natural environments in which early intervention services shall appropriately be provided, including a justification of the extent, if any, to which the services will not be provided in a natural environment;
6. The projected dates for initiation of services and the anticipated duration of the services;
7. The identification of the service coordinator from the profession most immediately relevant to the infant's or toddler's or family's needs (or who is otherwise qualified to carry out all applicable responsibilities under this part) who will be responsible for the implementation of the plan and coordination with other agencies and person; and
8. The steps to be taken to support the transition of the toddler with a disability to preschool or other appropriate services (20 U.S.C. 1400.636[d][1–8]).

Children who are between the ages of 3 and 5, at the request of their family, can have an IFSP written instead of an Individualized Education Program (IEP), which is the document usually written for children ages 3 through 21 (see Chapter 16) (34 CFR § 300.342[c]).

As noted above, for each IFSP written, there must be a person designated as the service coordinator who is responsible for ensuring the implementation of the IFSP and coordination of care with other service providers (AOTA, 1999; 20 U.S.C. 1400.636[d][7]). If the infant or toddler's needs are best served by intervention from an occupational therapist (e.g., an infant with cerebral palsy or a toddler who had a stroke), then the occupational therapist can serve as the service coordinator. As service coordinator, the occupational therapist would be the person responsible for completing all notice and consent forms as well as the IFSP. The order in which the required information appears on the IFSP document may vary from state to state or agency to agency.

Documentation for services provided under an IFSP minimally consists of the notice and consent forms (see Chapter 14) and the IFSP document. In some states and under some circumstances (such as when a third-party payer is involved) additional documentation may be required. When birth through age 2 services are provided in a child's home, it is common for the occupational therapist to also write visit notes that describe what occurred during the intervention session and recommendations for follow-through (i.e., home programs). These notes can be written in either a narrative or a SOAP format.

Exercise 15.1

Get on the Internet and look up the rules governing how services are delivered to infants and toddlers with disabilities in your state. The rules may be posted by your state Department of Education, Department of Human Services, Department of Health, Department of Public Health, Department of Health and Human Services, Department of Children and Families, Department of Public Instruction, or State Board of Education. Read the section on IFSP services. If you live in a state that mandates or recommends use of a particular form for writing the IFSP, download it to look at as you work your way through the rest of this chapter.

▼ EVALUATION ▼

The evaluation is the first step in preparing the IFSP (after consent to evaluate is obtained). Based on the results of the evaluation, the IFSP is developed and implemented. The occupational therapist and other members of the IFSP team use the evaluation to develop statements of the present level of performance in the areas of "physical development (including vision, hearing and health status), cognitive development, communication development, social or emotional development, and adaptive development" (34 C.F.R. § 303.344[a]).

If the occupational therapist is the service coordinator for a particular child and family, he or she will be responsible for ensuring the quality of the evaluation process (Stephens & Tauber, 2001). This means that the occupational therapist has to ensure that the evaluation process meets certain criteria (AOTA, 1999; Stephens & Tauber, 2001):

- The evaluation is conducted by qualified personnel;
- It is based on the criteria established by the state;
- The child's medical and health histories are included;
- The report includes levels of performance, unique needs of the child and family, and services recommended to improve the cognitive, physical, communication, social, and emotional development of the child; and
- The evaluation is conducted in the child's natural environment.

The service coordinator must also gather data about available family resources, family priorities, and the concerns the family has regarding the child's development (Stephens & Tauber; 30 C.F.R. 303.344[b]).

The evaluation process is conducted by members of a multidisciplinary team (AOTA, 1999). The evaluation must be completed within 45 days after the agency receives the referral for services (30 C.F.R. 303.321[a][2]). If an interim IFSP is developed, the child may begin to receive early intervention services prior to the completion of the evaluation process (AOTA; 30 C.F.R. 303.345).

▼ PRESENT LEVELS OF DEVELOPMENT ▼

Based on professionally acceptable objective criteria, the infant or toddler's physical, cognitive, communication, social or emotional, and adaptive (e.g., self-care skills) development are summarized using both descriptive and interpretive statements (34 C.F.R. 303.344[a]). These summaries identify the infant or toddler's present levels of performance and include both strengths and areas in need of improvement. It is important to note that not every child will have needs in every area. If an infant or toddler's development in an area is adequate, or is not a problem, then describe what he or she can do and state that development in this area is within normal expectations (Michigan Department of Education [MDE], 1998).

An example of a present level of development in the physical area:

Tylor is rolling to the right and left independently. At this time he requires assistance to move from prone to all fours and prone to sit. Once positioned, he can maintain the sitting position for up to a minute. He uses his whole hand to grasp objects and bring them to midline. He does not weight shift to reach objects, rather, he grasps objects within range of an outstretched arm.

Along with the present level of development, the writer of the IFSP identifies the child's needs [Massachusetts Department of Public Health [MDPH], 1998; Minnesota Department of Children, Families, and Learning [MDCFL], 1997). The need statement is a single sentence, although there may be more than one need statement for one area of the present levels of performance. For example, a need statement that would correlate with the above present level of performance could be "Tylor needs to be able to shift positions independently in order to explore, interact with, and learn from his environment." Another possible need statement could be "Tylor needs to improve hand use to enable play and learning." You can see how broad and sweeping these need statements can be.

However, it is possible to make need statements too broad. For example, if you said, "The child needs occupational therapy intervention," that would be inadequate. You have to link the need to a skill or function that is necessary to prepare a child to participate in school. In other words, the need statement needs to be educationally relevant. The present level of performance and accompanying need statements are used to develop outcomes.

Exercise 15.2

Place an "X" in front of the need statements below that you think are adequately written (MDCFL, 1997):

_____ Needs to improve sensory processing.
_____ Needs to navigate through the school without becoming lost or confused.
_____ Needs to increase range of motion to move more.
_____ Needs to improve writing skills.
_____ Needs to feed self independently so that he can eat lunch.
_____ Needs to sit in alignment to facilitate attention and ability to work.
_____ Needs to effectively use a writing instrument to produce timely and legible written work.

Exercise 15.3

Write a need statement for each of the present levels of performance below:

1. Sophie is a 2-year-old with Down syndrome

   Sophie has low muscle tone. She "w" sits while playing on the floor. She mouths a lot of her toys. She is beginning to walk behind push toys. She has a wide-based gait pattern. She feeds herself finger food by grasping the food between her thumb and index finger. There is a strong tongue thrust when she eats.

2. Erubio is a 6-month-old infant with VATER syndrome

   Erubio will grasp an object placed in his hand, but he does not make any movement to reach for an object. He will shake a rattle, but does not bring it to midline. He is starting to push up on elbows when in prone, but is not rolling or sitting. He has normal muscle tone.

▼ FAMILY INFORMATION, RESOURCES, AND CONCERNS ▼

In addition to what professionals identify as the present levels of performance and needs, the family's input is recorded on the IFSP. There is space to identify the resources that the family has, the family's priorities, and concerns the family has related to the child's development (AOTA, 1999; MDCFL, 2000; MDE, 1998; MDPH, 1998; Nebraska HHS, 1998; 34 C.F.R. 303.334[b]; 20 U.S.C. 1400.636[d][2]). Families contribute to identifying the child's strengths as well as desired outcomes of early intervention. Because this document is written for families as well as the providers of early intervention services, it can be helpful to use the parent's words to the extent that you can. Family resources can include people, skills, capacities, and assets (such as private health insurance) that can help the family of an infant or toddler with a disability. You can ask the family to share this information with you, but it would be unethical to pressure the family to divulging more than they want to. Whatever concerns, worries, or distresses the family expresses gets recorded on the IFSP. Other members of the team can identify concerns, but unless the family agrees with them, they are not recorded on the IFSP. The family determines the priorities for their infant or toddler. It is not necessary to prioritize every individual concern, only those that are of the greatest concern to the family right now.

I have seen some IFSPs that identify each member of the team working with the client, including school system personnel; physician; private physical, occupational, or speech therapists; county social workers; and others involved in the care of that child. This page is a wonderful resource for families because it lists names, addresses, and phone numbers of all these key people all on one page.

▼ OUTCOMES ▼

Next, the IFSP documents the expected outcomes for the child, based on input from both school system professionals and the family. These outcomes can be for either the child or the family (AOTA, 1999; MDCFL, 2000; Nebraska HHS, 1998; 20 U.SC. 1400.636[d][5]). The outcomes have to be specific and have criteria, procedures and a timeline for meeting them. While the outcomes are written annually, they are reviewed at 6-month intervals (AOTA; 34 C.F.R. 303.3422[b]). An outcome is a statement of change that the family will be able to see that relates to the infant or toddler's development. This requires using the family's language rather than professional jargon. For example, use the phrase "brothers and sisters" rather than "siblings" or "sit without support" instead of "improve muscle tone."

The exact format for wording the outcomes will vary from state to state, and perhaps within a state, from agency to agency. Usually, there is an annual outcome that identifies what the child will be doing 1 year from the start date of the IFSP, although some states use a 6-month timeframe instead (Nebraska HHS, 1998). An annual outcome is sometimes referred to as the annual goal. Below that, there are objectives or subgoals (Michigan uses the phrase "short-term instructional objectives [STIO]") that represent steps that will be taken to move toward meeting the annual goal.

One format for writing the annual goal includes both the starting and ending performance. For example, Ebony will appropriately play with a variety of toys, moving from simple manipulation of toys/objects to consistent intentional use of toys/objects as observed by the occupational therapist. Notice that this goal is worded differently than any of the formats talked about in Chapter 10. It does not include a measure of time. The time frame is implied since a new goal is written every year when the IFSP is rewritten. The subgoals/objectives are usually more measurable, although they do not usually contain a time frame. When the goals and objectives are reviewed, it is necessary to indicate whether they were met, need modifying or revising, or need to continue as written (MDCFL, 1997; 20 U.S.C. 1400.636[b]).

▼ MAJOR OUTCOMES ▼

Regardless of the wording, there are three components that must be present in the outcome statements: criteria, procedures, and timelines (MDE, 1998; MDCFL, 2000; MDPH, 1998; 34 C.F.R. § 303.344[c]). The criteria is the measurement that will tell the reader what level of skill is needed to say the outcome was met (MDE). It can be stated as a level of accuracy, a percentage or amount of assistance required. Procedures explain how the outcome will be measured, for example, whether the goal/objective will be measured by parent observation, provider observation, or formal testing. Finally, the timeline refers to the length of time estimated for achievement of the outcome (MDE). In some states, the timeline for the annual goal is implied (since annual means yearly) rather than stated explicitly.

The frequency and intensity of intervention provided by each service provider involved in that child's care must be explicitly stated (AOTA, 1999; MDCFL, 2000; 20 U.S.C. 1400.636[d][4]; 34 C.F.R. § 303.344[d][1][i][iii–iv]; 34 C.F.R. § 303.344[d][2][i]; 34 C.F.R. § 303.344[d][4]). Intensity is stated in terms of the average number of minutes per week the child will receive services and whether that time is spent in individual or group interventions (MDCFL; 34 C.F.R. § 303.344[d][2][i]). For example if you see a child twice a week for 30-minute sessions, then you would say that the child was receiving 60 minutes of service per week. On the other hand, if you see a child for 1 hour a month, you would state the minutes per week as 15.

Frequency refers to how often the child is seen (MDCFL, 2000; 34 C.F.R. § 303.344 [d][2][i]). In some school districts you differentiate between direct and indirect minutes. Direct minutes are those in which the service provider spends directly with the child. Indirect minutes are spent on a case but without working directly with the child; it could be time spent in observation and consultation with the child's parents or other caregivers.

The IFSP also includes a place to document proposed methods of intervention, the location of the services, and any payment arrangements that may affect or be affected by the services provided (AOTA, 1999; MDCFL, 1997; MDPH, 1998; 20 U.S.C. 1400.636[d][5]; 34 C.F.R. § 303.344[d][1][i][iii–iv]). The methods of intervention would be written just as the methods of intervention are written in clinical settings (see Chapter 11). Methods of intervention are the things you plan to implement when you are working with the child; they are your best guess as to what will work to move the child toward achievement of the established goals and objectives.

▼ ENVIRONMENTAL STATEMENT ▼

Location of service is exactly what it sounds like. You identify where each service will be provided. Often for young children, services are provided in the home, but they may also be provided in a clinic, a preschool, on the playground, in an early childhood classroom, or in a day care facility. IDEA does require that services to these young children be provided in natural environments or justification be provided explaining why the natural environment is not the best place to provide a service (MDCFL, 2000; MDE, 1998; MDPH, 1998; 20 U.S.C. 1400.636[d][5]; 34 C.F.R. § 303.344[d][1][ii]; 34 C.F.R. 303.12[b]). A natural environment is a setting that would be considered natural or normal for a child that age without disabilities (MDE; 34 C.F.R. § 303.344[d][1][ii]).

▼ STARTING DATE AND DURATION OF SERVICES ▼

The IFSP must include information about the date the plan will take effect and the anticipated length of time the plan will cover (almost always a year) (AOTA, 1999; MDCFL, 2000; MDPH, 1998; 34 C.F.R. § 303.344[f]). This task usually falls to the service coordinator.

▼ SERVICE COORDINATOR ▼

The IFSP must clearly name the person who will serve as service coordinator (34 C.F.R. § 303.344[g]). The service coordinator is responsible for seeing to the implementation of the plan as well as coordination of care provided by other service providers. If there will be other medical providers or financial assistance that the family needs but are not required by Part C of IDEA, they may be listed on the IFSP but it does not mean that the state agency will provide those services (MDE, 1998; 34 C.F.R. § 303.344[e]).

▼ TRANSITION TO PRESCHOOL SERVICES ▼

Finally, there must be documentation in the IFSP of steps that will be taken to help the child make the transition from home-based or center-based early intervention services to preschool or other appropriate services (AOTA, 1999; MDCFL, 1997, 2000; MDE, 1998; MDPH, 1998; 20 U.S.C. § 1436[d][8]; 34 C.F.R. § 303.344[h][1]). This plan needs to include how families will be involved in this process (AOTA; MDCFL; 34 C.F.R. § 303.344[h][2]).

▼ OTHER DOCUMENTATION ▼

Since the natural environment for most infants and toddlers is the home, most IFSP services are provided in the home. Rarely will these services be provided on a daily basis; once or twice a week is usually adequate. However, in providing services only a couple times a week, the occupational therapist may want to see some kind of follow-through on the infant's program by the family or personal care attendant. That is where a visit note comes in.

The occupational therapist can use a visit note to communicate with the child's family. The occupational therapist can document what happened during the intervention session, how the child reacted, and what the family can do to supplement or enhance the occupational therapy program. The note can be written in either narrative or SOAP format.

While the law does not require this documentation, it is recommended because it does create a paper trail should there ever be questions about how a family was instructed. If an occupational therapist does write visit notes, it is a good idea to do it on "magic-carbon" (NCR) paper so that both the family and the occupational therapist can both retain a copy.

Preprinted exercise/activity sheets can also be given to families to help them follow through on occupational therapy programs. These may be in addition to or in place of visit notes. Several vendors sell reprintable handouts. Be careful not to copy and distribute pages of books or journal articles that are copyright protected (see Chapter 7).

SUMMARY

The IFSP is written annually to show the child's current level of performance, set goals to move the child's development forward, and determine the frequency and intensity of services. Since an infant or toddler is totally dependent on his or her family, the family takes a big role in the development and implementation of the IFSP. The IFSP must be written in words the family will understand. The goals (outcomes) established in the IFSP can be for the child or the family to achieve. The IFSP contains specific information on what services will be provided, who will provide them, who will pay for them, where they will be provided, and the frequency and duration of those services.

An occupational therapist can be the service coordinator for birth to age 2 services. A service coordinator is the person responsible for the development, coordination, and implementation of the plan. Writing the IFSP is a team effort, with the family included as part of the team. While much of the IFSP is similar to an intervention plan in a clinical setting, it differs in that it is written for the family rather than being written for other professionals or third-party payers as the primary audience. While an intervention plan usually represents the services of one provider, an IFSP represents the integrated plan of everyone working with that child.

REFERENCES

American Occupational Therapy Association. (1999). *Occupational therapy services for children and youth under the Individuals with Disabilities Education Act* (2nd ed.). Bethesda, MD: Author.

Massachusetts Department of Public Health. (1998). *Early intervention services operational standards.* Retrieved March 28, 2003, from *http://www.state.ma.us/dph/bfch/shn/early/eiopstnd.pdf*

Michigan Department of Education. (1998). *Early on® Michigan: Guidelines for completing individualized family service plans (IFSPs).* Retrieved March 28, 2003, from *http://www.michigan.gov/documents/1998-01_IFSP_Guidelines_38486_7.pdf*

Minnesota Department of Children, Families, and Learning. (1997). *Occupational therapy and physical therapy services in the schools: Minnesota state guidelines for practice.* St. Paul, MN: Author.

Minnesota Department of Children, Families, and Learning. (2000). IEP *IFSP planning standards.* Retrieved October 24, 2002, from *http://www.cfl.mn.us*

Nebraska HHS. (1998). *Early intervention program: Nebraska individualized family service plan.* Retrieved November 8, 2002, from *http:// nncf.unl.edu/ifspweb/pdf/EI-1.pdf*

One Hundred Fifth Congress of the United States of America. (1997). *HR5: An act to amend the Individuals with Disabilities Education Act.* Retrieved March 24, 2003, from *http://www.ideapractices.org/law/downloads/Idea97.pdf*

Stephens, L. C., & Tauber, S. K. (2001). Early intervention. In J. Case-Smith, (Ed.), *Occupational therapy for children* (4th ed., pp. 708–729). St. Louis, MO: Mosby.

CHAPTER 16

Individualized Education Program

INTRODUCTION

The Individualized Education Program (IEP) is the guiding document for special education and related services for children with special needs. It is written for children with special needs ages 3–21 and administered by the school district. The Individuals with Disabilities Education Act (IDEA) (20 U.S.C. 1400 et seq.) allows children between the ages of 3 and 5 to have an IFSP written instead of an IEP as long as the IFSP contains the same information as would be contained in an IEP (34 C.F.R. §303.342[c]). Because the IEP is individualized, it takes a great deal of planning and interdisciplinary coordination to produce and implement the document. Specific information on the content of the IEP is found in Part B of IDEA (AOTA, 1999).

The IEP has some similarities to the IFSP: Both are written by a team of professionals and include input from the parents of the child involved; both are written annually and both start with an evaluation of the child. Both require parent notification, consent (see Chapter 14), and involvement throughout the process. There are also some differences. While the IFSP is family-centered, the IEP is student-centered. The IFSP looks at the overall development of the child; the IEP looks at levels of educational development, the ways in which a student's disability affects the child's ability to participate in learning (20 U.S.C. 1400.614[b][2][A]; 20 U.S.C. 1400.614[d][1][A][i][I]; 34 C.F.R. §300.347[a][1]).

Occupational therapy is considered a related service under Part B of IDEA (AOTA, 1999; Office of Special Education Programs (OSEP), 2000; 20 U.S.C. 1400.602[22]). That means that usually, the occupational therapist would not be the service coordinator, but rather would be a contributor to the IEP process. In this instance, the child must first qualify for special education before receiving occupational therapy. An IEP is not a guarantee that the maximum amount of service will be provided; it identifies the necessary services to allow the student to participate in learning. In other words, it provides need-to-have services, not want-to-have services.

Every IEP must include certain information. While IDEA does not mandate the use of one particular form or format, it does mandate the content required in each IEP. Figure 16.1 shows the minimum content required by IDEA (34 C.F.R. §300.347). The order in which the information appears in the IEP document is irrelevant. Essentially, the minimum content can be summarized as

- Present level of educational performance
- Annual goals
- Special education and related services
- Participation with nondisabled children
- Participation in state- and district-wide tests
- Starting date and location of services
- Transition services
- Measurement of progress

(a)   The IEP for each child with a disability must include—

    (1)   A statement of the child's present levels of educational performance, including-

        (i)   How the child's disability affects the child's involvement and progress in the general curriculum (i.e., the same curriculum as for nondisabled children); or

        (ii)   For preschool children, as appropriate, how the disability affects the child's participation in appropriate activities;

    (2)   A statement of measurable annual goals, including benchmarks or short-term objectives, related to—

        (i)   Meeting the child's needs that result from the child's disability to enable the child to be involved in and progress in the general curriculum (i.e., the same curriculum as for nondisabled children), or for preschool children, as appropriate, to participate in appropriate activities; and

        (ii)   Meeting each of the child's other educational needs that result from the child's disability;

    (3)   A statement of the special education and related services and supplementary aids and services to be provided to the child, or on behalf of the child, and a statement of the program modifications or supports for school personnel that will be provided for the child—

        (i)   To advance appropriately toward attaining the annual goals;

        (ii)   To be involved and progress in the general curriculum in accordance with paragraph (a)(1) of this section and to participate in extracurricular and other nonacademic activities; and

        (iii)   To be educated and participate with other children with disabilities and nondisabled children in the activities described in this section;

    (4)   An explanation of the extent, if any, to which the child will not participate with nondisabled children in the regular class and in the activities described in paragraph (a)(3) of this section;

    (5)   State or district-wide assessment

        (i)   A statement of any individual modifications in the administration of State or district-wide assessments of student achievement that are needed in order for the child to participate in the assessment; and

        (ii)   If the EP team determines that the child will not participate in a particular State or district-wide assessment of student achievement (or part of an assessment), as statement of—

            (A)   Why that assessment is not appropriate for the child; and

            (B)   How the child will be assessed;

    (6)   The projected date for the beginning of the services and modifications described in paragraph (a)(3) of this section, and the anticipated frequency, location, and duration of those services and modifications; and

    (7)   A statement of—

        (i)   How the child's progress toward the annual goals described in paragraph (a)(2) of this section will be measured; and

        (ii)   How the child's parents will be regularly informed (through such means as periodic report cards), at least as often as parents are informed of their nondisabled children's progress of—

            (A)   Their child's progress toward the annual goals; and

            (B)   The extent to which that progress is sufficient to enable the child to achieve the goals by the end of the year.

(b)   Transition services. The IEP must include—

    (1)   For each student with a disability beginning at age 14 (or younger, if determined appropriate by the IEP team), and updated annually, a statement of the transition service needs of the student under the applicable components of the student's IEP that focuses on the student's courses of study (such as participation in advanced-placement courses or a vocational education program); and

FIGURE 16.1   Required Content of the IEP. *(Source: 20 U.S.C. 1414(d)(1)(A) and (d)(6)(A)(ii))*

(2)   For each student beginning at age 16 (or younger, if determined appropriate by the IEP team), a statement of needed transition services for the student, including, if appropriate, a statement of the interagency responsibilities or any needed linkages.

(c)   Transfer of rights. In a State that transfers rights at the age of majority, beginning at least one year before a student reaches the age of majority under State law, the student's IEP must include a statement that the student has been informed of his or her rights under Part B of the Act, if any, that will transfer to the student on reaching the age of majority, consistent with §300.517.

(d)   Students with disabilities convicted as adults and incarcerated in adult prisons. Special rules concerning the content of IEPs for students with disabilities convicted as adults and incarcerated in adult prisons are contained in §300.311 (b) and (c).

FIGURE 16.1   (Continued)

Exercise 16.1

Get on the Internet and look up the rules governing how services are delivered to children with disabilities in your state. The rules may be posted by your state Department of Education, Department of Human Services, Department of Health, Department of Public Health, Department of Health and Human Services, Department of Children and Families, Department of Public Instruction or State Board of Education. Read the section on IEP services. If you live in a state that mandates or recommends use of a particular form for writing the IEP, download it to look at as you work your way through the rest of this chapter.

▼ EVALUATION PROCESS ▼

The IEP process begins with an evaluation. For a student receiving services under an IEP, a reevaluation is done at least every 3 years (AOTA, 1999; 20 U.S.C. 1400.614[a][2][A]). The initial evaluation is done to determine the child's disability and educational needs (AOTA; and 20 U.S.C. 1400.614[a][1][B][i–ii]). Subsequent evaluations identify the child's current level of performance, determine whether the child continues to have a disability, whether the child continues to need special education services, and whether changes or additions to the special education and related services the child receives are needed to enable participation in the general curriculum (AOTA; 20 U.S.C. 1400.614[c][1][B][i–iv]). The evaluation process is driven by the needs of the student and covers all areas related to the student's potential disability (Massachusetts Department of Education [MDE], 2001) or exceptionality (Louisiana Department of Education [LDOE], 2000). Generally, a student's performance in academic/cognitive, behavior, communication, motor, self-help, social, and vocational areas may be evaluated (LDOE; Texas Department of Education, 2002; 34 C.F.R. §300.532[g]).

IDEA contains legal requirements for conducting an evaluation of a child (20 U.S.C. 1400.614[b][2][A–C]):

a. Use a variety of assessment tools and strategies to gather relevant functional and developmental information, including information provided by the parent, that may assist in determining whether the child is a child with a disability and the content of the child's individualized education program, including information related to enabling the child to be involved in and progress in the general curriculum or, for preschool children, to participate in appropriate activities

b. Not use any single procedure as the sole criterion for determining whether a child is a child with a disability or determining an appropriate educational program for the child; and

c. Use technically sound instruments that may assess the relative contribution of cognitive and behavioral factors, in addition to physical or developmental factors.

In addition, IDEA requires tests and evaluation materials to be nondiscriminatory or contain racial or cultural bias and be administered in the child's native language whenever feasible (20 U.S.C. 1400.614[b][3][A]). Standardized tests have to be valid for the purposes they are being used for, be administered by someone who is knowledgeable and trained in the use of the test, and be administered according to the instructions provided by the test producer (20 U.S.C. 1400.614[b][2][B]). Besides standardized tests, other evaluation methods include information provided by the parents, observation, work samples, interviews, and a review of the student's cumulative educational record (MDE, 2001; OSEP, 2000).

In some states, the evaluation report is a separate document from the IEP. The evaluation report is written as a team document. An occupational therapist contributing to this report would need to explain the degree to which something is a problem for the child and be explicit in relating the functional deficit to performance in school (N. Scott, personal communication, October 24, 2002). The occupational therapist, along with the other members of the team, signs the evaluation report (MDCFL, 2002a). In some states, the occupational therapist and other team members may indicate whether or not they are in agreement with the conclusions of the team (MDCFL, 2002a).

If the results of the evaluation show that the child qualifies for special education services, the school then has 30 calendar days in which to meet with the parents to discuss evaluation findings and write the IEP (OSEP, 2000; 34 C.F.R. §300.343[b][2]). Often the sharing of results of the evaluation and writing the IEP occur at the same meeting (MDE, 2001).

▼ PRESENT LEVEL OF EDUCATIONAL PERFORMANCE ▼

In other states, the results of the evaluation are incorporated into the IEP, usually in the section on present level of educational performance. IDEA is quite specific about the kind of information that must be included in the IEP. In the section of the IEP that discusses the present level of educational performance, federal law requires the IEP to consider five components: the strengths and concerns of parents, recent evaluation results, communication needs, student behavior that could impede learning, and assistive technology needs (AOTA, 1999; 34 C.F.R. 300.346[a][1][i–iii]; 34 C.F.R. 300.346[a][2][i–v]). Present levels of educational performance reflect what the student is able to do now, regardless of what that child was able to do or not do in the past. In this sense, it is very different than a summary of the client's progress or pertinent history in a clinical setting.

The strengths of a child are determined through the evaluation process. The occupational therapist, along with other members of the team including the parents, contributes information on motor, sensory, perceptual, psychosocial and cognitive, and environmental factors (Case-Smith, Rogers, & Johnson, 2001).

Recent evaluation results are shared with the IEP team (including parents/guardians). The specific areas that an occupational therapist looks at are listed above. The evaluation results need to show any identified deficits that interfere with the education process. If no connection to the educational needs of the child can be drawn, then occupational therapy services may not be necessary in the school setting. That does not mean that occupational therapy services would not in some way benefit the child, it simply means that those services would not be part of the IEP services provided by the school. An example would be that a child has deficits in tying her shoe. Tying one's shoes is not essential for participating in school. The child could wear slip-ons or shoes with Velcro® closures. Occupational therapy to work on shoe tying would not be educationally relevant, so it would not be part of the IEP. However, the child could receive occupational therapy services to work on shoe tying from another provider (other than the school district). If the occupational therapist can make a connection between the child's inability to motor plan the act of tying her shoes to the inability to motor plan in other situations that are necessary for learning (such as handwriting), then occupational therapy services might be justifiable. It is the responsibility of the occupational therapist to show how the deficits identified in the evaluation process have the potential to interfere with the learning process and that occupational therapy services are necessary to help the child overcome those deficits.

Communication is an essential skill for children in the school setting. They have to be able to receive instructional messages and respond to them. Federal law requires that if a child has difficulties in communication because of deafness, hard of hearing, blindness, or has limited proficiency in English, the school must consider those needs in developing the IEP (AOTA, 1999; Delaware Department of Education [DDOE], 2000; MDCFL, 2000; Oregon Department of Education [ODE], 2000).

Anyone who has spent any time in a school or preschool classroom will tell you that a student's behavior can interfere not only with that child's learning, but the learning of other students in the room as well. In the present level of performance section, a clear and specific description of observed behaviors and how they may interfere with learning must be documented (AOTA, 1999; DDOE, 2000; MDCFL, 2000; ODE, 2000). For example, you observe that a child is repeatedly getting up and down off his chair, moving around his chair, and jumping up and down whenever he is asked to stand in line. This is distracting to other children in the room, and the teacher questions whether the boy is paying attention when he moves around like that. The present level of educational performance would reflect exactly what the behavior looks like and a statement of need related to that behavior would be written.

Finally, the present level of performance looks at whether a child has assistive technology needs (AOTA, 1999; DDOE, 2000; MDCFL, 2000; ODE, 2000). Following the evaluation process, team members will have a good idea of whether the child will need assistive technology to participate in learning. The team may not know exactly which piece(s) of assistive technology will be needed until they try out a couple options, but they will know if something should be tried. The IEP must contain explicit information on both the assistive technology needs and what accommodations/supports are recommended.

As discussed in Chapter 15, the present level of performance can include both a description of the performance and the occupational therapist's interpretation of that performance. The Massachusetts Department of Education (2001) uses the following examples to show proper wording of a present level of educational performance:

Less than helpful: Joe is not committed to his school program.

More helpful: Joe submits fewer than half of his required homework assignments. He starts most assignments but lacks the organizational skills to complete them by the required due dates (p. 18).

Less than helpful: Jill has a short attention span.

More helpful: Jill typically interrupts the work of others five times per hour. She interrupts when she requires teacher assistance (p. 18).

Exercise 16.2

Write a more helpful present level of educational performance for each less helpful statement below.

1. Less helpful: Omar has difficulty cutting with a scissors.
   More helpful:

2. Less helpful: Lucinda does not respect the personal space of other students.
   More helpful:

3. Less helpful: Bethany is very messy and careless with supplies.
   More helpful:

On the IEP, there are annual goals, with shorter-term specific objectives or benchmarks that will lead to achievement of the annual goal. These short-term objectives or benchmarks help the IEP team, including the parents, to measure the child's progress throughout the year. Short-term objectives break an annual goal down into smaller steps (OSEP, 2000). Benchmarks describe expected progress at a given point in the year. Unlike the IFSP (Chapter 15), the goals and objectives/benchmarks are written to describe only what the student will do; they cannot be written to address family needs (LDOE, 2000).

The annual goals must relate to the child's needs that result from the child's disability (OSEP, 2000). They must enable the child to participate in and make progress in the general education curriculum (34 C.F.R. §300.347[a][2]). They can relate to the child's needs in the areas of behavioral skills, communication, self-determination skills, job-related skills, independent living skills, or social skills (OSEP, 2000). If a child only needs modifications or accommodations in an area in order to progress in the general curriculum, the IEP does not need to include goals or objectives/benchmarks in that area (OSEP, 2000).

How the goals are worded will vary by state, and to some degree, the school district you work for. You may be the member of the team to draft the wording of the goal/objectives, or your services may be provided under a goal/objectives written by other members of the team. Either way, the occupational therapist has input into the goal-writing process.

The main components of an IEP annual goal are the behavior or skill to be performed, the direction of the change, and the level of performance expected at the end of the year (12 months from when the goal is written) (MDCFL, 1999). All goals must be measurable (OSEP, 2000). The present level of performance may be explicit or implied (MDCFL). For example, if the performance level is explicit, an annual goal might read: Jalena will decrease self-stimulating behavior from 10 episodes per day to two episodes per day. If the performance level is implied, the goal could be: Jalena will decrease self-stimulating behavior to two episodes per day. The advantage of making it explicit is that if the goal page gets separated from the rest of the IEP document, you will know where you started from and be better able to identify progress. The advantage of making it implicit is that it takes fewer words to write it.

Case-Smith, in her book *Occupational Therapy for Children* (2001) describes three kinds of approaches to goal writing: developmental, functional curriculum, and ecological. A developmental goal focuses on skills that are acquired in a specific and predictable sequence or pattern. For example, the goal might focus the development of higher-level grasp patterns, or development of social skills. A functional curriculum approach looks at skills required for community or vocational participation. Such goals might address a child's need to don and doff his jacket to participate in recess, or to learn work behaviors such as being on time to a job. An ecological approach looks at the various environments that are important to the child's learning and the priority behaviors that need to occur in those environments. This kind of goal can address behavior on the playground, or in the lunchroom, classroom, restroom, library, gym, or auditorium. An example of this kind of goal could have the child improving her ability to copy accurately from the blackboard onto lined paper, or to maintain her balance on a variety of uneven surfaces on the playground and surrounding grassy areas.

Once the annual goal has been established, the objectives or benchmarks can be developed. While there is no federal legal requirement regarding the number of objectives/benchmarks per goal, two to four seems to be a good range. One objective seems insufficient to allow step-wise progression toward an annual goal, but more than four seems like too many steps to accomplish in 1 year.

Here is an example:

Goal: Anna will consistently maintain her balance while walking on uneven surfaces from walking in a high-guard position and losing her balance five times in 50 feet, to walking in medium-guard without losing her balance at all in 50 feet.

Objective 1: Anna will consistently walk from the playground, up over a curb, to the grassy area around the playground while holding on to an assistant with one hand as observed by teacher or occupational therapist.

Objective 2: Anna will walk from the playground, up over a curb, to the grassy area around the playground without assistance but with arms in high-guard position as observed by the teacher or occupational therapist.

Objective 3: Anna will consistently walk up and down the hill next to the school with arms in high-guard but without assistance as observed by the teacher or occupational therapist.

You may have noticed that the objectives in the above examples contained the phrase "as observed by the teacher or occupational therapist." Not every state or school district requires that the objectives include procedures for evaluation, but some do. In general, objectives need to include the conditions under which the behavior or activity occurs, what behavior is to be performed, and the criteria (measurement) for the performance (MDCFL, 1999). The conditions can include the environment(s), specialized instruction or cuing, specialized materials or equipment, and any assistance needed. The behavior to be performed needs to be observable; it can be qualitative or quantitative. The criteria has to show how the student will demonstrate successful completion of the goal, which means there has to be a measurement, and in some states, who will evaluate the student's performance and document it (MDCFL; ODE, 2000). Figure 16.2 shows a sample goal page from an IEP.

In some states, the goal statement may be generally written, while the objectives must contain certain specific content. In Illinois, for example, the short-term objective/benchmark must specify the percent of accuracy or the number of successful executions out of how many attempts (Illinois State Board of Education [ISBE], 2001). There is space to use other evaluation criteria, but it must be clearly and explicitly stated (ISBE, 2001). Evaluation procedures (log of observation, chart, tests, or other [specify]) and the schedule for determining achievement (daily, weekly, quarterly, semester, or other [specify]) are also indicated by placing a checkmark in a box next to the appropriate criteria (ISBE, 2001).

Exercise 16.3

For each goal, list two objectives that would help the student meet the goal.

Goal 1: Keyshawn will improve his penmanship so that he can write his name legibly on unlined paper, as observed by his regular classroom teacher.

Objective 1a:

Objective 1b:

Goal 2: Miriam will improve her attention to task from going off task eight times during a 15-minute task to going off task once during a half-hour of task participation, as observed by her special education teacher.

Objective 2a:

Objective 2b:

Goal 3: Paul will improve scissors use from hand over hand assistance to independently cutting along a curved line, as observed by the occupational therapist.

Objective 3a:

Objective 3b:

Individualized Education Program for: <u>Tran Vang</u>
IEP Dates: from <u>Sept. 29, 2003</u> to <u>Sept. 29, 2004</u>   DOB: <u>July 17, 1995</u>

Current Level of Performance/Measurable Annual Goals/ Benchmarks

Goal # <u>3</u>
Educational need area: _____ Academic/cognitive _____ Behavior _____ Communication
<u>X</u> Motor _____ Self-help _____ Social _____ Vocational

Current Level of Performance:
Tran uses a rolling walker to move around inside the school building, and a wheelchair for longer distances out of doors. He has very high muscle tone in all four limbs. When he gets excited, he throws his head back, arches his back, and straightens his arms and legs. He uses a whole hand grasp with large-diameter writing utensils. His writing is illegible; the letters are misshapen, letters do not rest on the bottom line, letter size varies.

Measurable Annual Goal:
Tran will write his name (first and last) legibly, on a line 80% of the time, as observed by his classroom teacher.

Benchmark/Objectives:
1) Tran will write his first name legibly, on a line 50% of the time, as observed by the occupational therapist.
2) Tran will write his first name legibly, on a line, 80% of the time, as observed by the occupational therapist.
3) Tran will write his last name legibly, on a line, 50% of the time, as observed by the occupational therapist.

Methods of intervention:
Tran will practice writing his name on a large scale, such as on the white board, in sand in a sandbox, and other types of materials.
Tran will be instructed in techniques for forming letters.
Tran's sitting posture will be modified to decrease muscle tone in his trunk and arms.
Tran will try different types of writing utensils and papers (with and without raised lines) to see which feels best to him and which yields the best results

Location of intervention:
In his regular education classroom and in the occupational therapy room.

Assistive technology needs:
Various writing utensils
Assorted writing papers
Keyboard with key guard for beginning computer use

FIGURE 16.2   Sample IEP Goal Page

▼ SPECIAL EDUCATION AND RELATED SERVICES ▼

The IEP must specifically state the type and amount of special education and related services a child will receive (DDOE, 2000; MDCFL, 2000, 2002b&c; ODE, 2000). This is so that both parents and IEP team members are clear on the level of the agency's commitment of resources (OSEP, 2000). School districts will vary in how they want the frequency stated; most will want the number of minutes per week. Often, the minutes per week or per session will be further specified as either direct or indirect (MDCFL, 2002c) or as individual, group, or consultative (ODE). The amount of service may be stated as a range (e.g., 30–45 minutes per week) only if the IEP team deems that to be the most appropriate way to serve the child's needs. It cannot be stated as a range because of staffing uncertainties or shortages.

The IEP must also include information on supplemental aids and supports. Any aids or supports must be focused on helping the student succeed in school (MDE, 2001; OSEP, 2000).

When appropriate for the unique needs of a child, the IEP includes a statement of whether or not the child will need an extended school year or other calendar modification (MDE, 2001; OSEP, 2000). Because of special health needs or other reasons, some students may need shorter school days or a shorter school year. Most school districts will have guidelines that explain under what conditions (how to justify it) this service is offered. Federal regulations require that school districts do not limit this option to any particular category of disability or the type, amount, or duration of those services (34 C.F.R. §300.309[a]).

Sometimes the recording of the details of this section occurs on the same page as the goals; in other cases it may appear on a page that lists services and supports. Since each school district has forms or a format for what information goes where in the IEP, simply follow the form. Follow the school district's lead in terms of how specific or general to be in describing the intervention plans.

▼ PARTICIPATION WITH NONDISABLED CHILDREN ▼

IDEA requires that the IEP contain specific information on the extent to which a child with a disability will participate with children without disabilities in a regular classroom, the general curriculum, and extracurricular/nonacademic activities (OSEP, 2000). The IEP must explain why, if participation in the above-mentioned activities is limited in any way, full participation is not possible (OSEP). Under IDEA, the preference is that the student spend as much time as possible with nondisabled peers (MDE, 2001), which means that IEP team members must have good reasons for providing services outside of the regular classroom. The IEP team must determine whether the child could participate in a regular classroom with the use of supplementary services and aids (OSEP). Removing a child from a regular classroom cannot be done only because of needed modifications in the curriculum (OSEP). The child's transportation needs can be addressed in this section or on a separate page. While the occupational therapist is not usually the person on the team responsible for documenting this, her knowledge and experience in adaptation of tasks and environments make her a great contributor to this process.

▼ PARTICIPATION IN STATE- AND DISTRICT-WIDE TESTS ▼

The IEP needs to explain why the unique needs of that child would make participation in state- or district-wide tests inappropriate (OSEP, 2000). If the child cannot participate in the state- or district-wide testing, the IEP states the way in which the child will be assessed. Additional rules for which children can be exempt from state- or district-wide tests can be found in the "No Child Left Behind" legislation, President George W. Bush's education reform law.

▼ DATES AND PLACES ▼

The date the IEP takes effect and the location of the services provided is identified in writing. The IEP needs to specify whether the child will receive special education and related services in the regular classroom, special education or other separate room, or a separate setting, such as a hospital, special school, or home (DDOE, 2000; MDCFL, 2002c; OSEP, 2000). Decisions about the location of services require discussion of the "least restrictive environment" (LRE) (AOTA, 1999; OSEP). The least restrictive environment refers to the place were a child with a disability has the greatest exposure to children without disabilities, yet where the child with a disability can get his or her needs met. For many children, that means they spend some portion of their day in a regular classroom, some in a separate location. The occupational therapist must make a recommendation to the IEP team as to whether occupational therapy intervention will happen in a regular classroom, in a separate room, or both.

▼ TRANSITION ▼

Transition planning and services typically begin when a child is age 14 (MDCFL, 2000). These services are designed to help the child move from school to life after school, such as preparing for a job and independent living (AOTA, 1999; LDOE, 2000). These services are based on the student's wants, needs, and preferred lifestyle. Again, the expertise of an occupational therapist can be of great help in planning for such a move. While the occupational therapist may not write this part of the IEP, she will have good ideas to contribute to the planning process.

▼ MEASURING PROGRESS ▼

If you set goals, it stands to reason that you would want to do some evaluation of the child's progress toward meeting those goals throughout the year. The IEP team must have a method of reviewing progress and communicating that progress to the child's parents and/or guardians (OSEP, 2000). If the child is not making the progress that was expected, the IEP must be revised to address that lack of progress (OSEP, 34 C.F.R. §300.343[c][2][i]). Both the occupational therapist and occupational therapy assistant participate in this process.

SUMMARY

The Individual Education Program (IEP) is the guiding document for services provided by school system personnel, including occupational therapy. Careful wording of goals and objectives or benchmarks is essential. Goals and objectives/benchmarks often follow a specific formula for wording. Goals are the outcomes the child is expected to meet a year from when they are written. Objectives are steps to help the child meet the goals. Occupational therapy practitioners contribute to many parts of the IEP, but are usually not responsible for writing the entire document.

All of this demonstrates just how explicit school system documentation is. Nothing can be assumed. Be clear and direct because not everyone reading the IEP will have the same level of education and understanding of the material as you do.

Because of the amount of specificity in goal setting, specifying minutes per week for every service provider involved with the child in the school, identifying the least restrictive environment, and listing curricular, environmental, and programmatic modifications, the IEP can become a lengthy document. Once you participate in writing one, you will be glad to only do one per year per child. You will also be grateful for a chance to revise your goals and objectives at midyear.

REFERENCES

American Occupational Therapy Association. (1999). *Occupational therapy services for children and youth under the Individuals with Disabilities Education Act* (2nd ed.). Bethesda, MD: Author.

Case-Smith, J. (Ed.) (2001). *Occupational therapy for children* (4th ed.). St. Louis, MO: Mosby.

Case-Smith, J., Rogers, J., & Johnson, J. (2001). School-based occupational therapy. In J. Case-Smith (Ed.), *Occupational therapy for children* (4th ed., pp. 757–779). St. Louis, MO: Mosby.

Delaware Department of Education. (2000). *Individualized education program.* Retrieved October 29, 2002, from *http://www.doe.state.de.us/exceptional_child/NewIEP/newIEP. doc*

Illinois State Board of Education. (2001). *Individual education program.* Retrieved March 28, 2003, from *http://www.isbe.state.il.us/spec-ed/PDF/iepform01.pdf*

Louisiana Department of Education. (2000). *Individualized education program* [Online]. Retrieved March 28, 2003, from *http://www.doe.state.la.us/DOE/PDFs/Bulletins/1530.pdf*

Massachusetts Department of Education. (2001). *IEP process guide.* Retrieved March 28, 2003, from *http://www.doe.mas.edu/sped/iep/proguide.pdf*

Minnesota Department of Children, Families, and Learning. (1999). *Goal writing tutorial: K–12.* Retrieved October 29, 2002, from *http://cfl.state.mn.us/dmc/sem/K-12IEPGoalWritingTutorial.pdf*

Minnesota Department of Children, Families, and Learning. (2000) *IEP/IFSP Planning.* Retrieved October 24, 2002 from *http://www.cfl.mn.us*

Minnesota Department of Children, Families, and Learning. (2002a). *Evaluation report.* Retrieved October 29, 2002, from *http://cfl.state.mn.us/dmc/sem/Evaluation%20Report.pdf*

Minnesota Department of Children, Families, and Learning. (2002b). *Individualized education program.* Retrieved October 29, 2002, from *http://cfl.state.mn.us/dmc/sem/IEP.pdf*

Minnesota Department of Children, Families, and Learning. (2002c). *Informal record review checklist.* Retrieved October 29, 2002, from *http://cfl.state.mn.us/dmc/sem/PartCRecordReview9.pdf*

Office of Special Education Programs. (2000). *A guide to the individualized education program.* Retrieved November 7, 2002, from *http://www.ed.gov/offices/OSERS/OSEP/Products/IEP_Guide*

Oregon Department of Education. (2000). *IEP guidelines* [Online]. Retrieved October 29, 2000, from *http://www.ode.state.or.us/sped/docpub/forms/IEPGuidelines.pdf*

Texas Department of Education. (2002). *Full and individual evaluation.* Retrieved October 31, 2002, from *http://framework.esc18.net/Documents/05_Initial _Eval.htm*

SECTION V

Administrative Documentation

▼ INTRODUCTION ▼

In addition to clinical or school-based documentation, there is documentation related to administrative tasks such as getting paid for services, documenting workplace injuries, writing policies and procedures, and similar functions. Some of these documents may be written by anyone in the department; they are not necessarily the sole domain of supervisory personnel.

Administrative documentation varies greatly from facility to facility and setting to setting. The chapters in the section deal with several different types of administrative documentation, but these are by no means the only administrative documentation that gets done. Specifically, documents like productivity reports and staffing reports are so individualized by each facility/setting, it would be impossible to do justice to them here, therefore, they are not included in this book. As you read the chapters in this section, realize that the information is intentionally general. You can expect modifications in form and content by the facility/setting.

▼ STRUCTURE OF THIS SECTION OF THE BOOK ▼

Chapter 17 deals with incident reports. Incident reports are written whenever there is an injury, no matter how slight, to a client, visitor, or a staff member. Incident reports are used by the facility to help learn from accidents or errors in an effort to prevent them from happening again.

Chapter 18 discusses ways to word appeal letters. Appeal letters are used when an occupational therapist or client thinks that a third-party payer (like Medicare or an HMO) has denied reimbursement unjustly. These letters explain why occupational therapy services are needed for a particular client.

Chapter 19 presents various ways to take minutes at a meeting. It has been said that if it was not documented, it did not happen. One way to demonstrate that a supervisor provided instruction to staff or that a policy was reviewed is to document it in meeting minutes. The minutes need to be retained in such a fashion that they can be easily retrieved and that everyone in the department has access to them.

Chapter 20 deals with grant writing. Grants are funds made available to an organization for a specific purpose, such as developing a new program or to fund services for clients who do not have the financial resources to pay for services (like scholarships for occupational therapy intervention). Usually grants are awarded to facilities, departments, or nonprofit organizations. Grant money does not need to be repaid, but there are usually conditions for the award of the money. There is always a process for applying for grant money. This chapter discusses a common process for requesting grant money, but there may be details that are unique to particular funding sources that are not covered here.

Finally, Chapter 21 presents a format for writing policies and procedures. Policy and procedure manuals are used to guide employees in their on-the-job performance. They explain what must be done and how it must be done. Following policies and procedures is essential for the orderly conduct of the workplace. When an occupational therapy practitioner fails to follow policy and procedure, he or she weakens his or her defense if a client should decide to sue.

CHAPTER 17

Incident Reports

INTRODUCTION

Imagine this scene:

> An occupational therapist is working on toilet transfers with an elderly man who recently had a stroke. The client is much taller than the clinician, and when he starts to lose his balance, the occupational therapist tries in vain to lower him gently to the floor. Instead, he falls and hits his head on the sink, causing a gash on his forehead before landing in a heap on the floor with the occupational therapist still holding on to his transfer belt. The occupational therapist immediately pulls the emergency cord in the bathroom to summon help.

After attending to the immediate medical needs of the client and the occupational therapist (if he or she is hurt during this event), it will be necessary to document this incident. Generally, the facility will have a form, usually called an incident report, to be completed by the occupational therapist or whatever staff was involved in the incident. Often after the occupational therapist completes this form, a supervisor will review the form, and may complete a section of the form designed for supervisor input. The form is then routed to the person designated by the facility as the risk management coordinator (may be called by another, similar title). It will be used to help the facility investigate possible corrective actions to prevent such incidents, sometimes called "adverse events" (Scott, 1997). Do not place a copy of the incident report in the clinical record, or mention the form in any other clinical document. Just what should be documented in the clinical record will be discussed later in this chapter.

Schools also require incident reports if a student, faculty, or staff member is injured on school property. If the incident took place on school property, the principal usually needs to be notified as soon as possible, in addition to the designated risk manager for the school district. Schools may also require incident reports to be completed for incidents of fighting, bullying, cheating, or weapons violations. In these cases, the incident reports may become part of the educational record (Hollis/Brookline High School, 2003).

▼ LEGAL CONSIDERATIONS ▼

The facility's liability or property insurance provider often requires the incident report. Whenever a client, visitor, or employee is injured, there is the possibility of a lawsuit. The incident report is the primary source of documentation of what happened (Scott, 1997). However, if the case does go to court, the incident report itself is usually immune (exempt) from discovery by the person who files the lawsuit (plaintiff) and his or her attorney. To be exempt, the incident reports usually have to be clearly labeled as "'quality assurance/improvement documents' or a 'report prepared at the directions of the organization's attorney for possible use in litigation.'" (Scott, 1997, p. 70). If they are not labeled in that way, they can be considered business records (Southwick, 1988). If the plaintiff's attorney thinks that the incident report is essential for proving the case, and would be admissible as evidence in court, business records can be obtained before they are presented in court.

An incident report is completed whenever a client, visitor, or staff member is injured, no matter how big or how small the incident. There may be slightly different forms for when the injured party is a client/visitor or a staff member, but both forms will want similar information. I have always been told that an incident report should be completed for any injury, even a paper cut. One risk manager told me that what looks like a simple paper cut could get infected, and that could turn into a big problem, so always fill out the form.

In reality, many staff members fail to complete the report for such a small thing as a paper cut. In cold, dry climates, paper cuts can be a daily occurrence. If a staff member filled out an incident report for each cut, he or she would be doing it several times a week. It seems like a waste of paper and a waste of time. You cannot prevent paper cuts. However, you need to follow the policies and procedures of the facility. If the person in charge of risk management at your facility says it is not necessary to complete an incident report for a paper cut, then that is fine. If the risk manager says that incident reports are necessary regardless of the size of the injury, then you have to do it.

▼ RECORDING INFORMATION ON AN INCIDENT REPORT FORM AND CLIENT RECORD ▼

Any lawyer I've ever talked to has told me that if I am ever questioned about an event that has occurred, simply answer the questions and do not volunteer additional information. I think it would be wise to view the incident report in the same way. Answer the questions directly, but do not volunteer additional information. The more information you provide, the more likely you are to add embellishments, exaggerations, and extraneous information that could be turned against you by a skilled attorney. As concisely as possible, simply provide the necessary facts on the incident report itself. If you are concerned that the incident could wind up in court, there is nothing that prohibits you from recording a more thorough description of what transpired, including your impressions (as opposed to facts), for your own records, as long as you protect the confidentiality of those involved in the incident.

That said, you still have to provide enough evidence to adequately describe what happened. You must be objective. Remember the "Descriptive, Interpretive, and Evaluative" discussion from the chapter on evaluation reports? Keep it descriptive, but avoid interpretive or evaluative statements. Do not make it seem like you are taking the blame or blaming someone else for the incident (Scott, 1997). Only record what you experienced, not what others tell you that they saw, unless you put the other statements in quote marks and identify the statement as hearsay. If there are witnesses, you may be asked to name them (Elkin, Perry, & Potter, 2000). You will also be asked to specify the time, to the nearest minute, that the incident occurred.

Let's look at another case:

Korpo is an occupational therapy assistant who was born in Somalia and immigrated to this country 10 years ago. She has been assigned to work with a man who recently suffered a head injury, dislocated right shoulder, and two cracked ribs as a result of a motorcycle accident. He is in an agitated state, but needs to relearn grooming, hygiene, and dressing skills. He is a large man with many tattoos and body piercings.

When Korpo enters the room, he immediately begins name-calling and refusing to cooperate. His exact words are "Get out of here, you bitch! I don't do nothin' for n-g---s!" As she brings him a warm, wet washcloth, he hurls it at her, and then shoves the overbed table into her stomach, knocking her down hard. His face gets red, his eyes are open wide, his teeth are bared, and the veins in his neck are standing out. He picks up the phone on the bedside table and throws it at her, hitting her in the head. She crawls out of the room, a small cut on her forehead.

What would be documented in the medical record, and what would be recorded in the incident report? Here is one possibility.

In the medical record, a narrative note might read:

2/4/03, 10:00 AM. Patient refused to participate in self-care training at bedside. He swore and threw things at the occupational therapy assistant. Will attempt to work with him again bedside tomorrow as per the plan of care. Korpo Bohla, OTA/L

A SOAP note might look like this:

S: "Get out of here, you b---h! I don't do nothin' for n-g---s!
O: Client refused occupational therapy self-care training at bedside. He swore and threw the telephone at the occupational therapy assistant.
A: Client is agitated and uncooperative.
P: Continue to attempt bedside intervention 12/5/03.

Korpo Bohla, OTA/L

In the narrative portion of the incident report, you would see:

When I entered the room, he immediately began name-calling and refusing to cooperate. His exact words were "Get out of here, you b---h! I don't do nothin' for n-g---s!" When I brought him a warm, wet washcloth, he hurled it at me, and then shoved the overbed table into my stomach, knocking me down hard. His face got red, his eyes were open wide, his teeth were bared, and the veins in his neck were standing out. He picked up the phone on the bedside table and threw it at me, which hit me in the head. I crawled out of the room. There was a small cut on my forehead. The cut was cleaned, antibiotic cream was applied, and the wound was closed with steri-strips.

There are some obvious differences between what gets written in the clinical record and what is written in the incident report. The progress note (narrative or SOAP format) is very concise, only the bare minimum of information is written (Distasio, 2000; Scott, 1997). While the progress notes do not convey the entire picture, you do get some sense of the anger expressed by the client. In a client recovering from a brain injury, this is a predictable phase that many clients go through. It is essential that the agitation and anger be documented. Notice that neither progress note mentions the incident report form.

If the incident results in a client needing medical intervention, that intervention must be documented in the client's clinical record (Elkin et al., 2000). If you are working in a setting without a clinical record, such as at a school, then the incident report may be the only document you write on, depending on the facility's (school's) policy. Of course, in either case, you need to talk to your supervisor as soon as possible after the incident, and in a school, you need to notify the principal as well.

The question that remains is, if a trigger for the explosive behavior can be identified, should it be documented? One side of the issue, using this case as an example, is if the trigger is identified, it can be avoided in the future, cutting down on the risk of injury to staff (Distasio, 2000). On the other hand, what if the trigger is identified, but it casts the client in a negative light? For example, what if the trigger in this case is that the client is prejudiced against people of color. To decrease agitation, one could make an argument that only white staff should work with the client. But that would be discriminatory, and might cause staff of all colors to dislike the client. This is a really delicate issue. Most facilities have policies on discrimination. Whether or not to document the trigger would not be a decision that occupational therapy staff would make alone.

Clearly, what is written in the incident report is more detailed. The incident report addresses what happened to the staff person whereas a progress note in a client's record would not. As stated earlier in this chapter, do not even make a reference to completing an incident report in the client's record (Scott, 1997).

An incident report is also likely to include some checklists for the employee to mark. There may be a checklist that asks the writer to check off what precautions were taken, where the incident occurred, what kind of medical attention was required, and what measures could be taken to prevent further incidents. Of course, with any checklist, there is usually a space for "other" with a blank to fill in where the writer could add to the list something that had not been considered before.

Exercise 17.1

1. Using the case from the beginning of this chapter (post-stroke client during toilet transfer training), write a narrative progress note and a narrative entry for the incident report.

   Narrative progress note:

   Incident report:

2. Using the following case, write a SOAP note and a narrative entry for the incident report.

   You are working in a community-based program for persons with mental health disorders. The program focuses on development of job skills. The client you are working with on completing job applications begins to get frustrated with the number of errors she is making. On the second application, she begins to scribble across the whole page saying "Dammit" repeatedly. You calm her down and have her try again. This time, about halfway through, she picks up the application and begins to tear it into pieces while yelling, "I quit. I can't do this. I'm never going to get a job." Before you can stop her, she gets a paper cut. Then she starts cursing, "F---ing S---, A--hole moron, S---" and then more of the same. You interrupt her tirade to tell her she has a cut, and when she sees it, she stops and stares at it. You take her to the sink, run it under cold water for a bit, gently dry it off, and then put an adhesive bandage on it. You have her sit calmly for a while before engaging her in another task.

   S:

   O:

   A:

   P:

   Incident report:

3. Write either a SOAP or narrative progress note and a narrative portion of an incident report about the following scene.

   You are an occupational therapist working in a preschool transition program. You are co-leading a group of 3-year-olds. It is snack time. There will be sliced apples and peanut butter. While you are putting peanut butter on the plates, the special ed teacher is sitting at the table with the children, showing them what the inside of an apple looks like. She is using a 10" cook's knife to cut the apple. Her hands are getting sticky from the apple's juice, so she gets up to get a napkin, setting the knife down on the table. You are at the other end of the table. Just as you are about to remind the teacher to take the knife with her, 3-year-old Tyla picks it up by the blade end, cutting the palm side of three fingers. The special education teacher never saw anything; her back was turned, so she tells you that you have to fill out the paperwork. You take the screaming child to the sink, but realize the child will need medical attention. You wrap up the hand in a clean towel while the special education teacher calls the child's mom and you keep pressure on the wound.

Progress note:

Incident report:

SUMMARY

When the unexpected happens, it needs to be documented in two ways. First, a concise note explaining the event is written in the client's record. The narrative or SOAP/DAP note must contain objective information that does not lay blame on anyone. Then there is the incident report. You need to provide all the relevant facts on an incident report, but do not volunteer any extra information. Do not lay blame or accept blame anywhere on an incident report. The information you provide may be used by the facility for quality or risk management purposes.

REFERENCES

Distasio, C. A. (2000). Workplace violence: Part II: Documentation and reporting—how to paint the picture. *Maryland-Nurse, 1*(2), 12.

Elkin, M. K., Perry, A. G., & Potter, P. A. (2000). *Nursing interventions and clinical skills* (2nd ed.). St. Louis, MO: Mosby.

Hollis/Brookline High School. (2003). *Safe school policy: Incident report.* Retrieved April 7, 2003, from *http://www.Hollis/BrooklineHighSchool.k12.nh.us/equitycouncil/harassme.htm*

Scott, R. (1997). *Promoting legal awareness in physical and occupational therapy.* St. Louis, MO: Mosby.

Southwick, A. F. (1988). *The law of hospital and health care administration* (2nd ed.). Ann Arbor, MI: Foundation of the American College of Healthcare Executives.

CHAPTER 18

Appeal Letters

INTRODUCTION

It is not unusual for an occupational therapist and a third-party payer to disagree about a client's need for services. In some cases, the occupational therapist may not know until after the service is delivered that the payer does not think that occupational therapy services were medically necessary (or whatever that payer's standard is). Most occupational therapy services must be paid for in order for the provider to stay in business, to continue to serve other clients. If the occupational therapist thinks that a client needs services, and that those services reasonably fall within the scope of what the payer customarily pays for, he or she can appeal the decision not to pay for services. In addition to providing additional clinical documentation (if there is any that was not submitted with the initial claim), the occupational therapist writes an appeal letter that explains the rationale for occupational therapy for that particular client and an explicit request to overturn the denial.

▼ APPEAL LETTERS AS OPPORTUNITIES TO EDUCATE ▼

It is critically important that the appeal letter is clear, to the point, and states what you want done about the original denial. In some cases, the person reading the appeal letter may be the same person that wrote the denial in the first place, so you have to be very careful to appear professional and respectful of the initial decision. In other cases, there may be levels of review, and a nurse, an occupational therapist, or a physician may conduct the second or third review.

I think it is helpful to look at an appeal as a learning process for the reviewer. If the reviewer is not an occupational therapist, this is an opportunity for you to teach him or her something about it. As unbelievable as it sounds in this day and age, there are still people out there who think occupational therapists only work with hand function or only provide diversional therapy. I have heard of some insurers who only pay for physical therapy on an outpatient basis for clients with hand injuries, not occupational therapy, even if the occupational therapist is a certified hand therapist.

Not so many years ago, when I called an insurance company to check on coverage for an outpatient, I was told the insurer did not cover occupational therapy services for outpatients (only for inpatients) because "who needs underwater basket weaving anyway?" After a few calming breaths and a couple more phone calls to the insurer and the client's employer (the insurance was through the client's work), the insurer did pay for occupational therapy, explaining that it had inadvertently left occupational therapy out of the policy. Since it was not listed specifically as an excluded service, they had to cover it.

You have a fighting chance of getting coverage for occupational therapy if the insurance policy is silent on occupational therapy coverage. The insurer can be convinced of the need for occupational therapy and save face by saying the omission of occupational therapy was simply an oversight. If the policy specifically says that occupational therapy services are excluded from coverage, then it is hard to get the insurer to pay for occupational therapy services no matter how strong your arguments are.

You are working with an elderly man in his home. He has coverage through Medicare. The Medicare fiscal intermediary determines that occupational therapy services are no longer medically necessary and should have been discontinued. You had continued to work with the man until you heard that the last 2 weeks of occupational therapy were not paid for. He is recovering from a hip replacement on his left side (6 weeks ago), complicated by a below-knee amputation of his left leg (5 years ago), diabetic neuropathy (decreased sensation in all remaining limbs), and cataracts in both eyes. Occupational therapy services have been provided twice a week for 6 weeks to improve self-care skills. Physical therapy has also been involved with this client, working on ambulation and transfers. Physical therapy had discontinued services, saying the client has plateaued; he is not making any more progress. You want to continue to see the client in his own home to work on more kitchen skills, lower-extremity dressing, and problem solving related to day-to-day challenges he faces. He lives with his wife of 60 years who has been his caretaker but has recently begun to show signs of Alzheimer's. Their children live 3 hours away and do not visit often. You have seen the client make good progress in all areas. Since it is inappropriate for you to write about another person in your client's documentation, you have not documented his wife's deteriorating cognitive state. Your client is cognitively intact. However, you know that the client needs to learn to cook because he has expressed concern about his wife leaving the gas stove on when cooking is done, burning food, and misplacing food items. You decide to appeal this decision.

▼ WRITING AN APPEAL LETTER ▼

In the above case, you are privy to information that the intermediary does not know. The intermediary has read all your intervention plans, but is unaware of other environmental factors affecting this case. You have done a good job documenting the client's progress in the stated need areas. The intermediary has assumed that since the client reached a plateau in physical therapy, a plateau in occupational therapy cannot be far behind. In your letter you will outline progress made so far, what additional progress you expect in the next 4 weeks, and justify it by explaining the social environmental factors that affect this case. Your letter will be formal and professional. Figure 18.1 shows an example of what it might look like.

▼ MEDICARE APPEALS ▼

Under Medicare rules, a provider or client has 120 days to appeal a coverage determination (Department of Human Services, 2002). The first level of appeal usually is at the intermediary or carrier level. Depending on the state in which you provided the service, the carrier or intermediary will vary. You need to follow the procedures established by your carrier or intermediary. This usually involves completing some kind of form and attaching support materials. Your explanation for wanting a review of the coverage decision needs to be detailed, succinct, and factual.

If you are still not satisfied with the outcome, an appeal, referred to as a request for review of a Part B Medicare claim, is done on a form called CMS-1964 (downloadable on the Internet from *www.cms.gov/forms/cms-1964.pdf*) and submitted to the local Social Security Office (Centers for Medicare and Medicaid Services [CMS], 2000). A copy of the form is in Appendix G of this book. The form requests identifying information, the reasons for disagreeing with the initial determination, and a description of the illness or injury. You are required to attach a copy of the Explanation of Medicare Benefits (or a description of the service, the dates of service, and the physician's name) and you may attach additional evidence before sending the form (with attachments) to the carrier or to a local Social Security Administration office. Always make a copy of all documents associated with the appeal to keep for your records.

Part B Reviewer
Best Deal Intermediary
1234 Tightwad Street
New Money, NJ 07666-7666

April 15, 2004

Dear Reviewer,

I am the occupational therapist working with Mr. J. Doe, case #246810. I am writing to request that the decision to deny further occupational therapy services be reversed based on the following additional information.

Mr. Doe has been making steady gains in lower extremity dressing, meal preparation and cleanup, and problem solving. He has progressed from being totally dependent in lower extremity dressing to needing minimal assist and adaptive equipment. Meal preparation has progressed from needing step-by-step instruction to Mr. Doe initiating meal planning and preparation. He still has difficulty transporting food from the stove to the table or counter and opening some packaging. He uses a tall stool to sit on when washing or drying the dishes. He provides instruction to his wife in cleaning up after meals. Mr. Doe has expressed concern for allowing his wife to use the stove. She is showing significant episodes of memory loss and confusion about daily chores leading to some dangerous situations in the kitchen. Mr. Doe wants to take over some of her kitchen responsibilities. Teaching Mr. Doe to plan and prepare meals is essential in order for the Does to live in their own home safely.

In addition to the plans of care you have already reviewed, I am enclosing copies of the visit notes for each of the occupational therapy sessions from the last 6 weeks. If I can provide you with any additional information, please let me know.

Sincerely,

Carin Provider, OTR/L
Carin Provider, OTR/L

FIGURE 18.1 Sample Appeals Letter

In wording your reasons for appealing the decision, be clear and direct. Do not imply anything, say it explicitly. If the Explanation of Medicare Benefits says that your services are not medically necessary, say that you feel the services are medically necessary because the client needs to be able to feed herself or she will not eat. Or you could say that the services are medically necessary because the client is at risk of developing contractures if serial casting does not continue, or whatever it is that makes your services necessary for that particular client.

▼ APPEALS TO PRIVATE INSURERS (INCLUDING HMOs) ▼

Insurers have appeals processes written into each of their health plans (and worker's compensation plans, auto insurance plans, etc.). If it is at all possible, a good first step is to contact the insurer and find out exactly why the claim was denied (Appeal Solutions, 2002). Find out what the insurer's definition of medical necessity is and build your arguments for covering the service around that definition. For example, some insurers routinely deny coverage for sensory integration intervention. They say it is experimental (often insurers say experimental procedures are not medically necessary), that there is not conclusive evidence that it is an effective, medically acceptable intervention. I know of one insurer who will deny an entire claim if even one unit of sensory integration intervention shows up on a claim, even if there are other procedures used during the same intervention session.

The occupational therapist could do one of two things here. One is that she could find as much evidence in the literature supporting the use of sensory integrative techniques and attach those to her letter of appeal. This could be a lengthy process, and you have no guarantee the reviewer will read any of the supporting literature since it does not relate specifically to this case. But it is better than doing nothing. Another would be to make an argument that the other procedures used during that intervention session are reasonable and necessary for the child's condition, and that the insurer has paid for those services in the past. In this case you might get paid for some of the session, but probably not the whole session. If I were going to fight an insurer who considers sensory integration to be experimental, I would also enlist the support of the parent and referring physician, asking them to write letters explaining the potential benefits of the denied services.

If you find out that the denial is for all services of a type, such as sensory integration, you can enlist the support of your state occupational therapy association (if you are a member). The association can try to work with the insurer's medical director to change corporate policy. The American Occupational Therapy Association also has resources for members to help in challenging insurance companies.

Exercise 18.1

Give reasons to overturn a coverage decision for each of the two cases below.

Case 1: Nomi

Nomi is a 6-year-old child with fetal alcohol syndrome seen for occupational therapy at an after-school program. She has trouble concentrating and is quite active. She is tactilely defensive and fearful of movement through space when both feet are not on the ground (i.e., swings, slides, etc.). She does receive special education services at school, but there are reports that she hits other children and frequently gets off her chair to walk around when she should be sitting and listening. At the after-school program, you have observed her improve at sitting for longer stretches of time, up to 5 minutes sometimes. She has been in the program for 2 months. She is beginning to appear more relaxed on a swing, as long as her feet can touch the ground and she can control the distance the swing goes with her feet. Just yesterday she allowed the swing to go back and forth gently twice before stopping it. She was scribbling on a coloring book page when she first came to the program, but now she attempts to stay roughly within the lines.

The insurance company said that the services of an occupational therapist are not medically necessary. They say that the services could be provided by lesser-skilled personnel.

Case 2: Seiki

Seiki is an elderly man who had a brain tumor removed from the right side of his brain 2 weeks ago. He is now at a long-term care facility for rehabilitation and then plans to return home to his farm after 4 to 6 weeks of rehab. He has a grandson who is looking after his cows for him. His grandson lives on a neighboring farm. As a result of the surgery, Seiki has some limitation in the movement and coordination of his left arm and side. He also has left side neglect. He is beginning to accept that he has a neglect, but at the time of the last evaluation report/plan of care the neglect was strong and he denied he had it. His left arm is flaccid, but in the last 2 days you have noticed some spasticity has set in. Seiki is making steady gains in dressing, feeding, grooming, and hygiene. His wife visits everyday, but she is a worrier, and says they will have to give up the farm if he does not get better. This agitates Seiki. He is sure that he will recover and be able to go back to farming. In fact, he says that where there is a will, there is a way, and he will rig something up to help him do the work. He has always been a bit of an inventor, and has invented several helpful farm implements in his day. You gave your word to Seiki that you would help him come up with some adaptation that would allow him to do some of the work he used to do in the barn. Then the denial notice came.

The Medicare intermediary says that Seiki's potential for recovery is poor at best. The intermediary says that Seiki should move to a lower RUG level with fewer therapy minutes.

SUMMARY

You have the right to appeal any payer's decision to deny coverage for occupational therapy services. Each payer will have a process for appealing such a decision. Writing a letter of appeal requires tact, clarity, and the powers of persuasion. You have to remain respectful regardless of how angry the decision makes you. You have to clearly state your reasons for wanting a coverage determination to be overturned. You have to construct sound arguments for the necessity of occupational therapy interventions in this specific case. Well-written appeal letters are extremely important to getting a denial overturned. You cannot overturn a denial unless you appeal it.

REFERENCES

American Occupational Therapy Association. (2001). *Medicare coverage decision: HCFA announces new process for coverage decisions.* Retrieved January 5, 2001, from *http://www.aota.org/members/area5/links/LINK60.asp?PLACE=/members/area5/links/link60.asp*

American Occupational Therapy Association. (2002). *Medicare appeals checklist.* Retrieved November 21, 2002, from *http://www.aota.org/members/area5/links/LINK18.asp?PLACE=/members/area5/links/link18.asp*

Appeal Solutions. (2002). Case study: Responding to insurance denials due to lack of medical necessity. *The Appeal Letter.* Retrieved November 21, 2002, from *http://www.appealsolutions.com/tal/medical-necessity-case-study/htm*

Centers for Medicare and Medicaid Services. (2002). *Outpatient physical therapy comprehensive outpatient rehabilitation facility and community mental health center manual.* Retrieved November 21, 2002, from *http://cms.hhs.gov/manuals/09_opt/op600.asp*

Department of Human Services, Centers for Medicare and Medicaid Services. (2002). Medicare program: Changes in Medicare appeals procedures based on section 521 of the Medicare, Medicaid, and SCHIP benefits improvement and protections act of 2000. *Federal Register, 67*(194), 62478–62482.

CHAPTER 19

Meeting Minutes

INTRODUCTION

As has been said many times before, if it isn't documented, it didn't happen. While taking minutes may make some meetings feel more formal than the actual tone of the meeting, it is necessary to keep a record of what was discussed. When surveyors of any type (JCAHO, CARF, Department of Health, Department of Education, etc.) come to evaluate a facility or department, they usually ask to see copies of meeting minutes. Sometimes they are looking to verify that staff have been instructed in certain policies and procedures; other times they may be looking to see that continuing education has occurred. Meeting minutes also "give all group members the chance to see how issues that were discussed were finally resolved" (Mosvick & Nelson, 1987, p. 169).

▼ OVERVIEW OF MEETING MINUTES ▼

Most facilities, departments, or organizations have an already established system for taking minutes. For the sake of tradition, that system is continued. This is fine most of the time, but occasionally a new note taker will look for a different system. This chapter presents a couple of systems. Which system is used is often a reflection of the management style of that facility, department, or organization.

Meeting minutes can also be used as evidence in legal proceedings. There may be a question of when staff was informed about an administrative decision or policy change. Often, if there is a question about the level of training received by staff, meeting minutes can be used to see how much training (i.e., about a new policy or procedure) was provided and when.

Sometimes, the minutes are documentation of decisions made by a department, facility, or organization. It is not unusual for a topic of discussion that is raised today to have been discussed last year or a couple years ago. By going back over the minutes, time can be saved and the results of the last discussion shared. If there is nothing new to add, the group can move on to the next topic.

▼ COMMONALITIES ▼

All meeting minutes contain certain information, but the format may vary. One very important piece of information on every meeting minute is the date, including the year. Meeting minutes are not much good if you cannot tell when the meeting occurred. Minutes should also reflect who was present at the meeting. If the names of attendees and the date of the meeting are documented, then there is proof that a particular person was informed of whatever the topic was on that date. That person cannot claim ignorance as a means of defending him- or herself.

Topics of discussion are a main component of meeting minutes. Obviously, minutes are more than just a listing of people and dates. They have to contain something of substance. Some minutes try to capture the entire discussion, some summarize the discussion. How much of the discussion is captured in the minutes will vary from place to place.

Finally, the action items are included in the minutes. Action items are the tasks that people must do as a result of the discussion. Examples of action items include:

- Ellie will clean the refrigerator and Chris will clean the microwave.
- Jane will meet with the nursing staff to present our program revisions for post-mastectomy patients.
- Arica will represent the department on the interdisciplinary quality improvement team looking at improving customer service.
- Tanya will contact the vendor for splinting materials about presenting an in-service for the department.

▼ TAKING MINUTES ▼

If you are the person taking minutes at a meeting, the recorder, you have some special responsibilities. Because of the amount of concentration that it takes to record the discussion, it is difficult for one person to both lead a discussion and write minutes at the same time. The recorder is responsible for asking for clarification when discussions seem confusing or start going off on tangents (Mosvick & Nelson, 1987). The recorder can ask the group to verify the conclusions or summaries he or she draws at the end of a discussion. At the same time, the recorder needs to be ready to read back portions of the minutes to the group at the request of a group member. If you are the recorder, be prepared with proper materials and be on time. Be careful that your opinions on a particular subject do not color the minutes that you are taking. Use as few adjectives and adverbs as possible; it is fine if the minutes are dull to read (basic-learning.com, 2003). Words that signal that your opinions are surfacing include "inspiring," "interesting," "wonderful," "proud," or "antagonistic."

You may take minutes by writing longhand, using a laptop computer, or by tape recording the meeting and transcribing it later. If you take minutes with paper and pen, be sure to number your pages. If you have a tendency to abbreviate words or use your own cryptic system, be sure to transcribe the minutes into usable form as soon as possible after the meeting. If you wait too long, you may not be able to make sense of your own minutes. If the minutes refer to other documents, be sure to attach these documents to the official set of minutes or state where the documents can be found (effectivemeetings.com, 2003).

While you may make copies of minutes to distribute to each person who attended or should have attended the meeting, there is usually one set of minutes that is kept as the official record of the meeting. In some places, it may be a three-ring binder kept in the office. In others, it may be a website or folder on a shared drive on a computer. If a paper copy of the minutes is kept, some organizations require that the official minutes contain the signature of the minute-taker. In some organizations, the minutes do not become official until the Board of Directors or the membership of the committee approves them.

▼ FORMATS ▼

The simplest, but perhaps the wordiest way to take minutes is to keep a narrative record of the meeting. In this format, after the date and list of attendees, the minute-taker writes down as much of what happened at the meeting as possible. It may include who said what. The paragraphs may be numbered when they represent a new topic.

Figure 19.1 shows an example of narrative minutes of a department meeting.

You can see that taking minutes like this could lead to writer's cramp. It is a lot of writing, and not all of it is important to note. Perhaps some things would be better left undocumented (i.e., getting cut out of parking spaces by an aggressive lab employee) in departmental meeting minutes. On the other hand, if someone in the department missed the

Date: 11-25-03
Present: E. Bay, J. Kay, G. Whiz, and A. Ging

1. Announcements
   • Ellie announced that she would be taking Friday off and a sub would be called in.
   • Jane announced that the United Way fund drive would be starting next week.
   • Gina reminded staff that rounds this week are changed to Thursday at 9:00 AM.

2. New patient transportation policy
   Jane presented the proposed new hospital policy on patient transportation. Rehabilitation thera-pies are to send the next day's schedule to each nursing unit, medical imaging, the lab, and the transportation pool by 3:00 each day. Unless otherwise noted on the schedule, nursing will have the patients dressed, in a wheelchair, with hearing aids and glasses on as needed by the sched-uled pick-up time. Transportation pool personnel will transport those patients who are ready at their appointed time. If a patient is not ready, the transporter may wait for up to 5 minutes. If the patient is still not ready, then nursing will be responsible for finding a volunteer or aide to do the transporting. Patients must be finished with therapy at the time they are scheduled to go back to their rooms (or to other appointments), the transporter can only wait up to 5 minutes if the patient is not ready. After that, therapy is responsible for finding a volunteer or aide to do the transport-ing. Jane said the new policy was designed to encourage everyone to try to stick to the sched-ule. The policy is expected to go into effect in 30 days unless there is overwhelming negative feedback. The transportation improvement team is accepting written comments for the next 2 weeks. Gina asked if compliance to the policy would be tracked. Jane said yes, there would be forms that transporters fill out whenever they complete a transportation. Jane asked for a show of hands of people who were supportive of the proposed new policy. The department gave unan-imous support to the policy. The policy is attached to these minutes.

3. Infection control
   Jane conducted the annual review of infection control policies and procedures for the depart-ment. We reviewed hand washing, and each member was asked to demonstrate proper tech-nique. We discussed cleaning of supplies and equipment, including which cleaning solution is used for which items we clean and which items need to be sent to central sterile supply to be cleaned. We reviewed policies for working with patients in isolation rooms, when to wear protec-tive gear (gloves, masks, and gowns), and proper technique for donning and doffing them. Fi-nally, universal precautions were reviewed in detail. Each member of the department signed an annual review of infection control training confirmation sheet. Jane will forward these to the human resources department for placement in employee files.

4. Parking
   Jane asked for a volunteer to serve on a task force looking into issues regarding employee park-ing. Parking complaints have risen dramatically in the last year. Everyone in the department agrees that parking has gotten worse lately. Ellie said she tries to get to work 20 minutes early to find a decent spot. Arica said she has noticed that some employees get really competitive about parking spaces and that she has been cut out of a space on several occasions by an aggressive parker who works in the lab. The task force will look at existing parking options and consider al-ternatives for parking in the future. Arica volunteered to serve on the task force. The first meeting is next Friday at 2:30.

5. Budget request
   Ellie asked if there was any room in the budget for buying the newest revision of the Peabody Motor Scales. The test has new norms and a few new test items. Our competitors have all switched to the newer version. We use the test about 2–3 times per month, more often in sum-mer. It would be a good investment. Jane said that she would need more information about the cost of the test and ordering information. There is some money in the budget, but there may not be enough for the test kit. We may have to delay or eliminate other expenses if we want it this year. If we cannot fit it in this year's budget, we should make it a priority for next year's budget.

FIGURE 19.1   Sample Narrative Meeting Minutes

meeting, he or she could have a pretty good idea of what transpired at the meeting simply from reading the minutes.

Another way to take minutes also involves a narrative format, but it uses summaries instead of trying to capture everything that was said. Figure 19.2 is an example of the same meeting, but a different format for the minutes.

You can see that minutes like this take up less space, but they also have less information. The summary format gives minimal information about what was discussed. It is enough to get the essence of what was discussed, but nothing is very substantial.

Minutes can use different numbering systems. Sometimes a typical outline format is used (I., A., 1., a.), but numerical systems are also used (1., 1.1., 1.1.2.). While I have seen minutes that were not numbered at all, a numbering system of some kind does make it easier to refer back to specific items.

Another format is to list agenda items at the top of the page, and then only document action items. This format definitely saves space. It is sort of a "Just the facts ma'am" kind of format. If the minutes from the above meeting were done in an action format, they would look something like Figure 19.3. You can see what a sparse format this is. It is best used for very long meetings.

Date: 11-25-03
Present: E. Bay, J. Kay, G. Whiz, and A. Ging

1. Announcements
   a. Ellie announced that she would be taking Friday off and a sub would be called in.
   b. Jane announced that the United Way fund drive would be starting next week.
   c. Gina reminded staff that rounds this week is changed to Thursday at 9:00 AM.

2. New patient transportation policy
   Jane presented the proposed new hospital policy on patient transportation, which was designed to encourage everyone to try to stick to the schedule. The policy is expected to go into effect in 30 days unless there is overwhelming negative feedback. The transportation improvement team is accepting written comments for the next 2 weeks. Jane asked for a show of hands of people who were supportive of the proposed new policy. The department gave unanimous support to the policy. Policy is attached.

3. Infection control
   Jane conducted the annual review of infection control policies and procedures for the department as per hospital policy. We signed annual review of infection control training confirmation sheets, which Jane will forward to the human resources department for placement in employee files.

4. Parking
   Jane asked for a volunteer to serve on a task force looking at issues around employee parking. The task force will look at existing parking options and consider alternatives for parking in the future. Arica volunteered to serve on the task force. The first meeting is next Friday at 2:30.

5. Budget request
   Ellie asked if there was any room in the budget for buying the newest revision of the Peabody Motor Scales. Jane said that she would need more information about the cost of the test and ordering information. If we cannot fit it in this year's budget, we should make it a priority for next year's budget.

FIGURE 19.2   Example of Summary Format Meeting Minutes

```
Date: 11-25-03
Present: E. Bay, J. Kay, G. Whiz, and A. Ging

1. Agenda
    1.1. Announcements
    1.2. New patient transportation policy
    1.3. Infection control
    1.4. Parking
    1.5. New budget request

2. Announcements
    2.1. Ellie announced that she would be taking Friday off and a sub would be called in.
    2.2. Jane announced that the United Way fund drive would be starting next week.
    2.3. Gina reminded staff that rounds this week is changed to Thursday at 9:00 AM.

3. Action Items
    3.1. New patient transportation policy
        3.1.1. The department gave unanimous support to the policy.
        3.1.2. See attached policy
    3.2. Infection control
        3.2.1. We reviewed and signed annual review of infection control confirmation sheets,
               which Jane will forward to the human resources department for placement in em-
               ployee files.
    3.3. Parking
        3.3.1. Arica volunteered to serve on the task force.
    3.4. Budget request
        3.4.1. Ellie will provide Jane with ordering information for the new Peabody Motor
               Scales.
        3.4.2. It will be ordered if it fits within the department's budget.
```

FIGURE 19.3   Sample Action Format Minutes

Another format is a combination of the last two. It summarizes a topic, and then identifies the action item. For example, the parking discussion might look like this:

4. Parking
Jane asked for a volunteer to serve on a task force looking at issues around employee parking. The task force will look at existing parking options and consider alternatives for parking in the future.
Action: Arica volunteered to serve on the task force.

The last format that will be presented here is using a preprinted form. Figure 19.4 shows an example of this format. This form requires some preparation before the meeting, but simplifies taking minutes during the meeting (meetingwizard.org, 2001). Names of the people expected to attend the meeting can be listed on the form and a checkmark placed in front of the ones who attended the meeting (effectivemeetings.com, 2003).

There are many other formats. Some facilities have forms that get filled out with columns for discussions and action items. There can be lots of other variations. When taking minutes, the important thing is to listen for the most important information and record it accurately.

OT Department Meeting Minutes
Date/Time: 11-25-03/3:00 P.M.
Members Present: _____ E. Bay _____ J. Kay _____ G. Whiz _____ A. Ging

Topic	Discussion	Action	Person Responsible
Announce-ments	Ellie announced that she would be taking Friday off and a sub would be called in. Jane announced that the United Way fund drive would be starting next week. Gina reminded staff that rounds this week is changed to Thursday at 9:00 AM.	N/A	N/A
New Policy	The proposed new hospital policy on patient transportation was presented. It was designed to encourage everyone to try to stick to the schedule. The policy is expected to go into effect in 30 days unless there is over-whelming negative feedback. The transportation improvement team is accepting written comments for the next 2 weeks.	The department gave unanimous support to the policy (attached).	Jane
Infection Control	The annual review of infection control policies and procedures for the department as per hospital policy was conducted.	We signed annual review of infection control training confirmation sheets that will be forwarded to HR for placement in employee files.	Jane
Parking	The hospital is looking for a volunteer to serve on a task force looking at issues around employee parking; existing parking options and consider alternatives for parking in the future.	Arica volunteered to serve on the task force.	Arica
New Budget Request	A request was received to buy the newest revision of the Peabody Motor Scales.	Ellie will find information about the cost of the test and order-ting information. Jane will see if it fits in this year's budget.	Ellie and Jane

FIGURE 19.4   Sample Meeting Minutes Form

Summarize the following meeting topics using the combined format (the last one presented).

Riva gave an update on the actions of the committee that is planning the 50th anniversary celebration of the hospital. The celebration committee is looking for success stories for a weeklong series (a 4-minute segment each day) on the 11:00 local news. They would like to highlight a different department each day, but they cannot cover every department in the 5-day series. Rhonda suggested Mr. Sayed who recovered from Guillian-Barré syndrome 2 years ago. He still sends a holiday card each year. Rolanda suggested Mr. Hernandez who had extensive rehab following a head injury, but eventually went home and back to work part time. Robert suggested Mrs. Hellenberger who lost six toes and three fingers to frostbite. The committee is also planning an open house in the cafeteria, and each department can put together a display table promoting programs in the department. After much discussion, the department agreed to talk with the other departments in the rehabilitation area about sharing a segment on Mr. Hernandez. Rhonda volunteered to work with the occupational therapy fieldwork students on a display table for the open house.

1. 50th Anniversary Committee Report

Action:

The head of the department, Barb, said she had noticed a decrease in productivity lately. There has been a downward trend over the last 6 weeks. The company's financial picture is not looking as good as was hoped. Ours is not the only department that is falling below projections. The president of the company is asking each department to develop a plan for cutting expenses for the rest of the year by 10%. Barb would like input from the staff as to what cuts would be the least painful to make. Bob suggested that we could cut out doughnuts and coffee for the morning department meetings. Belinda suggested that we could use coupons and buy generic brands for the occupational therapy kitchen. Becky suggested being more careful about walking off with each other's pens, and try to conserve paper. Bob suggested that they be more conscientious about remembering to bill for adaptive equipment. Barb said those were good suggestions, but they wouldn't come anywhere near 10% of the budget. She asked each person to meet with her privately to discuss other possibilities.

1. Budget

Action:

SUMMARY

Taking accurate meeting minutes is an essential function of any occupational therapy department. There is a delicate balance between recording too much information and too little. The names of the people present at the meeting, the date of the meeting, and the outcomes of the meeting in terms of actions and decisions need to be recorded. There are several formats for recording these meetings. While each has some advantages and disadvantages, choose one that fits your facility's needs.

REFERENCES

Basic-learning.com. (2003). *Bull's eye business writing tips: Getting to your writing target.* Retrieved April 7, 2003, from *http://www.basic-learning.com/wbwt/tip134.htm*

Effectivemeetings.com. (2003). *Meeting basics, how to record useful meeting minutes.* Retrieved April 7, 2003, from *http://www.effectivemeetings.com/meeting/basics/minutes.asp*

Meetingwizard.org. (2001). *Writing meeting minutes—Useful tips* Retrieved April 7, 2003, from *http://www.meetingwizard.org/meetings/taking-minutes.cfm?re=11*

Mosvick, R. K., & Nelson, R. B. (1987). *We've got to start meeting like this! A guide to successful business meeting management.* Glenview, IL: Scott, Foresman.

CHAPTER 20

Grant Writing

INTRODUCTION

Occupational therapy services are generally paid for by third-party payers such as Medicare and managed care companies. However, these sources of payment are often inadequate to cover the costs of providing occupational therapy services. While many occupational therapy programs may be part of not-for-profit organizations, that does not mean that the program can afford to continue year after year without at least breaking even financially. Without covering at least the cost of providing services, it is hard for an organization to make the investment needed to develop new programs or expand existing ones. Perhaps there are clients who cannot afford needed services or equipment. Grants can be written to help underwrite the costs of new programs or to set up fund accounts to help clients pay for services and/or equipment. Rarely will grants be awarded to cover ongoing expenses of existing programs.

▼ WHAT GRANTS ARE ▼

Grants are awards of specific amounts of money for specific purposes. Grants can be awarded by either governmental agencies or private organizations. Regardless of the source of the grant, grants are only awarded to those who apply for them. Grants may be awarded to school districts, hospitals or other medical facilities, rehabilitation agencies, community-based organizations, and other for-profit or not-for-profit organizations (Prabst-Hunt, 2002). The organization requesting the grant must demonstrate in writing that there is a purpose and a plan for using the funds.

▼ WHERE TO FIND GRANT OPPORTUNITIES ▼

There are several places to look for grant funding opportunities. The Internet has literally hundreds of thousands of sites related to grant writing. Some sites focus more on tips for writing grants, but many others contain specific instructions for applying for particular grants. Table 20.1 lists selected web sites and the type of information found on those sites.

If you work at a facility that has a development office, the people working in that office can also be of great assistance. Hospitals and nonprofit corporations often have development offices. The staff of these offices can help you locate funding sources, help you write the grant, and in some cases, actually solicit funds for you. These people have lots of experience working with funding agencies. They know the tricks of the trade. It helps to have a friendly working relationship with development staff if you are going to be seeking grant money from any source. Few things make development staff angrier than staff from other departments going out and seeking funds without their knowledge. It is critical that development staff be aware of every time an outside source is asked to make a donation or fund a grant so they can know which funding agency has been asked for what contribution this year. In this sense, they act as gatekeepers for soliciting funds.

TABLE 20.1   Grant-Related Web Sites

Web Site Address	Agency or Organization	Type of Content
www.cbd.cos.com	Federal Government	Searchable listing of government contracts Limited access unless you subscribe to this service
www.fdncenter.org	Foundation Center	Directory of foundations Offers online and classroom training programs on seeking foundation money Has subscription service Has a foundation finder Free tutorials on grant seeking Online library has a glossary of terms used in grant-writing process
www.fundsnetservices.com/grantwri.htm	Grant Writing Resources	Fundraising and grant-writing resources Grant applications Proposal writing guides
www.tgci.com	The Grantsmanship Center	Grant information and grantsmanship training Includes grant sources by state search engine
web.cfda.gov/federalcommons/employment.html	Federal Government	Links to government contracts
www.niaid.nih.gov/ncn/write/index.htm	National Institutes of Health (Federal Gov't)	Lots of information on applying for NIH grants
www.ssrc.org/programs/publications_editors/publications/art_of_writing_proposals.page	Private Foundation	Lessons and tips for writing grant proposals
www.unl.edu/nepscor/newpages/noframes/pubs/winners/writing.html	University of Nebraska	Colorful handbook for proposal writing Includes chapter on how proposals are read
www.middlebury.edu/~grants/ tips_advice.html	Middlebury College	Provides advice on grant preparation Links to sites with information on grant writing

(continued)

TABLE 20.1 Continued

Web Site Address	Agency or Organization	Type of Content
www.jcdowning.org/ resources/generalguide. html	J. C. Downing Foundation on grant writing (private)	Provides general guidance See also *www.jcdowning/org /funding/grantmaking.html*
web.gisd.k12.mi.us/gisd/ Grants/GrantWritingTips. html	Genesee Intermediate School District in Michigan	Links to grant writing re- sources Dos and don'ts of grant writing

▼ GENERAL GRANT WRITING TIPS ▼

The awarding of grants is a competitive process. Granting organizations usually have less money to award than the total amount requested by grant applicants. This means there will be criteria established to help guide the decision making. It is critical that anyone applying for a grant know exactly what criteria will be used to determine who will receive the grant, and then to use that information in writing the grant (Fazio, 2001).

The two most important things to remember when applying for a grant are to follow the instructions and to proofread, proofread, and then proofread some more. While these seem like simple and obvious tips, they are absolutely critical to the grant application process. Granting agencies provide instructions to those interested in applying for grants. There is usually a good reason why they instruct applicants to organize the grant applica- tion in a certain way, so even if the applicant thinks it would look better if organized differ- ently, the instructions, as written, have to be followed. You want the reader of your grant proposal to look favorably at your proposal. A proposal that does not follow the grant agency's instructions may be discarded without being reviewed (J. C. Downing Foundation, 2000; Middlebury College, 2000).

Proofreading will ensure there are no typos, no grammatical or spelling errors, and no sloppy formatting or bad copies (i.e., printer running low on ink). As mentioned several times in this book, people form impressions of you and your program based on your written work. To be seen as competent and able to implement the proposed program, you have to write like a competent and polished professional. Not only does the proposal writer need to proofread the proposal, but it is a good idea to get a couple other people to proofread it as well. You want the application to look good. Be careful to choose words that the funding agency will understand. The person reading your grant request will probably not be an oc- cupational therapist.

While specific instructions for the organization of the grant application will vary, most will expect a cover letter as the first thing the granting agency will read. A cover letter needs to provide enough information to interest the reader and make the reader want to read the rest of the proposal. Be sure your cover letter is addressed to the right person. A phone call to the funding agency can tell you who to address the letter to (name, creden- tials, and title) and how to correctly spell that person's name (Genesee Intermediate School District [GISD], 2000). Be sure the cover letter is on appropriate letterhead and is signed by the person in the highest authority as possible for your program/employer. Strive to keep the letter to one page (J. C. Downing Foundation, 2000; SeaCoast Web Design, 1999). The layout and visual qualities of this page can set the tone of the reader's disposition toward your proposal.

Begin your grant application with an abstract or executive summary (GISD, 2000). The abstract describes the need your proposal intends to meet, what the project involves, who will benefit from this project, why this project is important, and the total cost of the project in greatly condensed form. This is a lot of information to squeeze into one or two pages, but it can be done if you are clear, direct, and do not elaborate on anything. You have the rest of the proposal to do that.

- What do you want to do? (description)
- Why do you want to do it? (rationale)
- How are you going to do it? (method)
- How much will it cost? (financing)
- Why are you (or your organization) the one to do it? (self-evaluation)
- What good will come from it? (benefit)
- How will you show that it's been done and evaluate its success? (program evaluation)

FIGURE 20.1   Key Topics for a Grant Proposal. *Source: Middlebury College, 2000.*

▼ WRITING A GRANT TO FUND A NEW PROGRAM ▼

According to Middlebury College (2000), in general there are seven key topics that are addressed in the narrative portion of the grant application, as shown in Figure 20.1.

In your proposal, you need to describe what it is you hope to accomplish in a few sentences without oversimplifying and avoiding jargon (Middlebury College, 2000). Make it easy for the readers to understand what you want to do. You may want to include subheadings to make it easier to find certain information. Suggested section headings include:

- Program Description
- Goals and Objectives
- Operational Plans
- Financial Plans
- Marketing Plans
- Supplemental Materials

Program Description

It is important to establish why you want to do what you are proposing to do. You need a reason to do what you are proposing, and it has to be better than "Because no one else has done it before." A needs assessment can be used to demonstrate the need for this project. Show data that supports your claim of need (GISD, 2000). Describe how you became aware of the need. Do not make any claims of need that you cannot support. Be sure that the need you hope to address is not so huge that your proposed program could not make a reasonable dent in it. In other words, as a quality improvement coordinator used to tell me, "You can't boil the ocean one teaspoon at a time."

In addressing how your proposal will meet an existing need, you will need to explain what steps you will take to implement your plan. Explain the mission of the program. By reading the mission and a description of the proposed program, the reader should have a good idea of what you are hoping to accomplish. Include a timeline for which activities will be done by what date leading up to and including providing the services you propose (GISD, 2000; Middlebury College, 2000).

In your grant proposal, you need to explain why you are the one(s) to do it (Middlebury College, 2000). Here is where you clearly state your commitment to the proposal. Do not assume the readers will know much about your agency or organization, so tell them why you are in a position to address the stated need (GISD 2000). If you have developed other similar projects in the past, explain the success you have had with them. It can be helpful to demonstrate how some aspect of the proposed program could be continued after grant funding ends.

You need to explain what good will come from this proposed program (Middlebury College, 2000). This is where it is helpful to know what the mission and goals of the funding agency are. You can explain what would happen if the proposal is not funded. Most funding agencies need to know that their money is going to support an activity that will benefit some portion of society in some way. It is up to you to clearly demonstrate that your proposed program will do that.

Goals and Objectives

The goals and objectives of the proposed program need to be clearly articulated (Prabst-Hunt, 2002). The goals are overarching, long-range program goals, while objectives are specific and measurable. These will be the yardsticks by which your program's success or failure will be measured. They can be written in ABCD, FEAST, RHUMBA, or SMART format (see Chapter 10). For example, if you are developing a program for musicians with hand injuries, your goal might be to provide musicians with a program to help their recovery that is sensitive to their unique needs for very precise finger movements. The objectives of the program might be:

- 90% of the musicians participating in the program will rate their satisfaction with the program as very helpful or outstanding.
- 85% will report a decrease of pain while playing of at least two points on 1–10 scale.
- The reinjury rate will be 20% or less 6 months after intervention ends.

This would be an appropriate place to describe any program evaluation activities you plan to conduct, and how the data you collect will be used. Explain how you will use this information to modify the project during the grant period and beyond (GISD, 2000). Make sure the evaluation plan relates to the goals and objectives stated earlier in your proposal. Be specific about who will do what as part of the evaluation process.

Exercise 20.1

Write a measurable goal for the following programs.

1. Your clinic is developing a summer program for school-age children who will not be receiving school-based services during the summer break. It will focus on handwriting, movement, and socialization skills.

2. You want to start a not-for-profit agency to help adults with developmental disabilities develop work skills.

3. The hospital would like you to develop a program for women who have had mastectomies and breast reconstruction surgeries.

Operational Plans

Operational plans include information on space, supplies and equipment, staff, and methods of service delivery. Specify any space, equipment, and supplies that you will need. If you already have any supplies or equipment that will help in the implementation, describe them (Middlebury College, 2000). You can be general and lump similar items into a category. For example, for the musician's rehabilitation program, you could say you need assorted splinting materials and various intervention modalities. This is usually sufficient for small items. For higher-priced items, such as test materials, list them separately. Describe your space needs in terms of square feet required and the purpose for each required space. If you are so inclined, you can describe your vision of how the space will look.

Include information that demonstrates the training and experience (related to the program) of staff that will be involved in the program (GISD, 2000). Full resumes of staff can be included in an appendix, so just summarize here. If you are going to use the grant to fund the salaries for the start of the program, explain how salaries will be paid in future years when the grant money is gone.

Financial Plan

The budget section of the grant needs to include dollar amounts requested as well as a justification for those amounts (GISD, 2000; Middlebury College, 2000). The funding agency may require budget forms to be submitted with the proposal. Every budget item for which you request funding needs to be justified in the narrative portion; there should be no surprises on the budget forms. Your budget is an estimate of costs to deliver the program to consumers. As an estimate, you do not need to record costs down to the last penny; you can round to the nearest dollar, or if you are dealing with large amounts of money, the nearest $100. If some items of the budget for the proposed program will be paid for in some other way (not from the grant), explain the source of that funding. When calculating salaries, remember to include benefits such as health insurance, paid time off, and so on. Do not include any unexplained budget items such as "miscellaneous" or "other" expenses. Never ask for more money than you realistically need.

Marketing Plan

You will have to explain how you will spread the word about your program. If someone is going to fund a program, they want to know that the program will have participants. This means that you have to explain how referral sources will find out about your program and how the public will find out about it.

Supplemental Materials

In addition to whatever forms are required by the funding agency and the narrative proposal, you may want to supplement your proposal with supporting materials. These materials belong in appendices at the back of the proposal package. Some of the kinds of items that might be helpful to include in appendices are included in Figure 20.2.

- Documents showing the type of business (for-profit, not-for-profit, charitable, etc.) the proposed program will be operated as. This could be in the form of an IRS determination letter to verify tax-exempt status, certificate of incorporation, and by-laws of the organization.
- Listing of corporate officers and board of directors
- Financial statement for the last completed fiscal year
- Current operating budget
- Resumés or biographies of key personnel
- Letters of support from people outside the organization (only a couple)
- Floor plan for space that will be used for the program
- Equipment and supply lists in detail (summarized in body of proposal)

FIGURE 20.2   Suggested Contents for Appendices. *Source: SeaCoast Web Design, 1999.*

Obviously, it takes careful planning and lots of time to put together a solid grant proposal. The more work you can do before you start writing, the better off you will be in the long run. Understand what the funding agency is looking for in a proposal. If possible, read the proposals of programs the agency has funded in the past. Do not hesitate to ask the funding agency questions throughout the process. Always keep copies of everything you send out. A paper copy is usually preferred to an emailed or faxed one; however, a paper copy can take longer than you think to reach the funding agency. Always allow twice as much time as you think you will need for a paper proposal to be delivered to the funding agency.

▼ WRITING OTHER TYPES OF GRANTS ▼

Other types of programs for which you might write a grant include setting up a fund for clients who have no insurance to pay for services or a fund to help families buy needed equipment that third-party payers will not pay for. You might write a grant to enable your clinic to purchase a particularly expensive piece of equipment. A grant request for these purposes would be less cumbersome to write than a grant to fund a new program.

As with a new program grant, you would begin by following the funding agency's grant application process. You would want to choose your words carefully so that any reader will understand the purpose of your grant. A cover letter and executive summary would accompany the narrative part of your proposal.

The narrative portion of the grant proposal for funding noncovered services or equipment would be shorter than a new program grant. You will be asking for a lump sum of money, so there will not be a need for any kind of detailed budget. Instead, you would explain why you think the amount of money you are asking for will be sufficient to meet the need. If the grant will enable your clinic to purchase a particular piece of equipment, be sure to include the cost of shipping, handling, and any training required to use it. There may be less of a need to create a marketing plan, unless the new equipment will allow you to provide some kind of service that you currently do not provide. Usually, if there is a fund to help cover the cost of services for the uninsured or underinsured, it is not advertised to the public. You may or may not let referral sources know that you have such a fund. The reason is that if you make too big of a deal about having this fund, you may find yourself overwhelmed with people who need your services.

The narrative of these types of grants should explain the need for creating the fund or buying the piece of equipment. Provide whatever data you can collect that demonstrate a demand for the services or equipment. You may make both arguments of fact (based on data) and emotions (based on feelings, appealing to the heartstrings) in demonstrating the demand. For example, if you are trying to create a fund for uninsured clients, you could argue based on the percentage of people without insurance in your community, the number of clients who were unable to pay for services. You could also argue that without access to your services, these clients will live in pain, may be more likely to reinjure themselves, and may become a burden to their families.

Since organizations donating money for grants want to know what benefit to the community will result from granting their money to your program, you will need to be very explicit in stating the benefits expected. Perhaps the new equipment will enable you to be more precise in your measurements of dysfunction. Perhaps the fund will enable families to purchase custom-made seating devices for children with multiple disabilities. Perhaps the fund will allow a client to be fully rehabilitated before going back to work, decreasing the likelihood of reinjury.

Rather than setting specific objectives and conducting a comprehensive program evaluation, these kinds of grants require less accountability. Setting an overall goal may be sufficient. Instead of a comprehensive program evaluation system, it may be enough to collect data on how the money was spent during the year, a simple accounting of expenditures.

Exercise 20.2:

Which of the following statements are true and which are false, relative to the grant-writing process?

1. _____ In the abstract, take the time to thoroughly explain the purpose of your proposal.
2. _____ Address all the review criteria established by the funding agency in your proposal.
3. _____ It is a good idea to ask lots of questions throughout the process.
4. _____ It is better to present a good-looking proposal than one that is well written.
5. _____ The timeline can be general rather than specific.
6. _____ Goals can be broad and not measurable.
7. _____ Objectives need to meet RHUMBA criteria.
8. _____ You must demonstrate that your project will have an impact on the target population.
9. _____ Program evaluation criteria need to be as detailed as the rest of the proposal.

SUMMARY

When seeking grant money to fund a new program, it is important to present a well-written, thorough, and specific proposal. The proposal needs to contain the information that the funding agency is requesting. While there are some general similarities in the information and format that most funding agencies want, each has some unique requirements and the proposal needs to be tailored to fit the funding agency. It is vital that someone applying for a grant follow the instructions of the grant funding agency. A cover letter can help create interest on the part of the funding agency in your proposed program. Somewhere in your proposal, you have to be explicit in what you propose to do, why you propose to do it, how you will do it, why you are the one(s) to do it, and how much it will cost to do it. A grant proposal has to be tailored to the funding agency and to the type of grant being requested.

REFERENCES

Fazio, L. S. (2001). *Developing occupation-centered programs for the community: A workbook for students and professionals.* Upper Saddle River, NJ: Prentice Hall.

Genesee Intermediate School District — Grants and Development Department. (2000). *Grants development summary: Dos and don'ts of grant writing.* Retrieved May 5, 2000, from *http://web/gisd.k12.mi.us/gisd/Dos_and_Donts_Chart.htm*

J.C. Downing Foundation. (2000). *General guidance.* Retrieved May 5, 2000, from *http://www.jcdowning.org/resources/generalguide.htm*

Middlebury College. (2000). *Grant preparation advice: Questions your grant proposal must address.* Retrieved May 5, 2000, from *http://www.middlebury.edu/~grants/advice.htm*

Prabst-Hunt, W. (2002). *Occupational therapy administration manual.* Albany, NY: Delmar.

SeaCoast Web Design. (1999). *Grant writing guide: 10-point plan for standard grant funding proposal.* Retrieved May 5, 2000, from *http://www.seacoastweb.com/resource/grant1.htm*

CHAPTER 21

Policies and Procedures

INTRODUCTION

In any organization there is a need for everyone to understand what is expected of him or her. People need to know what company policy is, and the acceptable ways to do things. This is where policy and procedure manuals come in. They help employees to know what the company wants employees to do without them having to ask a superior before doing anything. A policy and procedure manual can be used as a training tool and as a resource when any problems or questions arise (Kenny, 2000).

When facilities, agencies, or programs are credentialed (licensed, certified, or accredited), the surveyors who make the recommendation on credential status will always ask to see policy and procedure manuals. The manuals show that the organization has communicated with employees, in writing, regarding expectations in the workplace. Large organizations have multiple policy and procedure manuals. Often, they will have one for human resource policies and procedures, and then one for each department. Smaller organizations may have one manual that has sections for various departments.

A member of the occupational therapy staff may serve on a committee drafting policies and procedures. Occupational therapy staff usually write their own departmental policies and procedures. There is likely some sort of approval process for the development of new policies and procedures.

▼ POLICIES ▼

Policies tell employees what the company's position is on a particular issue. Some policies are required by law or by the credentialing agency. For example, federal law requires that employers have policies on nondiscrimination. A credentialing agency may require a policy on infection control.

In addition to explaining what is expected, policies often state who is responsible for complying with the policy. Individual names are not used, but it might list a job title or state that all employees are responsible for compliance. For example, a policy on infection control would be the responsibility of all employees while a policy on calibration of electronic equipment may be the responsibility of an electrical engineer.

Usually, policies also explain the purpose of the policy. The purpose of a policy on safety may be to protect the health of employees. The purposes of a policy on scheduling of clients are to be fair to both clients and staff and to make the most efficient use of resources (staff and space). The purpose is not always explicitly stated. If the policy is the result of a law or a credentialing requirement, the number of the law or standard can be cited in the purpose statement.

Finally, each policy needs an effective date. Any policy revisions also need to be dated. Sometimes, there is a signature page at the front or back of the manual that the department head or head of the organization signs to indicate that all the policies and procedures have been approved by the organization.

▼ PROCEDURES ▼

Procedures explain, in great detail, what steps need to happen to comply with the policy. A procedure for infection control would include instructions on hand washing, use of protective clothing (masks, gowns, gloves), disposal of infected waste, cleaning up blood or body fluid spills, and so on. A procedure for scheduling would describe how clients are assigned to a particular staff person, where the schedule is recorded, how appointments are made and canceled, and so on. A policy tells what, a procedure tells how. Because of occupational therapy practitioners' background in task analysis, they are good at breaking down the steps of a task, a necessary skill in writing procedures.

▼ WRITING POLICIES AND PROCEDURES ▼

It is essential that policies and procedures be written clearly, explicitly, and thoroughly to avoid any misinterpretations of policy. Readers should be able to find the important information as quickly and easily as possible. As technology and laws change, it is necessary to revise the policy and procedures. Figure 21.1 shows a sample policy and procedure for timeliness of documentation.

Notice that the sample policy and procedure is written in straightforward, simple terms. The policy addresses the rule, while the procedure describes the tasks required to meet the rule (University of California, Santa Cruz [UCSC], 1994). Make sure you avoid words or names that can become quickly outdated. Any words that may not be understood by a reader (especially a new employee) need to be defined right in the policy.

Timeliness of Documentation
Occupational Therapy Department

Policy: Documentation will be completed in a timely fashion according to the schedule below.

Responsible party: All occupational therapists and occupational therapy assistants.

Purpose: To ensure timely completion of the medical record.

Effective date: January 1, 2004

Procedure:
1. Orders will be acknowledged in the client's medical record by an occupational therapist within 24 hours of receipt of the order.
2. Evaluation summaries will be completed by an occupational therapist and filed in the medical record within 48 hours of the first client visit.
3. Progress notes are written at time of the visit by either the occupational therapist or the occupational therapy assistant, whoever conducted the visit.
4. Missed visits will be documented on the same day as the missed visit by the occupational therapist or occupational therapy assistant who was scheduled to work with the client.
5. Reevaluations/revised plans of care will be written by the occupational therapist at least every 30 days.
6. Discontinuation summaries will be written by the occupational therapist and filed in the medical record within 48 hours of discontinuation.
7. Occupational therapy documentation may be filed by any member of the occupational therapy department or by the unit coordinator on the nursing station.

FIGURE 21.1 Sample Policy and Procedure

Exercise 21.1

Write a procedure for the following policy.

Policy: Occupational therapy personnel will wash their hands between client visits.

Responsible party: All occupational therapists and occupational therapy assistants.

Purpose: To try to prevent the spread of infectious diseases.

Effective date: January 1, 2004

Procedure:

Exercise 21.2

Write a policy for the following procedure.

Policy:

Responsible party: All occupational therapists and occupational therapy assistants.

Purpose: To ensure that documentation meets with regulatory standards.

Effective date: January 1, 2004

Procedure:

1. Document each individual intervention session.
2. An occupational therapist or occupational therapy assistant may write and file the visit/contact note
3. The visit/contact note must include a description of the activities or techniques engaged in along with the degree of participation by the client.
4. The visit/contact note must include a description of any adaptive equipment, prosthetic or orthotics device that is provided to the client and whether the client or client's caregiver appeared to understand instructions in the use and care of the devices.
5. All notes must be signed with first initial, full last name, and credentials of the writer.
6. All notes must be dated and the time it was entered into the record noted.
7. All notes must be written in black ink.

SUMMARY

Policies and procedures tell employees what to do and how to do it. They need to be kept up to date. They are written in simple, direct, and clear wording. Any member of an occupational therapy department may be asked to write a policy and procedure. Some policies and procedures are required by law or by credentialing standards. In addition to complying with laws and standards, policy and procedure manuals can be used as training tools and as resources for questions or problems.

REFERENCES

Kenny, C. J. (2000). Policy and procedure manual should portray well-organized system. *ADVANCE for Medical Laboratory Professionals* (March 13, 2000). Retrieved December 5, 2002, from *http://www.deltasci.com/kenny3.htm*

University of California Santa Cruz, (1994). *Guide to writing policy and procedure documents.* Retrieved December 5, 2002, from *http://www.ucsc.edu/ppmanual/pdf/guide.pdf*

Answers to Selected Exercises

▼ EXERCISE 1.1 ▼

1. Jennifer attended three sessions this week. She needed encouragement to participate in the group discussion. She rarely made eye contact with the therapist or other group members. She mumbled incoherently and occasionally picked at something unseen in the air around her. When given a sorting task to do, she refused to participate. Her attention span was less than 2 minutes. She smiled while listening to classical music, and the mumbling and picking at the air stopped. When asked specific questions at different times on different days, she was not oriented to person, place, or time.

2. Chrissy was seen for a 45-minute session today. First she laid across the 30″ ball and proceeded to rock back and forth. Then she went to the bolster swing and moved it around in circles. She alternated between these two activities for 15 minutes. Next, she asked to draw in the shaving cream on a mirror for 10 minutes before washing and drying her hands. Next, she wrapped herself in a parachute. Finally, she quietly played with puzzles. She is demonstrating improved tolerance to touch and movement activities. The plan is to continue working on sensory integration activities to normalize her reactions to sensations, as outlined in the plan of care.

▼ EXERCISE 1.2 ▼

1. Jacques had surgical repair of tendons around his Ⓡ first MCP joint 4 weeks ago. He wears a thumb immobilizer splint, but is now allowed to remove it three times a day for 5 minutes of movement, within 20° of midline in flexion/extension and abduction/adduction. He reports that pain has decreased during Ⓡ thumb movements. No swelling is evident; the wound has healed. He has begun to swing a bat, gripping it fully with his left hand and gripping with his fingers only, thumb immobilized with his right. Maintaining upper arm strength is important for him to be able to return to finish the baseball season (he plays outfield for the Chicago Cubs). Plan to continue ROM exercises as prescribed, ice, and electrical stimulation.

2. Andrea has been referred to OT for work on self-care skills, following a TBI and fractured Ⓛ clavicle, humerus, and pelvis. Visited Andrea in her room to introduce her to OT and explain the schedule of visits. She has no memory of the accident or first week in the hospital. In the 5 minutes I spent with her, she asked my name six times. She knows she is married, but cannot remember the names of her four children. She appears to tire easily, yawning often. She is agreeable to therapy, but states she has no idea what she'd like to accomplish in OT; does not know what would be realistic for short-term goals. For a long-term goal, she would like to go home and live life like she did before her accident.

▼ EXERCISE 2.1 ▼

A	Combing one's hair
C	Elbow range of motion
A	Wheelchair mobility
P	Making one's needs known
C	Hand strength
A	Career exploration
C	Time-management
C	Understanding nonverbal communication
P	Posture
P	Endurance
A	Knitting
A	Balancing a checkbook
P	Making eye contact

▼ EXERCISE 3.1 ▼

1. **No,** *this would be appropriate for the biomechanical frame of reference. To be consistent with Bobath, the goal would address patterns of movement.*
2. **Yes**
3. **Yes**
4. **Yes**
5. **No,** *with this frame of reference you would expect goals related to expression of feelings.*
6. **No,** *with this frame of reference, goals would describe client expression of self-worth or use of stress management techniques.*

▼ EXERCISE 4.1 ▼

Case 1

C: What is there is clear, free from jargon, spelling and grammar seem OK.

A: Probably is accurate, but it seems incomplete; interpretations not clearly separate from findings.

R: It is unclear how anything in this note is relevant to her goals; it jumps around a lot.

E: Documented refusal on an activity (slide).

Case 2

C: OK, good use of an example to clarify.

A: Seems accurate, although some generalizing.

R: Note holds together well, seems relevant given the type of program it is.

E: No exceptions noted; there may not have been any to document.

Case 3

C: This note is not very clear. Probably meant hand therapy not hard therapy. How much progress is steady progress? What can he do now that he could not do at the time of his last note?

A: There are no good measurements in the note, but there may be in the flow sheet. It is OK to do this.

R: Note is relevant to client's condition.

E: No exceptions noted; there may not have been any to document.

▼ EXERCISE 5.1 ▼

1. If the wording of the release is limited to the discontinuation summary, this is a breach. In addition, providing such subjective information would leave the hospital occupational therapist open to allegations of defamation of character or slander.
2. This is OK, the case manager is contracted to the insurer.
3. This is a breach of confidentiality.

▼ EXERCISE 6.1 ▼

1. Probably carelessness
2. Carelessness
3. Fraud
4. Fraud
5. Fraud and carelessness

▼ EXERCISE 7.1 ▼

1. In client-centered therapy, the client actively participates in the evaluation and intervention processes (Schwartzberg, 2002).
2. When an occupational therapist countersigns any documentation, he or she is essentially taking responsibility for that intervention (T. Gutheil, as cited in Bailey & Schwarzberg, 1995).
3. A client's written consent is required before releasing any medical record information to anyone outside the intervention team (Fremgen, 2002).
4. Freud is credited with developing classical psychoanalysis in the early 1900s (Hagedorn, 1997).
5. Wordiness and the use of jargon can interfere with the reader's ability to understand the message (APA, 1994).
6. Occupational therapy helps people do the things that are important to them when circumstances create barriers to getting them done (Niestadt & Crepeau, 1998).

▼ EXERCISE 8.1 ▼

1.

7-10-04	Date of referral	Dr. Sara Bellar	Name of physician
Gertrude Silverstein	Name of client	daily	Frequency
one week	Duration	twice a day	Intensity

She had a stroke and needs to work on ADLs and IADLs   Reason for referral

Is this an adequate referral?   (yes)   no

Why or why not?

It contains the necessary information and it is appropriate for occupational therapy to work with a client who has had a stroke and needs help with ADLs and IADLs.

2. | __May 31, 2002__ | Date of referral | __Dr. Don Touchme__ | Name of physician |
    | __Jonathan Apple__ | Name of client | __unknown__ | Frequency |
    | __unknown__ | Duration | __unknown__ | Intensity |

<u>Work on ADLs.</u>   Reason for referral

Is this an adequate referral?   yes   (no)

Why or why not?

There is not enough information. Judging by the age of the client, Medicare may be the payer. In that case, more detailed information is needed. It would be OK to do the evaluation and then call the physician with a recommendation for clearer orders. Having the physician sign the plan of care provides written evidence that the physician certifies that the plan is appropriate. I would not provide any intervention beyond the evaluation without written or oral orders from the physician.

▼ EXERCISE 8.2 ▼

1. Typically, a minimal screening would be done; chart review and meet the client.
2. OK
3. This would be questionable. Before doing the screenings, decide if you have the knowledge and expertise to work with this population and know who would provide the services should they be needed.
4. OK

▼ EXERCISE 9.1 ▼

1. Descriptive
2. Interpretative
3. Evaluative
4. Descriptive, although more professional wording could be used.
5. Interpretive
6. Interpretive
7. Descriptive
8. Descriptive
9. Descriptive
10. Interpretive

▼ EXERCISE 9.2 ▼

1. R
2. R
3. I
4. R
5. I
6. I

▼ EXERCISE 9.3 ▼

1. *Interpretation:* Client is at risk for choking with thin liquids. Client needs to slow down his eating, swallow after chewing each bite, and learn to use utensils.

2. *Interpretation:* Client has limited range of motion in her left shoulder and elbow, and no range of motion in her left forearm, wrist, or fingers. She is unable to use her left arm in daily activities.

▼ EXERCISE 9.4 ▼

OCCUPATIONAL THERAPY EVALUATION REPORT

BACKGROUND INFORMATION
Date of report: 1-15-04   **Client's name or initials:** Jacob Olsen
Date of birth &/or age: 6-25-84   **Date of referral:** 1-14-04
Primary intervention diagnosis concern: Tendonitis of ⓡ thumb; neck, back, and ⓡ arm pain
Secondary diagnosis concern: Depression
Precautions/contraindications: Thumb immobilized until 1-28-04
Reason for referral to OT: Immobilization of thumb interferes with daily life tasks
Therapist: Rula LaRue, OTR/L

Assessments Performed: Observation and interview, UMOT interest inventory, ergonomic assessment of dorm room chair and desk, and the Multiple Dimension Hand Assessment.

FINDINGS

Occupational Profile: Jake is a student-athlete. He is a junior and is the starting forward on the university's basketball team. He lives in the athlete's dorm on campus. Jake spent many hours a day playing computer games with a joystick resulting in cumulative trauma to the thumb joints. Prior to this injury, Jake participated fully in occupations that supported his participation in all aspects of his life. Currently, any occupations that require Jake to use his ⓡ thumb are problematic. He is also at risk of future similar injuries if he does not make adaptations to his environment or the manner in which he participates in repetitive tasks. Since his injury, he reports being bored; that he has nothing to do with all the time on his hands. Being occupied is important to him. Prior to his injury, basketball and computer games were his only hobbies. He prefers hobbies that he can do alone. Jake would like to play in the NBA when he graduates. He would like to stay a bachelor for at least the next 10 years.

Occupational Analysis:

    Areas of occupation: Jake is independent in bathing, bowel and bladder management, dressing (sweats, no fasteners), eating, feeding, functional mobility, personal hygiene and grooming, sexual activity, sleep/rest, and toileting. Jake reports that he currently requires assistance with note taking and word processing. He did not identify any leisure interests beyond computer games and basketball. He says he is bored just watching TV and watching practice all day. He attends his classes, but is unable to write with his nondominant hand.

    Performance skills: Posture is poor, especially when sitting. Thumb is immobilized temporarily. Overall coordination, strength and effort, and energy are good, although the pain medication is making him a bit lethargic. Knowledge and temporal organization is good. Dorm room furniture has not been adapted to fit his needs; Jake said he did not know how to make adjustments to his environment to fit his needs. Communication skills are sufficient to meet his needs.

    Performance patterns: Jake reports a habit of playing computer games for hours nonstop, even when he experiences pain. He says it makes him uncomfortable to just watch practice and not play.

    Activity demands: Desk and chair do not fit his body, resulting in poor posture. Repetition of thumb movements caused injury to his thumb (as reported by physician). Basketball requires him to use his wrist, thumb, and fingers in repetitive motions.

(continued)

Client factors: Mental, sensory, cardiovascular, and respiratory functions intact. Right (dominant) thumb immobilized for 2 weeks. He has pain from his neck to his thumb/fingers on right side. He reports loss of appetite and energy. Jake says he can feel the anger of his teammates and coaches.

Contexts: *Temporal:* Middle of his basketball season, early in the semester. *Physical Environment:* Desk and chair are not fitted to his tall frame, resulting in poor sitting posture and neck, shoulder, and arm pain. Overuses his joystick (top button), which is not in an ergonomically placed position on his desk. Dorm room is shared with a teammate, it has a small kitchen, living room, bedroom, and bathroom. *Social/Cultural Environment:* Lives in dorm room, surrounded by males of similar age and interests. Family lives 6 hours away, visits a few times during basketball season home games. *Spiritual and Personal Environment:* 21-year-old college student, newly diagnosed. Limited personal interests (basketball and computer games).

INTERPRETATION
Supports and Hindrances to Occupational Performance

Hindrances include the current furniture in his dorm room, limited leisure interests resulting in boredom and lack of energy, dominating habit (computer games, difficulty terminating the activity), poor posture, and lack of support from his teammates and coaches.

Supports include encouragement from his family, independence in dressing and feeding, and a desire to get well. Except for his thumb, Jake is in good physical condition.

Prioritization of need areas:

Staying fit to enable return to basketball team.

Improving posture and modifying environment to decrease potential for future injuries.

Exploring alternative leisure interests.

PLAN

Mutually agreed on long-term goals:

1) Jake will return to the team, ready to play, in 2 weeks.

2) Jake will demonstrate two ways to adapt furniture to allow him to sit in an ergonomically correct positions in 2 weeks.

Mutually agreed-on short-term goals:

1a) Jake will do stretching exercises three times per day for each of the next 5 days.

1b) Jake will do a 1-mile run/walk twice a day for each of the next 10 days.

2a) Jake will verbally describe proper position for sitting in an ergonomically correct position by 1-22-04.

2b) Jake will verbally describe two strategies for safely raising the height of work surfaces by 1-25-04.

Recommended intervention methods and approaches: Promote problem solving, discuss and try out alternative leisure activities, exercises to stay fit for basketball, instruction in ergonomic principles.

Expected frequency, duration, and intensity: 3 x/wk for 2 weeks, 45-min sessions

Location of intervention: Occupational therapy clinic, Jake's dorm room

Anticipated D/C environment: Return to dorm life and basketball court.

Rula LaRue   *1-15-04*
Signature   **Date**

▼ EXERCISE 10.1 ▼

1. A: Client
   B: Prepare a meal
   C: Complete (meal), independently
   D: 3 consecutive days

2. A: Patient
   B: Bathe
   C: Using adaptive equipment if needed
   D: Less than 15 minutes

3. A: Bobby
   B: Retrieve tools
   C: Independently
   D: 3 out of 5 sessions

▼ EXERCISE 10.2 ▼

1. F: Use of a sharp knife
   E: Demonstrate safe
   A: Use of a sharp knife
   S: Without cuing
   T: June 1, 2004

2. F: Write
   E: Consistently
   A: Write
   S: Each letter correctly formed
   T: June 15, 2004

3. F: Going outside the house
   E: Will
   A: Retrieve from mailbox
   S: 3 consecutive days
   T: 4-17-04

▼ EXERCISE 10.3 ▼

1. R: Relates to using mouse with nondominant hand, result of the stroke
   H: By 1/2/05
   U: I would know what to do if I stepped in to work with this client
   M: Cut and paste 8 individual letters in 5 minutes or less
   B: Cutting and pasting is observable
   A: *You do not have enough information to answer this, but I assure you it is achievable.*

2. R: Relates to self-esteem, a symptom of depression
   H: By 6-26-04

U: I would know what to look for if I stepped in to work with this client

M: Each time (although it is vague) and consistently

B: Can observe if he catches himself

A: *You do not have enough information to answer this, but it seems achievable.*

3. R: Relates to motor development, which was presumably damaged during the near-SIDS event

H: By the end of the year

U: I could follow this goal if I had to step in for the usual occupational therapist

M: Independently sit without support for 10 minutes

B: Sitting is observable

A: *You do not have enough information to answer this, but it is achievable, trust me.*

▼ EXERCISE 10.4 ▼

1. S: This would make a significant impact on this client

M: 80% of opportunities to demonstrate proper lifting techniques

A: Seems achievable given what we know

R: Relates to back injury

T: By next week

2. S: This would make a difference in her life

M: Spilling two or fewer times per meal while using a fork or spoon

A: I think it is achievable in the time frame given

R: Relates to arthritis and vision difficulty

T: By April 22, 2004

3. S: This would make a difference in her life at school

M: Consistently cut within 1/4" of line

A: It is achievable

R: Relates to fine motor skills of children her age

T: By the end of the school year

▼ EXERCISE 10.5 ▼

1. **ABCD:** Client will independently don and doff splint within 2 days of receiving splint.
2. **FEAST:** The client will participate in a craft of her choosing for 10 minutes without moving around the room or shouting at other clients within 3 days.
3. **RHUMBA:** The client will maneuver her wheelchair from the front door of the school to her classroom without bumping into walls or people by 11-2-03.
4. **SMART:** By one month from now, the client will independently obtain a coffee mug on the bottom shelf of the above counter cabinet.

▼ EXERCISE 11.1 ▼

1. *Three suggested activities*: Roll and catch a 10" ball, build a block tower of three 3" blocks, and turn pages of a cloth book.

   Rationale: These activities require progressively finer coordination and approach age-appropriate level.

2. *Three suggested activities*: Practice feeding himself breadsticks or other large finger food, sort clothes for the laundry, and Velcro® checkers.

   Rationale: The more he uses it, the more comfortable he will be. May need to do both one-handed and two-handed activities.

3. *Three suggested activities*: Practice using a dressing stick, practice using long-handled shoehorn, and practice using a sock-aid.

   Rationale: Trying different adaptive equipment will allow client to see which is the most practical and useful.

4. *Three suggested activities*: Play games involving turn taking, require her to ask if she needs any tools in OT, role play casual conversations.

   Rationale: The more she talks with others, the more comfortable she will be.

▼ EXERCISE 11.2 ▼

Have an instructor or colleague read your plan and give you feedback.

▼ EXERCISE 12.1 ▼

1. _____ Ndebe appeared tired and listless.
2. _X_ Client said she is hearing voices telling her to cut her hair.
3. _____ Raësa got dressed by herself today.
4. _X_ Cyndee's mother said that Cyndee has not been sleeping well the past 3 nights.
5. _X_ "I am fat and ugly."
6. _____ Client is resistant to all suggestions.
7. _X_ "Where am I?"
8. _X_ Client made several lewd comments throughout the session, accompanied by sexually suggestive hand gestures.
9. _____ Saji's shirt was misbuttoned, untucked and stained.

▼ EXERCISE 12.2 ▼

1. _X_ The client's eyes were red and watery.
2. _____ Bob got angry.
3. _X_ He pushed away from the table and left the room.
4. _____ She said she hated strawberries.
5. _____ Pevitra wants to be recognized for good behavior.
6. _X_ Esai ate all of one food before eating the next food on his plate.
7. _____ The client appears bewildered when others get annoyed with him for invading their personal space.
8. _____ The client has a habit of twisting her ring around her finger during personal conversations.

▼ EXERCISE 12.3 ▼

L	Thumb	R
40	IP flexion	40
70	MCP flexion	30
55	Abduction	55

<table>
<tr><td colspan="3" align="center">Index finger</td></tr>
</table>

__50__	DIP flexion	__45__
__40__ (hyper)	DIP extension	__35__ (hyper)
__60__	PIP flexion	__85__
__50__	MCP flexion	__50__
__40__	MCP extension	__35__

Middle finger

__30__	DIP flexion	__50__
__60__	PIP flexion	__50__
__35__	MCP flexion	__30__
__40__	MCP extension	__30__

Ring finger

__30__	DIP flexion	__50__
__50__	PIP flexion	__40__
__35__	MCP flexion	__30__
__40__	MCP extension	__30__

Little finger

__0__	DIP flexion	__0__
__45__	PIP flexion	__30__
__35__	MCP flexion	__30__
__40__	MCP extension	__30__

Ulnar Drift

__20__	Index	__30__
__30__	Middle	__30__
__30__	Ring	__35__
__40__	Little	__40__

Finger	DIP flexion	DIP extension	PIP flexion	MCP flexion	MCP extension	Abduction	Ulnar drift
R Thumb	40			30		55	
L Thumb	40			70		55	
R Index	45	35-hyper	85	50	35		30
L Index	50	40-hyper	60	50	40		20
R Middle	50		50	30	30		30
L Middle	30		60	35	40		30
R Ring	50		40	30	30		35
L Ring	30		50	35	40		30
R Little	0		30	30	30		40
L Little	0		45	35	40		40

1. I think the list (the middle way) is the easiest to read and compare the two sides of the body. The narrative is by far the most difficult way to read and understand the information.

2. Present your idea to a colleague.

214 Appendix A

▼ EXERCISE 12.4 ▼

1. _X_ She has to be told to come out of her room.
2. _____ Client tried to use the TV remote control to call home.
3. _____ Client completed 75% of the task without assistance.
4. _X_ Usha does not interact with peers.
5. _X_ He can use public transportation independently.
6. _X_ Ashton can tolerate a moderately noisy environment for up to 10 minutes.
7. _X_ Client's statements are inappropriate to the situation.

▼ EXERCISE 12.5 ▼

1. A: Client has limited active range of motion in both hands. There is significant ulnar drift and swan neck deformity present in both index fingers. These limitations interfere with his ability to keyboard.
2a. A: Deshaun demonstrates sensitivity to tactile stimuli, but responds well to deep pressure and traction.
2b. A: Client denies he has left side neglect, yet he consistently ignores objects placed on his left side. He was unaware of his left hand coming off the golf club during the swing.

▼ EXERCISE 12.6 ▼

1. _P_ Practice writing his name three times per day.
2. _P_ Engage client in conversations about child care.
3. _____ She should be more careful in the kitchen.
4. _P_ Increase repetitions as tolerated.
5. _P_ Instruct in splint care and maintenance.
6. _____ Client needs to spend more time on leisure occupations.
7. _P_ Client will work on chewing food at least 10 times before swallowing.

▼ EXERCISE 12.7 ▼

Case 1: Client with severe arthritis

P: Construct splints and instruct in wear schedule and care of splints. Try alternative keyboards, mouse, and/or voice recognition software. Continue visit schedule as established in the plan of care.

Case 2: Client with sensory defensiveness

P: Alternate tactile stimulation activities with calming activities. Gently encourage touching toys with a variety of textures. Continue intervention as per plan of care.

Case 3: Client with left side neglect

P: Videotape client swinging a golf club and eating. Discuss evidence of left side neglect. Teach compensatory techniques. Continue 2x/wk home visits as per plan of care.

1. O
2. A
3. O
4. O
5. S
6. O
7. O
8. P
9. A
10. O

S: "What am I supposed to wear?"

O: The client sat on the side of the bed, waiting for dressing directions. While sitting there, she removed her nightclothes. When told what clothes to put on, she got dressed. The buttons on her blouse were not lined up. She put her anklets on under her TED stockings. She walked to the kitchen when dressed, carrying her purse, ready to go to day care.

A: The client is unable to initiate dressing, but when given cues she can dress herself with minor errors.

P: Clothing will carefully be placed in proper sequence and laid out the night before so she can see the clothes on the chair when she gets up. Continue to monitor functional status as per plan of care.

▼ EXERCISE 12.9 ▼

Case 1

S is OK.

O included some A terms by generalizing and analyzing performance.

A is supported by O.

P seems appropriate.

Case 2

S: Good

O: Needs to say whether he could demonstrate proper massage technique

A: Adequate

P: Good

▼ EXERCISE 12.10 ▼

Because of the variety of ways to write a progress note given the amount of information provided, it would be best to have a colleague or instructor look at your note and critique it. There is not one definitive way to write these progress notes.

▼ EXERCISE 12.11 ▼

Case 1

Kiki participated in occupational therapy twice daily, M–F and once on Saturday. She is showing increased visual tracking in both horizontal and vertical planes. Compared to last week, she gained 30° of horizontal tracking (now 90°). Last week she had 0° of vertical tracking, now it's 40°. She is no longer crying out with PROM of elbow, wrist or hand. She moved her ℞ elbow about 10° into flexion spontaneously, but not on command. Plan to continue to work with Kiki 2x/day M–F and 1x/day on Saturdays to increase Kiki's participation in life tasks.

Case 2

Client received OT for 45 minutes in a home visit today. She used a plastic bag hanging from her forearm near her elbow to collect supplies for a dinner salad and cottage cheese. She prepared the salad while seated on a tall stool at the counter. Client reported less fatigue than carrying one item at a time. Instructed client in use of bath bench. Client demonstrated proper use of the seat. She tried a sock-aid, she was successful in donning socks half the time. She said she was not sure she liked it but was willing to work with it for a couple of days. She was shown card holders, but did not like using either one. Plan to continue to work on meal prep, dressing, and leisure occupations 2x/wk at her home.

▼ EXERCISE 13.1 ▼

Case 1

Client received occupational therapy services as an outpatient 3x/wk for 3 wks and 2x/wk for 3 wks, for a total of 15 visits. Initially, she had severely limited shoulder flexion and abduction on her right side. She currently has nearly full range of motion in both directions. She was initially dependent in grooming and hygiene, now she is independent. When she started receiving occupational therapy intervention, she needed moderate assistance in feeding and dressing, now she is independent in these occupations. She is also now completing meal preparation on her own. She reports pain on movement of her right arm has decreased from a rating of 9 (on a 1–10 scale, 10 being excruciating) to a rating of 4.

Case 2

Client was seen in a work hardening program 4 hours/day, 5 days/wk. He initially demonstrated poor body mechanics when bending and lifting. He now consistently uses good body mechanics. He is reporting a significant decrease in pain both at rest (from 5 initially to 1 now, on a 1–10 scale with 10 being excruciating) and at the end of a therapy session (from 8 initially to 3 now). He is now independent in back strengthening exercises, which he reports doing twice each day. He is able to lift and carry 2 × 4s and nail them together to form a wall frame without complaining of pain, which he was not able to do prior to the work hardening program.

▼ EXERCISE 14.1 ▼

The information is different in every state.

▼ EXERCISE 14.2 ▼

1. To evaluate her performance in fine and gross motor skills such as using a pencil, paper, and scissors, throwing and catching a ball, and riding a tricycle necessary for full participation in school.
2. To determine if the way he is interpreting what he sees is different than other children his age.
3. To determine the ways in which her muscle tone and movement limitations interfere with her ability to play with peers and participate in school activities.

▼ EXERCISE 15.1 ▼

The information is different in every state.

▼ EXERCISE 15.2 ▼

1. _____ Needs to improve sensory processing.
2. _X_ Needs to navigate though the school without becoming lost or confused.
3. _____ Needs to increase range of motion to move more.
4. _____ Needs to improve writing skills.
5. _X_ Needs to feed self independently so that he can eat lunch.
6. _X_ Needs to sit in alignment to facilitate attention and ability to work.
7. _X_ Needs to effectively use a writing instrument to produce timely and legible written work.

▼ EXERCISE 15.3 ▼

1. Sophie needs to develop fine and gross motor skills that will enable her to play with same-age peers.
2. Bryan needs to be able to roll over, sit, reach, and grasp toys in order to interact with and learn from his environment.

▼ EXERCISE 16.1 ▼

The information is different in every state.

▼ EXERCISE 16.2 ▼

1. More helpful: Omar is able to make snips with a scissors, but not make successive cuts along a line. He moves the paper with the hand not using the scissors, rather than move the scissors to a new place to cut.
2. More helpful: Lucinda bumps into other children when they are standing in a line. She often will reach out and touch other children's hair or clothing, rubbing the hair or fabric between her thumb and index finger.
3. More helpful: Bethany frequently colors off the page, marking up her desk with paint, crayons, or markers. When supplies fall off her desk, she leaves them wherever they land. Her hands often get coated with paint or markers, leaving handprints on whatever she touches.

▼ EXERCISE 16.3 ▼

1. Objective 1a: Keyshawn will write his name on paper with raised or thick lines, with the first three letters formed and spaced correctly by December 1, 2003.

   Objective 1b: Keyshawn will write his name on a single line, forming each letter correctly and appropriately spaced by April 1, 2004.

2. Objective 2a: Miriam will attend to a fine-motor task for 5 minutes without going off task.

   Objective 2b: Miriam will attend to a group game for 20 minutes, going off task three or fewer times.

3. Objective 3a: Paul will cut single snips on short lines across a page without assistance by November 1, 2003.

   Objective 3b: Paul will cut an 8 1/2 × 11 piece of paper in half independently by March 1, 2004.

▼ EXERCISE 17.1 ▼

1. **Narrative progress note:**

   While practicing toilet transfers in the occupational therapy clinic bathroom the client fell, hitting his head on the sink. He returned to the unit under nursing care. Rest of session canceled today. Will resume intervention tomorrow.

   Incident Report:

   While attempting to teach the client a pivot transfer in the occupational therapy bathroom, the client fell, hitting his head on the sink. The client was wearing a transfer belt at the time, and I was holding on to it at the time of the incident. The client received a 1/2-inch cut on his forehead. Emergency call button activated, help came within 2 minutes. No loss of consciousness. I was not injured.

2. **SOAP note:**

   S: "I quit. I can't do this. I'm never going to get a job."

   O: Client made a number of errors while practicing filling out job applications. As she did so, her voice got louder and angrier. She cussed and began tearing up one of the applications. She got a paper cut. She stopped and stared at the cut for a while, then agreed to get it washed out in the sink and have a bandage put on it. She sat calmly for about 5 minutes after that, then engaged in a different task without interruption.

   A: Client got frustrated with the number of errors she was making.

   P: Discuss incident with client at next visit. Suggest alternative ways to express anger and frustration. Continue to pursue finding work as per plan of care.

   Incident Report:

   While working on completing job applications, client got agitated, swearing and tearing up the papers. She was unaware that she had cut herself until I pointed it out to her. The cut was on her right index finger, on the thumb side, near her MCP joint. It was less than a 1/2-inch long and very narrow. Edges were clean. Then she stared at it very calmly. I took her to the sink, ran it under cold water for a minute, and then applied an adhesive bandage.

3. **Note:**

Tyla was sitting at the table for snack time. She reached out and grabbed a knife by the blade end, cutting three of her fingers. The wounded hand was held under cold running water while help was summoned. Tyla's hand was wrapped in clean towels and pressure applied until her mom arrived. Plan to review safety precautions with children.

Incident Report:

The children were sitting at the table waiting for their snack. There were five children and two staff, one staff person sitting at either end of the table. The other staff member got up from the table, leaving a 10″ cook knife on the table. Before I could tell her to pick up the knife and take it with her, Tyla grabbed the blade end in her fist. She cut the palm side of three fingers. I picked her up and took her to the sink to run her hand under cold water. The other staff person called Tyla's mother. I wrapped Tyla's hand in towels and kept pressure on the wound until her mother could get there.

▼ EXERCISE 18.1 ▼

Case 1

1. The child is making good progress right now, so this is the best time for skilled intervention.
2. While she is making progress, she has not yet met her goals.
3. Providing graded sensory experiences requires the skilled judgment of an experienced occupational therapist.

Case 2

1. George is very motivated to go home, and going home would cost the government less money than keeping him in a nursing home.
2. To be able to go home, he needs skilled intervention from an occupational therapist in the areas of self-care skills, instrumental activities of daily living, and work.
3. With the use of adaptive equipment, it is possible that George could perform the tasks necessary to live at home and do some of the barn chores he has done all his life.
4. While the potential for recovery of all the body functions he had before the tumor is poor, his potential to participate fully in the life he chooses is great as long as he uses adaptive equipment and techniques to accomplish necessary tasks and activities. Many people have been able to run farms with the use of only one arm.

▼ EXERCISE 19.1 ▼

1. **50th Anniversary Committee Report**

The committee is looking for success stories that could be told in a 4-minute segment on the 11:00 news. After much discussion, we decided to speak to the other rehab departments about combining our efforts and tell the story of Mr. Hernandez (head injury). The committee is also looking for each department to put together a display table for the open house.

Action:

Rolanda will talk with the other rehab departments about combining our efforts and doing a story on Mr. Hernandez.

Rhonda will work with the fieldwork students on the display table.

2. **Budget**

The department needs to trim 10% of our expenses from the budget. We can trim some by being more conscientious about remembering to bill for adaptive equipment, conserving paper and food, and not walking off with each other's pens.

Action:

Each person needs to meet with Barb to discuss other ways to cut the budget.

▼ EXERCISE 20.1 ▼

1. By the end of each summer program, 95% of all children served will have met their program goals.
2. By the end of the first year of operation, the agency will place six participants into paid work situations.
3. Monthly client satisfaction surveys will show that 75% of women will say they were satisfied or very satisfied with the occupational therapy services they received.

▼ EXERCISE 20.2 ▼

1. __F__ In the abstract, take the time to thoroughly explain the purpose of your proposal. *Be thorough in the body of the proposal, not the abstract.*
2. __T__ Address all the review criteria established by the funding agency in your proposal.
3. __F__ It is a good idea to ask lots of questions throughout the process. *It is a good idea to ask questions as needed, but to not ask so many that you begin to be a bother to the agency.*
4. __F__ It is better to present a good-looking proposal than one that is well written. *While it is important to present a good-looking proposal, it is more important to present a well-written one.*
5. __T__ The timeline can be general rather than specific.
6. __T__ Goals can be broad and not measurable.
7. __T__ Objectives need to meet RHUMBA criteria.
8. __T__ You must demonstrate that your project will have an impact on the target population.
9. __T__ Evaluation criteria need to be as detailed as the rest of the proposal.

▼ EXERCISE 21.1 ▼

Procedure

1. Turn on warm water.
2. Wet hands thoroughly.
3. Use two squirts of soap from the dispenser, pushing the dispensing bar with the back of one's hand.
4. Massage hands with soap so that entire surface of both hands, front and back, and under nails are covered with soap suds. Keep massaging for 15 seconds.
5. Rinse hands under warm running water for 15 seconds, completely removing soap. Leave the water running.

6. Dry hands on paper towels. Use paper towels to turn off faucets.
7. Discard paper towels in waste basket.

Policy

Each client visit will be documented appropriately in the client's record.

▼ EXERCISE B.1 ▼

Corrected words are in **bold**.

calendar	**a lot**	definitely	sense	professor
accepted	**benefited**	necessary	against	develop
independent	maybe	**truly**	thoroughly	occasion
immediately	**until**	categorically	**tomato**	committee
noticeable	**chief**	**believe**	roommates	**apparently**

▼ EXERCISE B.2 ▼

Corrected versions are in **bold**.

Lake Superior
a monument to creativity   The Lincoln Memorial
The Bible   **a prayer book**
the school library   The Library of Congress
Occupational Therapy 101   **a foundations of occupational therapy course**
Professor Susan Jones   **Susan Jones, our professor**
my mother   Aunt Sylvia

▼ EXERCISE B.3 ▼

Wrong answers are in **bold**.

I am	**I were**	I was	**I are**	**I is**
We was	We are	**We is**	**We am**	We were
You are	**You am**	**You is**	You were	**You was**
He is	**She are**	**She were**	She was	**She am**
They were	They are	**They is**	**They was**	**They am**

▼ EXERCISE B.4 ▼

1. The client prepared a meal of toast and tea. **Yes**
2. The <u>balls was</u> placed into the container one at a time. **No**
3. The client is seated at the table with her feet on a footrest. **Yes**
4. After several tries, the <u>group make</u> a successful circle. **No**
5. The client's <u>family have</u> some concerns. **No**

▼ EXERCISE B.5 ▼

Errors are underlined and comments are in italics.

1. The client attended three occupational therapy sessions this week. She worked on sequencing the steps to making simple meals such as canned soup cooked on the stove, a frozen dinner cooked in a microwave, and a peanut butter and banana sandwich. The client <u>needed multiple</u> verbal cues <u>to</u> complete the tasks in the proper, safe sequence. She follows <u>one-step</u> directions only so far. Next week, will try <u>two-step</u> directions. *You do not need to use semi-colons, commas work fine when used the way they are in the second sentence.*

2. Bobby crawled <u>6</u> feet without assistance. He used a reciprocal <u>pattern</u> of arm and leg movement. He laughed when he finished and reached the toy. Bobby seems motivated. Then he tried to carry the toy back with him while he crawled but it kept falling, frustrating him. *You need an object for the third sentence; either Bobby, the client, or he could be used.*

3. R.L. stated that he slept well last night, but <u>was</u> still tired this morning. He completed 10 repetitions of shoulder stretches. Then <u>rested</u> for 5 minutes before repeating the exercise. He worked on his woodworking project with frequent rest periods. He <u>said</u> the pain is less than before. Plan is to continue to work on endurance, strength, and leisure skills. *This paragraph went from the past to the present to the past and then to the present tense. It should be entirely in one tense, and it does not matter whether you choose the present or the past.*

Grammar and Spelling Review

▼ INTRODUCTION ▼

All of us have read something that made us laugh because we misinterpreted the writer's intention. For example, a student of mine once wrote in a progress note "Patient was born at 36-week gestation with no significant pregnancy." While this is humorous to the reader, it is not funny when you are the one who wrote the laughable note in a client's official record. Then it's embarrassing. Beyond that, if it happens often enough the other professionals on the team may begin to think that you are not the brightest bulb on the tree. They may start to doubt your professional skills and knowledge. However, the impressions they form do not stop there. They may also view you as a typical representative of your profession or the academic program you attended. If they begin to doubt your professional skills and knowledge, they may project that and doubt the integrity of your profession or your alma mater. That is a heavy burden to bear.

Realistically, very few people are always accurate spellers or constantly grammatically correct. Occasional mistakes are normal. However, repeated mistakes need attention. Most colleges and universities have writing centers where students can go to get help with writing skills. There are also things you can do on your own to improve the quality of your writing.

I strongly recommend purchasing and keeping (do not sell this book at the end of the semester!) some kind of guide to writing. By this I mean a book like *The Everyday Writer* (Lunsford, 2001) or *Prentice Hall Handbook for Writers* (Kramer, Leggett, & Mead, 1995). Most occupational therapy journals use the American Psychological Association (APA) writing style, so using the *APA Publication Manual* (2001) is also a good resource. Find a book that explains and has examples of such things as punctuation and capitalization. A dictionary is also helpful to check your spelling.

In the next few pages, I will show you common errors in spelling and grammar and how they affect the way others perceive you. I will also show you a few simple rules to remember to help your writing look more professional.

Here are some examples of documentation gone bad, taken from *www.wwnurse.com.*

"On the second day the knee was better and on the third day it had completely disappeared." [*I assume the writer meant that the pain had disappeared, but that is not what the note says.*]

"Patient was released to outpatient department without dressing." [*This is not a pretty picture. Is the writer referring to dressing as in clothes, or dressing as in bandage?*]

"I have suggested that he loosen his pants before standing, and then, when he stands with the help of his wife, they should fall to the floor." [*The writer probably meant that the pants should fall to the floor, not the couple.*]

"Coming from Detroit, this man has no children." [*This is what happens when two unrelated ideas are put together in one sentence. The man comes from Detroit. He has no children. One statement does not have a causal link with the other.*]

"Patient was alert and unresponsive." [*I wonder what with this person was thinking. These would seem to be incompatible conditions.*]

"The patient lives at home with his mother, father, and pet turtle, who is presently enrolled in day care three times a week." [*Must be a talented turtle! Perhaps the writer meant that the patient goes to day care.*]

"I saw your patient today, who is still under our car for physical therapy." [*That must be some PT program! I can't imagine what the patient is doing there (strength training?) This is a problem with proofreading. Spell checkers would never catch this error.*]

The anonymous writers did not intend these to be funny. These are taken directly from medical records. A lawyer would have a field day in court with the writer of these statements, "And yet you claim to be competent at your job. . ."

▼ COMMON ERRORS ▼

Spelling and Proofreading

When one is writing quickly, it is very easy to drop a letter or blur two letters. As in the example of the patient "under our car" above, leaving the end "e" off of a word is a frequent occurrence. However, there is a big difference between car and care, mad and made, or scar and scare. Spell checkers on your computer will not catch these errors because all are real words. Only careful proofreading will catch this kind of error. Spell checkers do not catch misused words.

As found in *The Everyday Writer* (Lunsford, 2001), the rules you learned in grade school, such as "I before e, except after c, and when it sounds like an 'a' as in neighbor and weigh" still hold true today. Prefixes usually do not change the original spelling of a word. For example, by adding the prefix "un" to the word "necessary," it becomes "unnecessary." However, adding a suffix may change the last letter of the word to which it is added. When you want to make a noun ending in "y" into a plural, change the "y" to an "i" and add "es" (rather than simply adding an "s," unless the "y" is preceded by a vowel). For example, "key" becomes "keys" but "therapy" becomes "therapies." The silent "e" is dropped when adding a suffix that starts with a vowel, such as "ing," "able," or "istic." For example, "believe" becomes "believable." If the root word ends in a vowel–consonant combination, double the consonant before adding the suffix, but only if it is a single-syllable word or a word in which the last syllable is accented (Lunsford, 2001). If the accent is on another syllable, or the word ends in vowel–vowel–consonant or vowel–consonant–consonant, do not double the last consonant. For example, "stop" becomes "stopped," but "start" becomes "started."

Exercise B.1

Identify the words that are spelled correctly.

calander	alot	definitely	sense	professor
accepted	benifitted	necessary	against	develop
independent	maybe	truely	thoroughly	occasion
immediately	untill	categorically	tomatoe	committee
noticeible	cheif	beleive	roommates	apparantly

Homonyms are words that sound the same, but are spelled differently and have different meanings. The words in Figure B.1 are examples of some commonly confused homonyms.

I keep a small pocket dictionary next to my computer. If I am at all unsure whether a word is spelled with an "ea" or "ee," or if it ends with "able" or "ible," I look it up. When I am writing in a chart and I am unsure of a spelling, I will write the word a couple of differ-

accept/except	adapt/adopt	affect/effect	allusion/illusion
brake/break	buy/by/bye	capital/capitol	cite/site/sight
coarse/course	council/counsel	elicit/illicit	forth/fourth
its/it's	loose/lose	passed/past	hear/here
presence/presents	principal/principle	right/write/rite	patience/patients
their/there/they're	threw/through	to/too/two	than/then
weather/whether	who's/whose	your/you're	scene/seen

FIGURE B.1 Commonly Confused Homonyms

ent ways on a scratch piece of paper. Sometimes seeing it written two ways helps to find the right way. I do not depend on a spell checker to catch my errors.

There is a poem that was written by Jerrold H. Zar and has been widely adapted and circulated on the Internet, sometimes under the name "Ode to a Spelling Checker" or "Ann Owed Two the Spelling Checker" (*http://tenderbytes.net/rhymeworld/feeder/teacher/pullet .htm* on 5/8/02). Every word of this poem passes the computerized spelling checker programs but many of the words are used incorrectly. See how many errors you can find in the poem in Figure B.2. The author counted 127, more than half, of the words as incorrect, although they were all technically spelled correctly.

▼ CAPITALIZATION ▼

The first word of a sentence, names of people, cities, states, and countries are all capitalized. Names of companies, organizations, specific historical events, specific languages, and academic institutions are also capitalized (Lunsford, 2001). Names of seasons or professions are not capitalized (Lunsford, 2001). A common error that I've found in student writing is capitalizing the words "occupational therapy" in the middle of a sentence.

Exercise B.2

Which phrases are correctly capitalized?

Lake Superior	The Lincoln Memorial
A Monument to Creativity	A Prayer Book
The Bible	The Library of Congress
The School Library	a Foundations of Occupational Therapy
Occupational Therapy 101	Course
Professor Susan Jones	Susan Jones, our Professor
My Mother	Aunt Sylvia

▼ PUNCTUATION ▼

There are so many punctuation marks to choose from (,. /;: -!?). How do you know which one to use when? In clinical documentation, most sentences will end with a period. There are few instances where you would use an exclamation point or question mark, unless you are quoting a client.

It is easy to get confused about when to use commas, semicolons, and colons. Colons are used for three purposes: to introduce an explanation, a series or list, or to separate elements (Lunsford, 2001). According to APA style (APA, 2001), there should be one space after a colon, and it is usually not necessary to capitalize the first word after the colon. A

Candidate for a Pullet Surprise
by Jerrold H. Zar

I have a spelling checker,
It came with my PC
It plane lee marks four my revue
Miss steaks aye can knot sea.

Eye ran this poem threw it,
Your sure reel glad two no.
Its vary polished in it's weigh.
My checker tolled me sew.

A checker is a bless sing,
It freeze yew lodes of thyme.
It helps me right awl stiles two reed,
And aides me when eye rime.

Each frays come posed up on my screen
Eye trussed too bee a joule.
The checker pours o'er every word
To cheque sum spelling rule.

Bee fore a veiling checker's
Hour spelling mite decline,
And if we're lacks oar have a laps,
We wood bee maid too wine.

Butt now bee cause my spelling
Is checked with such grate flare,
There are know fault's with in my cite,
Of nun eye am a wear.

Now spelling does know phase me,
It does know bring a tier.
My pay purrs awl due glad den
With wrapped word's fare as hear.

To rite withy care is quite a feet
Of witch won should bee proud,
And wee mussed dew the bust wee can,
Sew flaw's are know aloud.

Sow ewe can sea why aye dew prays
Such soft wear for pea seas,
And why eye brake in two averse
Buy righting want too pleas.

FIGURE B.2   *Reprinted with permission. By Jerrold Zar, published Jan/Feb 1994 in the Journal of Irreproducible Results. Retrieved May 8, 2002 from http://www.tenderbytes.net/ rhymeworld/feeder/teacher/pullet.htm*

semicolon is used to link clauses of a sentence that are either closely related or joined by transitional phrases (Lunsford, 2001). Semicolons can also be used to separate words in a series that contain other punctuation, as in the example below:

The patient is independent in feeding; dressing, grooming and hygiene; meal preparation, serving, and clean up; and medication management.

Commas have multiple uses; however, in every case commas cause the reader to take a momentary break, a pause, in the sentence (Lunsford, 2001). Proper placement of a comma can change the whole meaning of a sentence. Here is an example (author unknown):

Woman, without her man, is nothing.
Woman, without her, man is nothing.

The words are the same, but the simple placement of a comma can change the entire meaning of a sentence.

▼ SUBJECT–VERB AGREEMENT ▼

Essentially, a subject is the primary noun in your sentence. It tells the reader who or what the sentence is about. The verb is the action part of the sentence. In a properly written sentence, the subject and verb will agree with each other in terms of the number of subjects and which person (voice) is being used (Lunsford, 2001). To help me remember, I recite little phrases like, "A person does what people do" or "I go where she goes." Here are some examples.

I am writing this sentence. (first person singular)
The committee is drafting a proposal. (third person singular)
The committee members are drafting a statement. (third person plural)
We are writing an interdisciplinary evaluation report. (first person plural)
You are writing an intervention plan for Ms. Rivera. (second person singular)

Exercise B.3

In the examples below, identify which verbs agree with which subjects.

I am	I were	I was	I are	I is
We was	We are	We is	We am	We were
You are	You am	You is	You were	You was
He is	She are	She were	She was	She am
They were	They are	They is	They was	They am

Exercise B.4

Identify which sentences have subject–verb agreement.

1. The client prepared a meal of toast and tea.
2. The balls was placed into the container one at a time.
3. The client is seated at the table with her feet on a footrest.
4. After several tries, the group make a successful circle.
5. The client's family have some concerns.

▼ VERB–TENSE AGREEMENT ▼

Within one sentence, as well as within one paragraph, the verb tenses should be the same (Lunsford, 2001). In other words, if the sentence or paragraph starts in the past tense it should stay there. You should not jump from present to past and back again. See if you can spot the verb–tense shifting in the following paragraph.

The client got out of bed unassisted and sits in her wheelchair. She pushes herself up to the sink and begins to adjust the temperature of the water. The water was too hot, so she turned down the hot water and turns up the cold water. Then she moistens the washcloth and adds soap. Next, she washed her face.

Changing tenses confuse the reader and are distracting when you are trying to make sense out of a note.

▼ PRONOUN–ANTECEDENT AGREEMENT ▼

Another common error is mixing singular and plural pronouns and antecedents in the same sentence (Lunsford, 2001). Pronouns are words that are used to replace other words (antecedents) in a sentence so that the sentence does not become repetitive (Lunsford, 2001). For example, in the sentence "The client sat down when he became tired," the pronoun "he" replaces the antecedent "the client." A pronoun should always agree with the antecedent in gender and in number (Lunsford, 2001). Here is an example of pronoun–antecedent mismatch: A *student* needs to be aware that *they* often have more homework than they anticipated. The corrected version is: Students need to be aware that they often have more homework than they anticipate. An alternative version would be: A student needs to be aware that he or she will often have more homework than anticipated.

When writing in the singular, choosing the right pronoun can become a challenge. The pronouns he, she, and one can be used. Some people object to the phrase "he or she" or "s/he" as cumbersome. Using "he" is viewed as gender insensitive, while "one" seems contrived or prim. As a writer, it is your prerogative to choose which word you use. Sensitivity does matter, so think things through thoroughly before you put pen to paper.

▼ PLACEMENT OF MODIFIERS ▼

Modifiers are used to clarify a sentence, adding important details or descriptions (Lunsford, 2001). However, when a modifier is used, where it is placed in the sentence can affect the meaning of the sentence. Here is another anonymous example of medical records humor (*www.wwnurse.com*): "Patient has chest pain if she lies on her left side for over a year." It sounds like she laid on her left side for a year. However, by moving the modifier, we can change the meaning of the sentence. *For over a year, the patient has chest pain if she lies on her left side.* It is still not a great sentence, but at least the meaning is clearer.

▼ INCOMPLETE SENTENCES ▼

As mentioned earlier in the chapter, a sentence must have a subject and a verb (Lunsford, 2001). If either one is missing, the sentence is incomplete. Find the incomplete sentence in the following paragraph:

> The client has been out of work for two months. She has difficulty maintaining a firm grasp on writing or eating utensils with her right hand. She can only use a keyboard for a few minutes at a time. Also comb her hair. Recovered mobility in her hand to dress herself with the use of adaptive equipment.

The incomplete sentence fits in the paragraph, it is just missing something. What about combing her hair? Can she do it or not? If she can comb her hair, how well does she do?

I heard an ad on the radio (presumably the speaker was reading from a script) where the store being advertised was trying to get shoppers to spend money in this particular store because of a great January sale. The speaker said something to the effect of "This year, resolute to save money, shop smart at our New Year's Sale." I think they meant to resolve to save money, make a resolution to save money. The word resolute is a real word, it just does not belong in the sentence in the way it was used.

There are many rules for speaking (and writing) English properly. They can be difficult to sort through. According to Lunsford (2001), the 20 most common errors in writing, listed in order of frequency, are:

1. Missing comma after an introductory element (i.e. In fact, the client. . .)
2. Vague pronoun reference (pronouns should refer to a specific antecedent in the same or previous sentence; if there is more than one possible antecedent, this can be confusing)
3. Missing comma in a compound sentence (i.e., when parts of a sentence could stand as a sentence on their own, but are joined by words such as "and," "but," or "or")
4. Wrong word (using improper homonyms or words with the wrong shade of meaning)
5. Missing comma(s) with a nonrestrictive element (an element not essential to the basic meaning of the sentence)
6. Wrong or missing verb ending (i.e., "ed" or "ing")
7. Wrong or missing preposition (i.e., "at" or "to")
8. Comma splice ("A comma splice occurs when only a comma separates clauses that could each stand alone as a sentence" [p. 16].)
9. Missing or misplaced possessive apostrophe (i.e., "client's" or "clients'")
10. Unnecessary shift in tense (i.e., from past tense to future tense in the same sentence)
11. Unnecessary shift in pronoun (i.e., from using "one" to using "you" or "I")
12. Sentence fragment (a part of a sentence is written as if it was a whole sentence)
13. Wrong tense or verb form (need to clarify whether the action is, was, or will be completed)
14. Lack of subject–verb agreement (subjects and verbs should agree in number and person; not every word that ends in "s" is a plural, so do not trust word-processing grammar-check programs)
15. Missing comma in a series (use commas to separate three or more items in a list)
16. Lack of agreement between pronoun and antecedent (i.e., "the client" and "they")
17. Unnecessary comma(s) with a restrictive element (a part of a sentence that is essential to its meaning)
18. Fused sentence (a run-on sentence with little or no punctuation)
19. Misplaced or dangling modifier (modifiers need to be as close as possible to the word they describe; a dangling modifier is one that does not seem to be attached to anything in the sentence)
20. Its/It's confusion (use an apostrophe only when you mean "it is" or "it has")

Not every reader of your documentation will be bothered by, or even recognize, each of these common errors (Lunsford, 2001). However, some readers might. If any item on this list seems unclear, that is probably a sign that a review of grammar rules would help your writing.

Exercise B.5

Find the errors in the notes below.

1. The client attended three occupational therapy sessions this week. She worked on sequencing the steps to making simple meals such as canned soup cooked on the stove; a frozen dinner cooked in a microwave; and a peanut butter and banana sandwich. The client need multipel verbal cues too complete the tasks in the proper, safe, sequence. She follows one step directions only so far. Next week, will try two step directions.

2. Bobby crawled six feet without assistance. He used a recipricol patter of arm and leg movement. He laughed when he finished and reached the toy. Seems motivated. Then he tried to carry the toy back with him while he crawled but it kept falling, frustrating him.

3. R.L. stated that he slept well last night, but is still tired this morning. He completed ten repetititions of shoulder stretches. Then rests for five minutes before repeating the exercise. He worked on his woodworking project with frequent rest periods. He says the pain is less than before. Continue to work on endurance, strength, and leisure skills.

SUMMARY

There are some general rules for grammar and spelling that are necessary for an occupational therapy practitioner to use in order to be perceived as a professional. Failure to write well can lead people to think the writer is incompetent. Proofreading one's writing is important. While proofreading, check for spelling, capitalization, punctuation, and word use. Watch out for incomplete sentences. Be careful with punctuation, subject–verb agreement, verb–tense agreement, and modifiers. There are many resources to help a person become a better writer, including dictionaries and grammar guides. Easy access to these resources is always helpful.

REFERENCES

American Psychological Association. (2001). *The publication manual of the American Psychological Association* (5th ed.). Washington, DC: Author.

Funny comments found in medical records. Retrieved May 6, 2002, from *http://www.wwnurse.com*

Kramer, M. G., Leggett, G., & Mead, C. D. (1995). *Prentice Hall handbook for writers* (12th ed.). Englewood Cliffs, NJ: Prentice Hall.

Lunsford, A. (2001). *The everyday writer* (2nd ed.). New York: Bedford/St. Martin's.

Zar, J. H. (1994). *Candidate for a pullet surprise.* Retrieved May 8, 2002, from *http://tenderbytes.net/rhymeworld/feeder/teacher/pullet.htm*

AOTA Standards of Practice for Occupational Therapy

▼ PREFACE ▼

The *Standards of Practice for Occupational Therapy* are requirements for the occupational therapy practitioner (registered occupational therapist and certified occupational therapy assistant) for the delivery of occupational therapy services that are client centered and interactive in nature (American Occupational Therapy Association [AOTA], 1995). The registered occupational therapist supervises the certified occupational therapy assistant, and both work together in a collaborative manner to meet the needs of the client. However, the registered occupational therapist is ultimately responsible and accountable for the delivery of occupational therapy services. This document identifies minimum standards for occupational therapy practice.

The minimum educational requirements for the registered occupational therapist are described in the current *Essentials and Guidelines of an Accredited Educational Program for the Occupational Therapist* (AOTA, 1991a). The minimum educational requirements for the certified occupational therapy assistant are described in the current *Essentials and Guidelines of an Accredited Educational Program for the Occupational Therapy Assistant* (AOTA, 1991b).

▼ DEFINITIONS ▼

Assessment. Specific tools, instruments, or interactions used during the evaluation process. An assessment is a component part of the evaluation process (Hinojosa & Kramer, 1998).

Client. A person, group, program, organization, or community for whom the occupational therapy practitioner is providing services (AOTA, 1995).

Evaluation. The process of obtaining and interpreting data necessary for understanding the individual, system, or situation. This includes planning for and documenting the evaluation process, results, and recommendations, including the need for intervention and/or potential change in the intervention plan (Hinojosa & Kramer, 1998).

Occupational therapy practitioner. Any individual initially certified to practice as an occupational therapist or occupational therapy assistant or licensed or regulated by a state, district, commonwealth, or territory of the United States to practice as an occupational therapist or occupational therapy assistant (AOTA, 1997).

American Occupational Therapy Association. (1998). *Occupational therapy standards of practice.* Retrieved January 5, 2001 from *http://www.aota.org/otsp.asp*

Performance areas. Broad categories of human activity that are typically part of daily life. They are activities of daily living, work and productive activities, and play or leisure activities (AOTA, 1994c).

Performance components. Elements of performance required for successful engagement in performance areas, including sensorimotor, cognitive, psychosocial, and psychological aspects (AOTA, 1994c).

Performance contexts. Situations or factors that influence an individual's engagement in desired and/or required performance areas. Performance contexts consist of *temporal* aspects (chronological, developmental, life cycle, disability status) and *environmental* aspects (physical, social, political, cultural) (AOTA, 1994c).

Screening. Obtaining and reviewing data relevant to a potential client to determine the need for further evaluation and intervention.

Transition. Process involving actions coordinated to prepare for or facilitate change, such as from one functional level to another, from one life stage to another, from one program to another, or from one environment to another.

▼ STANDARD I: PROFESSIONAL STANDING AND RESPONSIBILITY ▼

1. An occupational therapy practitioner delivers occupational therapy services that reflect the philosophical base of occupational therapy (AOTA, 1979) and are consistent with the established principles and concepts of theory and practice.

2. An occupational therapy practitioner delivers occupational therapy services in accordance with AOTA's standards and policies. The nature and scope of occupational therapy services provided must be in accordance with laws and regulations.

3. An occupational therapy practitioner maintains current licensure, registration, or certification as required by laws or regulations.

4. An occupational therapy practitioner abides by AOTA's *Occupational Therapy Code of Ethics* (AOTA, 1994a).

5. An occupational therapy practitioner assures continued competency by establishing, maintaining, and updating professional performance, knowledge, and skills.

6. A registered occupational therapist provides supervision for a certified occupational therapy assistant in a collaborative manner as defined by official AOTA documents and in accordance with laws or regulations.

7. A certified occupational therapy assistant seeks and follows supervision from a registered occupational therapist in the delivery of occupational therapy services.

8. An occupational therapy practitioner is knowledgeable about AOTA's *Standards of Practice for Occupational Therapy;* the *Philosophical Base of Occupational Therapy* (AOTA, 1979); and other AOTA, state, and federal documents relevant to practice and service delivery.

9. An occupational therapy practitioner maintains current knowledge of legislative, political, social, cultural, and reimbursement issues that affect clients and the practice of occupational therapy.

10. A registered occupational therapist is knowledgeable about research in the practitioner's areas of practice. A registered occupational therapist applies timely research findings ethically and appropriately to evaluation and intervention processes and discusses applicable research findings with the certified occupational therapy assistant.

11. A registered occupational therapist systematically assesses the efficiency and effectiveness of occupational therapy services and designs and implements processes to support quality service delivery.

12. A certified occupational therapy assistant collaborates with the registered occupational therapist in assessing the efficiency and effectiveness of occupational therapy

services and assists in designing and implementing processes to support quality service delivery.

▼ STANDARD II: REFERRAL ▼

1. A registered occupational therapist accepts and responds to referrals in accordance with AOTA's *Statement of Occupational Therapy Referral* (AOTA, 1994b) and in compliance with laws or regulations.
2. A registered occupational therapist accepts and responds to referrals for evaluation or evaluation with intervention in performance areas, performance components, or performance contexts when clients may have a functional limitation or disability or may be at risk for a disabling condition.
3. A registered occupational therapist refers clients to appropriate resources when the needs of the client can best be served by the expertise of other professionals or services.
4. An occupational therapy practitioner educates current and potential referral sources about the scope of occupational therapy services and the process of initiating occupational therapy services.

▼ STANDARD III: SCREENING ▼

1. A registered occupational therapist screens independently or as a member of a team in accordance with laws and regulations. A certified occupational therapy assistant may contribute to the screening process under the supervision of a registered occupational therapist.
2. A registered occupational therapist selects screening methods appropriate to the client's performance context.
3. A registered occupational therapist communicates screening results and recommendations to the appropriate person, group, or organization. A certified occupational therapy assistant may contribute to this process under the supervision of a registered occupational therapist.

▼ STANDARD IV: EVALUATION ▼

1. A registered occupational therapist evaluates performance areas, performance components, and performance contexts. A certified occupational therapy assistant may contribute to the evaluation process under the supervision of a registered occupational therapist.
2. An occupational therapy practitioner educates clients and appropriate others about the purposes and procedures of the occupational therapy evaluation.
3. A registered occupational therapist selects assessments to evaluate the client's level of function related to performance areas, performance components, and performance contexts.
4. An occupational therapy practitioner follows defined protocols when standardized assessments are used.
5. A registered occupational therapist analyzes, interprets, and summarizes assessment data to determine the client's current functional status and to develop an appropriate intervention plan. The certified occupational therapy assistant may contribute to this process under the supervision of a registered occupational therapist.
6. A registered occupational therapist completes and documents occupational therapy evaluation results within the time frames, formats, and standards established by

practice settings, government agencies, external accreditation programs, and payers. A certified occupational therapy assistant may contribute to documentation of evaluation results under the supervision of a registered occupational therapist and in accordance with laws or regulations.

7. A registered occupational therapist communicates evaluation results, within the boundaries of client confidentiality, to the appropriate person, group, or organization. A certified occupational therapy assistant may contribute to this process under the supervision of a registered occupational therapist.

8. A registered occupational therapist recommends additional consultations when the results of the evaluation indicate that intervention by other professionals would be beneficial.

▼ STANDARD V: INTERVENTION PLAN ▼

1. A registered occupational therapist develops and documents an intervention plan that is based on the results of the occupational therapy evaluation and the desires and expectations of the client and appropriate others about the outcome of service. A certified occupational therapy assistant may contribute to the intervention plan under the supervision of a registered occupational therapist.

2. A registered occupational therapist ensures that the intervention plan is documented within time frames, formats, and standards established by the practice settings, agencies, external accreditation programs, and payers.

3. A registered occupational therapist includes in the intervention plan client-centered goals that are clear, measurable, behavioral, functional, contextually relevant, and appropriate to the client's needs, desires, and expected outcomes. A certified occupational therapy assistant may contribute to this process.

4. A registered occupational therapist includes in the intervention plan the scope, frequency, duration of services, and the needs of the client.

5. A registered occupational therapist reviews the intervention plan with the client and appropriate others. A certified occupational therapy assistant may contribute to this process.

▼ STANDARD VI: INTERVENTION ▼

1. A registered occupational therapist implements the intervention plan through the use of specified purposeful activities or therapeutic methods that are meaningful to the client and are effective methods for enhancing occupational performance. A certified occupational therapy assistant may implement the intervention plan under the supervision of a registered occupational therapist.

2. An occupational therapy practitioner informs clients and appropriate others regarding the relative benefits and risks of the intervention.

3. An occupational therapy practitioner maintains or seeks current information on resources relevant to the client's needs.

4. A registered occupational therapist reevaluates during the intervention process and documents changes in the client's goals, performance, and needs. A certified occupational therapy assistant may contribute to the reevaluation process.

5. A registered occupational therapist modifies the intervention process to reflect changes in client status, desires, and response to intervention. A certified occupational therapy assistant may identify the need for modifications and may contribute to the intervention modifications under the supervision of a registered occupational therapist.

6. An occupational therapy practitioner documents the occupational therapy services provided within the time frames, formats, and standards established by the practice settings, agencies, external accreditation programs, and payers.

▼ STANDARD VII: TRANSITION SERVICES ▼

1. A registered occupational therapist prepares a formal transition plan that is based on identified needs. A certified occupational therapy assistant may contribute to the preparation of a formal transition plan.
2. An occupational therapy practitioner facilitates the transition process in cooperation with the client, family members, significant others, team, and community resources and individuals, when appropriate.

▼ STANDARD VIII: DISCONTINUATION ▼

1. A registered occupational therapist discontinues services when the client has achieved predetermined goals, has achieved maximum benefit from occupational therapy services, or does not desire to continue services. A certified occupational therapy assistant may recommend discontinuation of occupational therapy services to the supervising registered occupational therapist.
2. A registered occupational therapist prepares and implements a discontinuation plan that addresses appropriate follow-up resources. A certified occupational therapy assistant may contribute to the implementation of a discontinuation plan under the supervision of a registered occupational therapist.
3. A registered occupational therapist documents changes in the client's status between the initial evaluation and discontinuation of services. A certified occupational therapy assistant may contribute to the process under the supervision of a registered occupational therapist.
4. A registered occupational therapist documents recommendations for follow-up or reevaluation, when applicable.

REFERENCES

American Occupational Therapy Association. (1979). The philosophical base of occupational therapy. *American Journal of Occupational Therapy, 33,* 785.

American Occupational Therapy Association. (1991a). Essentials and guidelines of an accredited educational program for the occupational therapist. *American Journal of Occupational Therapy, 45,* 1077–1084.

American Occupational Therapy Association. (1991b). Essentials and guidelines of an accredited educational program for the occupational therapy assistant. *American Journal of Occupational Therapy, 45,* 1085–1092.

American Occupational Therapy Association. (1994a). Occupational therapy code of ethics. *American Journal of Occupational Therapy, 48,* 1037–1038.

American Occupational Therapy Association. (1994b). Statement of occupational therapy referral. *American Journal of Occupational Therapy, 48,* 1034.

American Occupational Therapy Association. (1994c). Uniform terminology for occupational therapy-Third edition. *American Journal of Occupational Therapy, 49,* 1047–1054.

American Occupational Therapy Association. (1995). Concept paper: Service delivery in occupational therapy. *American Journal of Occupational Therapy, 49,* 1029–1031.

American Occupational Therapy Association. (1997). Bylaws. Article III, Section 1. Bethesda, MD: Author.

Hinojosa, J., & Kramer, P. (Eds.). (1998). *Occupational therapy evaluation of clients: Obtaining and interpreting data.* Bethesda, MD: American Occupational Therapy Association.

AUTHOR

Commission on Practice
Linda Kohlman Thomson, MOT, OT(C), FAOTA, Chairperson
Adopted by the Representative Assembly 1998M15

NOTE: This document replaces the 1994 *Standards of Practice for Occupational Therapy.*

AOTA Guidelines for Documentation
of Occupational Therapy

Documentation is necessary whenever professional services are provided to a client. Occupational therapists and occupational therapy assistants under the supervision of an occupational therapist determine the appropriate type of documentation and document the services provided within their scope of practice. This document, based on the *Occupational Therapy Practice Framework: Domain and Process* (American Occupational Therapy Association [AOTA], 2002), describes the components and the purpose of professional documentation used in occupational therapy. AOTA's *Standards of Practice for Occupational Therapy* (1998) state: "An occupational therapy practitioner documents the occupational therapy services provided within the time frames, format, and standards established by the practice settings, agencies, external accreditation programs, and payers." In this document, *client* may refer to an individual, family/caregivers, group, or population.

The purpose of documentation is to:

- Articulate the rationale for provision of occupational therapy services and the relationship of this service to the client's outcomes
- Reflect the therapist's clinical reasoning and professional judgment
- Communicate information about the client from the occupational therapy perspective
- Create a chronological record of client status, occupational therapy services provided to the client, and client outcomes

▼ TYPES OF DOCUMENTATION ▼

The following box outlines common types of reports. Depending on the service delivery and setting, reports may be named differently or combined and reorganized to meet the specific needs of the setting. Occupational therapy documentation should always record the professional's activity in the areas of evaluation, intervention, and outcomes (AOTA, 2002).

American Occupational Therapy Association. (2003). *Guidelines for Documentation of Occupational Therapy*. Retrieved on June 27, 2003, from *http://www.aota.org/members/area2/docs/ra2.pdf*

Process Areas	Type of Report
I. EVALUATION	A. Evaluation or Screening Report
	B. Reevaluation Report
II. INTERVENTION	1. Intervention Plan
	2. Occupational Therapy Service Contacts
	3. Progress Report
	4. Transition Plan
III. OUTCOMES	5. Discharge/Discontinuation Report

▼ CONTENT OF REPORTS ▼

I. Evaluation
   A. Evaluation or Screening Report
      1. Documents the referral source and data gathered through the evaluation process. Includes:
         a. Description of the client's occupational profile
         b. Analysis of occupational performance and identification of factors that hinder and support performance in areas of occupation
         c. Delineation of specific areas of occupation that will be targeted for intervention and outcomes expected
      2. An abbreviated evaluation process (e.g., screening) documents only limited areas of occupation applicable to the client and to the situation.
      3. Suggested content with examples:
         a. Client information—name/agency, date of birth, gender, applicable medical/educational/developmental diagnoses, precautions, and contraindications
         b. Referral information—date and source of referral, services requested, reason for referral, funding source, and anticipated length of service
         c. Occupational profile—client's reason for seeking occupational therapy services, current areas of occupation that are successful and areas that are problematic, contexts that support or hinder occupations, medical/educational/work history, occupational history (e.g., patterns of living, interest, values), client's priorities, and targeted outcomes
         d. Assessments used and results—types of assessments used and results (e.g., interviews, record reviews, observations, and standardized or nonstandardized assessments), description of the client factors, contextual aspects or features of the activities that facilitate or inhibit performance, and confidence in test results
         e. Summary and analysis—interpretation and summary of data as it is related to occupational profile and referring concern
         f. Recommendation—judgement regarding appropriateness of occupational therapy services or other services
         Note: Intervention goals addressing anticipated outcomes, objectives, and frequency of therapy are listed on the Intervention Plan.
   B. Reevaluation Report
      1. Documents the results of the reevaluation process. Frequency of reevaluation depends upon the needs of the setting and the progress of the client.
      2. Suggested content with examples:
         a. Client information—name/agency, date of birth, gender, applicable medical/educational/developmental diagnoses, precautions, and contraindications

      b.   Occupational profile—updates on current areas of occupation that are successful and that are problematic, contexts that support or hinder occupations, summary of any new medical/educational/work information, and updates or changes to client's priorities and targeted outcomes

      c.   Reevaluation results—focus of reevaluation, specific types of assessments used, and client's performance and subjective responses

      d.   Summary and analysis—interpretation and summary of data as related to referring concern, and comparison of results with previous evaluation results

      e.   Recommendations—changes to occupational therapy services, revision or continuation of goals and objectives, frequency of occupational therapy services, and recommendation for referral to other professionals or agencies where applicable

II. Intervention

A. Intervention Plan

1. Documents the goals, intervention approaches, and types of interventions to be used to achieve the client's identified targeted outcomes based on results of evaluation or reevaluation processes. Includes recommendations or referrals to other professionals and agencies.

2. Suggested content with examples:

      a.   Client information—name/agency, date of birth, gender, precautions, and contraindications

      b.   Intervention goals—measurable goals and short-term objectives directly related to the client's ability to engage in desired occupations

      c.   Intervention approaches and types of interventions to be used—intervention approaches that include: create/promote, establish/restore, maintain, modify, and prevent; types of interventions that include: consultation process, education process, therapeutic use of activities to enhance occupation, and therapeutic use of self

      d.   Service delivery mechanisms—service provider, service location, and frequency and duration of services

      e.   Plan for discharge—discontinuation criteria, location of discharge, and follow-up care

      f.   Outcome measures—outcomes that include improved occupational performance, client satisfaction, role competence, improved health and wellness, prevention of further difficulties, and improved quality of life

      g.   Professionals responsible and date of plan—names and positions of persons overseeing intervention plan, date plan was developed, and date when plan was modified or reviewed

B. Occupational Therapy Service Contacts

1. Documents contacts between the client and the occupational therapist or the occupational therapy assistant. Records the types of interventions used and client's response. Includes telephone contacts, interventions, and meetings with others.

2. Suggested content with examples:

      a.   Client information—name/agency, date of birth, gender, diagnosis, precautions, and contraindications

      b.   Therapy log—date, type of contact, names/positions of persons involved, summary or significant information communicated during contacts, client attendance and participation in intervention, reason service is missed, types of interventions used, client's response, environmental or task modification, assistive or adaptive devices used or fabricated, statement of any training education or consultation provided, and the persons present

C. Progress Report

1. Summarizes intervention process and documents client's progress toward goals achievement. Includes new data collected; modifications of treatment plan; and statement of need for continuation, discontinuation, or referral.

2. Suggested content with examples:
   a. Client information—name/agency, date of birth, gender, diagnosis, precautions, and contraindications
   b. Summary of services provided—brief statement of frequency of services and length of time services have been provided; techniques and strategies used; environmental or task modifications provided; adaptive equipment or orthotics provided; medical, educational, or other pertinent client updates; client's response to occupational therapy services; and programs or training provided to the client or caregivers
   c. Current client performance—client's progress toward the goals, and client's performance in areas of occupations
   d. Plan or recommendations—recommendations and rationale as well as client's input to changes or continuation of plan

D. Transition Plan
   1. Documents the formal transition plan and is written when client is transitioning from one service setting to another within a service delivery system.
   2. Suggested content with examples:
      a. Client information—name/agency, date of birth, gender, diagnosis, precautions, and contraindications
      b. Client's current status—client's current performance in occupations
      c. Transition plan—name of current service setting and name of setting to which client will transition, reason for transition, time frame in which transition will occur, and outline of activities to be carried out during the transition plan
      d. Recommendations—recommendations and rationale for occupational therapy services, modifications or accommodations needed, and assistive technology and environmental modifications needed

III. Outcomes
   A. Discharge Report—Summary of Occupational Therapy Services and Outcomes
      1. Summarize the changes in client's ability to engage in occupations between the initial evaluation and discontinuation of services and make recommendations as applicable
      2. Suggested content with examples:
         a. Client information—name/agency, date of birth, gender, diagnosis, precautions, and contraindications
         b. Summary of intervention process—date of initial and final service; frequency, number of sessions, summary of interventions used; summary of progress toward goals; and occupational therapy outcomes—initial client status and ending status regarding engagement in occupations, client's assessment of efficacy of occupational therapy services
         c. Recommendations—recommendations pertaining to the client's future needs; specific follow-up plans, if applicable; and referrals to other professionals and agencies, if applicable

▼ APPENDIX A ▼

Fundamental Elements of Documentation

Each occupational therapy client has a client record maintained as a permanent file. The record is maintained in a professional and legal fashion (i.e., organized, legible, concise, clear, accurate, complete, current, grammatically correct, and objective). The following elements are present in all documentation:

1. Client's full name and case number (if applicable) on each page of documentation.
2. Date and type of occupational therapy contact.

3. Identification of type of documentation, agency, and department name.

4. Occupational therapist's or occupational therapy assistant's signature with a minimum of first name or initial, last name, and professional designation.

5. When applicable on notes or reports, signature of the recorder directly at the end of the note without space left between the body of the note and the signature.

6. Countersignature by an occupational therapist on documentation written by students and occupational therapy assistants when required by law or the facility.

7. Acceptable terminology defined within the boundaries of setting.

8. Abbreviations usage as acceptable within the boundaries of setting.

9. When no facility requirements are listed, errors corrected by drawing a single line through an error and by initialing the correction (liquid correction fluid and erasures are not acceptable).

10. Adherence to professional standards of technology, when used to document occupational therapy services.

11. Disposal of records within law or agency requirements.

12. Compliance with confidentiality standards.

13. Compliance with agency or legal requirements of storage of records.

REFERENCES

American Occupational Therapy Association. (2002). Occupational therapy practice framework: Domain and process. *American Journal of Occupational Therapy, 56,* 609–639.

American Occupational Therapy Association. (1998). Standards of practice for occupational therapy. *American Journal of Occupational Therapy, 52,* 866–869.

AUTHORS

Gloria Frolek Clark, MS, OTR/L, FAOTA
Mary Jane Youngstrom, MS, OTR/L, FAOTA
for
Commission on Practice
Sara Jane Brayman, PhD, OTR/L, FAOTA, Chairperson
Adopted by the Representative Assembly 2003M16

This document replaces the 1994 *Elements of Clinical Documentation* (previously published and copyrighted in 1995 by the *American Journal of Occupational Therapy, 49,* 1032–1035).

APPENDIX E

AOTA Code of Ethics

▼ PREAMBLE ▼

The American Occupational Therapy Association's Code of Ethics is a public statement of the common set of values and principles used to promote and maintain high standards of behavior in occupational therapy. The American Occupational Therapy Association and its members are committed to furthering the ability of individuals, groups, and systems to function within their total environment. To this end, occupational therapy personnel (including all staff and personnel who work and assist in providing occupational therapy services, (e.g., aides, orderlies, secretaries, technicians) have a responsibility to provide services to recipients in any stage of health and illness who are individuals, research participants, institutions and businesses, other professionals and colleagues, students, and to the general public.

The *Occupational Therapy Code of Ethics* is a set of principles that applies to occupational therapy personnel at all levels. These principles to which occupational therapists and occupational therapy assistants aspire are part of a lifelong effort to act in an ethical manner. The various roles of practitioner (occupational therapist and occupational therapy assistant), educator, fieldwork educator, clinical supervisor, manager, administrator, consultant, fieldwork coordinator, faculty program director, researcher/scholar, private practice owner, entrepreneur, and student are assumed.

Any action in violation of the spirit and purpose of this Code shall be considered unethical. To ensure compliance with the Code, the Commission on Standards and Ethics (SEC) establishes and maintains the enforcement procedures. Acceptance of membership in the American Occupational Therapy Association commits members to adherence to the Code of Ethics and its enforcement procedures. The Code of Ethics, Core Values and Attitudes of Occupational Therapy Practice (AOTA, 1993), and the Guidelines to the Occupational Therapy Code of Ethics (AOTA, 1998) are aspirational documents designed to be used together to guide occupational therapy personnel.

Principle 1. Occupational therapy personnel shall demonstrate a concern for the well-being of the recipients of their services. (beneficence)

A. Occupational therapy personnel shall provide services in a fair and equitable manner. They shall recognize and appreciate the cultural components of economics, geography, race, ethnicity, religious and political factors, marital status, sexual orientation, and disability of all recipients of their services.

B. Occupational therapy practitioners shall strive to ensure that fees are fair and reasonable and commensurate with services performed. When occupational therapy practi-

American Occupational Therapy Association. (2000). *Code of ethics–2000.* Retrieved on May 16, 2002 from *http://www.aota.org/general/coe.asp*

245

tioners set fees, they shall set fees considering institutional, local, state, and federal requirements, and with due regard for the service recipient's ability to pay.

C. Occupational therapy personnel shall make every effort to advocate for recipients to obtain needed services through available means.

Principle 2. Occupational therapy personnel shall take reasonable precautions to avoid imposing or inflicting harm upon the recipient of services or to his or her property. (nonmaleficence)

A. Occupational therapy personnel shall maintain relationships that do not exploit the recipient of services sexually, physically, emotionally, financially, socially, or in any other manner.

B. Occupational therapy practitioners shall avoid relationships or activities that interfere with professional judgment and objectivity.

Principle 3. Occupational therapy personnel shall respect the recipient and/or their surrogate(s) as well as the recipient's rights. (autonomy, privacy, confidentiality)

A. Occupational therapy practitioners shall collaborate with service recipients or their surrogate(s) in setting goals and priorities throughout the intervention process.

B. Occupational therapy practitioners shall fully inform the service recipients of the nature, risks, and potential outcomes of any interventions.

C. Occupational therapy practitioners shall obtain informed consent from participants involved in research activities and indicate that they have fully informed and advised the participants of potential risks and outcomes. Occupational therapy practitioners shall endeavor to ensure that the participant(s) comprehend these risks and outcomes.

D. Occupational therapy personnel shall respect the individual's right to refuse professional services or involvement in research or educational activities.

E. Occupational therapy personnel shall protect all privileged confidential forms of written, verbal, and electronic communication gained from educational, practice, research, and investigational activities unless otherwise mandated by local, state, or federal regulations.

Principle 4. Occupational therapy personnel shall achieve and continually maintain high standards of competence. (duties)

A. Occupational therapy practitioners shall hold the appropriate national and state credentials for the services they provide.

B. Occupational therapy practitioners shall use procedures that conform to the standards of practice and other appropriate AOTA documents relevant to practice.

C. Occupational therapy practitioners shall take responsibility for maintaining and documenting competence by participating in professional development and educational activities.

D. Occupational therapy practitioners shall critically examine and keep current with emerging knowledge relevant to their practice so they may perform their duties on the basis of accurate information.

E. Occupational therapy practitioners shall protect service recipients by ensuring that duties assumed by or assigned to other occupational therapy personnel match credentials, qualifications, experience, and scope of practice.

F. Occupational therapy practitioners shall provide appropriate supervision to individuals for whom the practitioners have supervisory responsibility in accordance with Association policies, local, state and federal laws, and institutional values.

G. Occupational therapy practitioners shall refer to or consult with other service providers whenever such a referral or consultation would be helpful to the care of the recipient of service. The referral or consultation process should be done in collaboration with the recipient of service.

Principle 5. Occupational therapy personnel shall comply with laws and Association policies guiding the profession of occupational therapy. (justice)

A. Occupational therapy personnel shall familiarize themselves with and seek to understand and abide by applicable Association policies; local, state, and federal laws; and institutional rules.
B. Occupational therapy practitioners shall remain abreast of revisions in those laws and Association policies that apply to the profession of occupational therapy and shall inform employers, employees, and colleagues of those changes.
C. Occupational therapy practitioners shall require those they supervise in occupational therapy-related activities to adhere to the Code of Ethics.
D. Occupational therapy practitioners shall take reasonable steps to ensure employers are aware of occupational therapy's ethical obligations, as set forth in this Code of Ethics, and of the implications of those obligations for occupational therapy practice, education, and research.
E. Occupational therapy practitioners shall record and report in an accurate and timely manner all information related to professional activities.

Principle 6. Occupational therapy personnel shall provide accurate information about occupational therapy services. (veracity)

A. Occupational therapy personnel shall accurately represent their credentials, qualifications, education, experience, training, and competence. This is of particular importance for those to whom occupational therapy personnel provide their services or with whom occupational therapy practitioners have a professional relationship.
B. Occupational therapy personnel shall disclose any professional, personal, financial, business, or volunteer affiliations that may pose a conflict of interest to those with whom they may establish a professional, contractual, or other working relationship.
C. Occupational therapy personnel shall refrain from using or participating in the use of any form of communication that contains false, fraudulent, deceptive, or unfair statements or claims.
D. Occupational therapy practitioners shall accept the responsibility for their professional actions which reduce the public's trust in occupational therapy services and those that perform those services.

Principle 7. Occupational therapy personnel shall treat colleagues and other professionals with fairness, discretion, and integrity. (fidelity)

A. Occupational therapy personnel shall preserve, respect, and safeguard confidential information about colleagues and staff, unless otherwise mandated by national, state, or local laws.
B. Occupational therapy practitioners shall accurately represent the qualifications, views, contributions, and findings of colleagues.
C. Occupational therapy personnel shall take adequate measures to discourage, prevent, expose, and correct any breaches of the Code of Ethics and report any breaches of the Code of Ethics to the appropriate authority.

D. Occupational therapy personnel shall familiarize themselves with established policies and procedures for handling concerns about this Code of Ethics, including familiarity with national, state, local, district, and territorial procedures for handling ethics complaints. These include policies and procedures created by the American Occupational Therapy Association, licensing and regulatory bodies, employers, agencies, certification boards, and other organizations who have jurisdiction over occupational therapy practice.

REFERENCES

American Occupational Therapy Association. (1993). Core values and attitudes of occupational therapy practice. *American Journal of Occupational Therapy, 47,* 1085–1086.

American Occupational Therapy Association. (1998). Guidelines to the occupational therapy code of ethics. *American Journal of Occupational Therapy, 52,* 881–884.

AUTHORS

The Commission on Standards and Ethics (SEC):
Barbara L. Kornblau, JD, OTR, FAOTA, Chairperson
Melba Arnold, MS, OTR/L
Nancy Nashiro, PhD, OTR, FAOTA
Diane Hill, COTA/L, AP
Deborah Y. Slater, MS, OTR/L
John Morris, PhD
Linda Withers, CNHA, FACHCA
Penny Kyler, MA, OTR/L, FAOTA, Staff Liaison
April 2000
Adopted by the Representative Assembly 2000M15

Note: This document replaces the 1994 document, *Occupational Therapy Code of Ethics (American Journal of Occupational Therapy, 48,* 1037–1038).
Prepared 4/7/2000

▼ **EXCERPTS FROM THE MEDICARE CORF MANUAL** ▼

251. Covered/Noncovered CORF Services

A. Covered CORF Services.—Covered services include:

- Physician services related to administrative functions;
- Physical therapy, occupational therapy, speech pathology services, and respiratory therapy;
- Social and psychological services;
- Nursing care provided by or under the supervision of a registered professional nurse;
- Prosthetic and orthotic devices, including testing, fitting, or training in the use of such devices;
- Drugs and biologicals which cannot be self-administered;
- Supplies, appliances, and equipment, including the purchase or rental of durable medical equipment (DME) from the CORF; and
- A single home visit to evaluate the potential impact of the home environment on the rehabilitation goals.

B. Noncovered Services.—The statute specifies that no service may be covered as a CORF service if it is not covered as an inpatient hospital service. This does not mean that the beneficiary must require a hospital level of care or meet other requirements unique to hospital care. This provision merely requires that the service be one that could be covered when provided in a hospital. Accordingly, coverage determinations for CORF services are based on established coverage guidelines.

CORF services are not covered if not reasonable and necessary for the diagnosis or treatment of illness or injury or to improve the function of a malformed body member. Thus, there must be potential for restoration or improvement of lost or impaired functions. For example, services involving repetitive services that do not require the skilled services of nurses or therapists, e.g., maintenance programs, general conditioning, or ambulation, are not covered. These services could be performed in the patient's residence by nonmedical personnel such as family members. It is not reasonable and necessary for such services to be performed in an ambulatory care setting by CORF personnel.

Excerpts from Comprehensive Outpatient Rehabilitation Facility Manual and the Medicare Program Integrity Manual.

252. Provision of Services

A. Place of Treatment.—In general, all services must be furnished on your premises. The only exceptions are the home evaluation (see §251) and, effective December 22, 1987, physical therapy, occupational therapy, and speech pathology services. There is no restriction on where these services may be furnished. They may be covered if furnished pursuant to the plan of treatment and if they do not duplicate services for which payment has otherwise been made under Medicare.

You must clearly identify each service performed off the premises of the facility so that your intermediary can easily differentiate between services provided at the facility and elsewhere. (See §416, item 94).

B. Personnel Qualification Requirements.—Services must be furnished or supervised by personnel who meet the requirements in 42 CFR 485.70.

C. Services Furnished Under Arrangements.—CORF services provided under arrangements are subject to the provisions of §202.

D. Referral for Treatment.—To become a patient of a CORF, the beneficiary must be under the care of a physician who certifies that the beneficiary needs skilled rehabilitation services.

The referring physician must advise you of the beneficiary's medical history, current diagnosis and medical findings, desired rehabilitation goals, and any contraindications to specific activity or intensity of rehabilitation services.

E. Plan of Treatment.—Your services must be furnished under a written plan of treatment established by a physician. The physician may be either a physician associated with you or the referring physician if he/she provides a detailed plan of treatment that meets the following requirements:
- The plan of treatment must contain the diagnosis, type, amount, frequency, and duration of services to be performed and the anticipated rehabilitation goals.
- The plan of treatment must be sufficiently detailed to permit an independent evaluation of the patient's specific need for the indicated services and of the likelihood that he/she will derive meaningful benefit from them.
- The plan of treatment must be reviewed by the CORF physician at least once every 60 days. Following the review, the physician must certify that the plan of treatment is being followed and that the patient is making progress in attaining the established rehabilitation goals. When the patient has reached a point where no further progress is being made toward one or more of the goals, Medicare coverage ends for that aspect of the plan of treatment.

F. Physician Certification and Recertification.—
1. Content of Physician Certification.—No payment may be made for CORF services unless a physician certifies that:
   - A plan for furnishing such services is or was established and periodically reviewed by a physician (see §252E);
   - The services are or were furnished while the patient was under the care of a physician (see §252D); and
   - The services are or were required because the patient needed skilled rehabilitation services.

Since the certification is closely associated with the plan of treatment, the same physician who establishes or reviews the plan must certify the necessity for the services. Obtain the certification at the time the plan of treatment is established or as soon thereafter as possible. A physician is a doctor of medicine, osteopathy (including an osteopathic practitioner), or podiatric medicine legally authorized to practice by a

State in which he/she performs the function. The services performed by physicians within this definition are subject to any limitations imposed by the State on the scope of practice.

2. Recertification.—A CORF physician must recertify at intervals of at least once every 60 days that:
   - The plan is being followed;
   - The patient is making progress in attaining the rehabilitation goals; and
   - The treatment is not having any harmful effect on the patient.

Obtain the recertification at the time the plan of treatment is reviewed since the same interval (at least once every 60 days) is required for the review of the plan. Recertifications are signed by the physician who reviews the plan of treatment. You may choose the form and manner of obtaining timely recertification.

3. Method and Disposition of Certifications.—There is no requirement that the certification or recertification be entered on any specific form or handled in any specific way, as long as the intermediary can determine, when necessary, that the certification and recertification requirements are met. Retain certification by the physician and certify on the billing form that the requisite certification and recertifications have been made by the physician and are on file when the request for payment is forwarded.

4. Delayed Certification.—Obtain certifications and recertifications as promptly as possible. Payment is not made unless the necessary certifications have been secured. In addition to complying with the usual content requirements, delayed certifications and recertifications are to include an explanation for the delay and any other evidence necessary in the case. You may choose the form and manner of obtaining delayed certifications and recertifications.

253. Specific CORF Services

253.1 Physician Services

253.2 Physical Therapy Services.—

253.3 Occupational Therapy Services.—

A. Definition.—Occupational therapy is medically prescribed treatment to improve or restore functions which have been impaired by illness or injury or, when function has been permanently lost or reduced by illness or injury, to improve the individual's ability to perform those tasks required for independent functioning. Such therapy may involve:
   - The evaluation and reevaluation (as required) of a patient's level of function by administering diagnostic and prognostic tests;
   - The selection and teaching of task-oriented therapeutic activities designed to restore physical function, e.g., use of woodworking activities on an inclined table to restore shoulder, elbow, and wrist range of motion lost as a result of burns;
   - The planning, implementation, and supervision of individualized therapeutic activity programs as part of an overall active treatment program for a patient with a diagnosed psychiatric illness, e.g., the use of sewing activities which require following a pattern to reduce confusion and restore reality orientation in a schizophrenic patient;
   - The planning and implementation of therapeutic tasks and activities to restore sensory-integrative function, e.g., providing motor and tactile activities to increase sensory input and improve response for a stroke patient with functional loss resulting in a distorted body image;

- The teaching of compensatory techniques to improve the level of independence in the activities of daily living, e.g., teaching a patient who has lost the use of an arm how to pare potatoes and chop vegetables with one hand, teaching an upper extremity amputee how to functionally utilize a prosthesis, or teaching a stroke patient new techniques to enable the patient to perform feeding, dressing, and other activities as independently as possible;
- The design, fabrication, and fitting of orthotic and self-help devices, e.g., making a hand splint for a patient with rheumatoid arthritis to maintain the hand in a functional position or constructing a device which enables an individual to hold a utensil and feed him/herself independently; and
- Vocational and prevocational assessment and training.

Only a qualified occupational therapist has the knowledge, training, and experience required to evaluate and reevaluate a patient's level of function, determine whether an occupational therapy program could reasonably be expected to improve, restore, or compensate for lost function, and, when appropriate, recommend to the physician a plan of treatment. However, while the skills of a qualified occupational therapist are required to evaluate the patient's level of function and develop a plan of treatment, the implementation of the plan may also be carried out by a qualified occupational therapy assistant functioning under the general supervision of the qualified occupational therapist.

NOTE: General supervision requires initial direction and periodic inspection of the actual activity. However, the supervisor need not always be physically present or on the premises when the assistant is providing the services.

B. Coverage Criteria.—To constitute covered occupational therapy for Medicare purposes, the services furnished to a beneficiary must be:
- Prescribed by a physician;
- Performed by a qualified occupational therapist or a qualified occupational therapy assistant under the general supervision of a qualified occupational therapist; and
- Reasonable and necessary for the treatment of the individual's illness or injury.
    1. Potential for Improvement.—Occupational therapy designed to improve function is considered reasonable and necessary for the treatment of the individual's illness or injury only if an expectation exists that the therapy will result in a significant practical improvement in the individual's level of functioning within a reasonable period of time. If an individual's improvement potential is insignificant in relation to the extent and duration of occupational therapy services required to achieve improvement, such services are not considered reasonable and necessary and are thus excluded from coverage. If a valid expectation of improvement exists at the time the occupational therapy program is instituted, the services are covered even though the expectation may not be realized. However, in such situations, the services are covered only up to the time at which it is reasonable to conclude that the patient's condition is not going to improve.
    2. Maintenance Programs.—Once a patient has reached the point where no further significant practical improvement can be expected, the skills of an occupational therapist or occupational therapy assistant are not required to carry out an activity and/or exercise program required to maintain function at the level to which it has been restored. Consequently, while the services of an occupational therapist in designing a maintenance program and making infrequent but periodic evaluations of its effectiveness are covered, the services of an occupational therapist or occupational therapy assistant in carrying out the program are not considered reasonable and necessary for the treatment of illness or injury and such services are excluded from coverage.

3. Temporary Condition.—Occupational therapy is not required to effect improvement or restoration of function when a patient suffers a temporary loss or reduction of function (e.g., temporary weakness resulting from prolonged bed rest after major abdominal surgery) which can reasonably be expected to spontaneously improve as the patient gradually resumes normal activities. Accordingly, occupational therapy furnished in such situations is not considered reasonable and necessary for the treatment of the individual's illness or injury and the services are excluded from coverage.

4. Psychiatric Services.—Occupational therapy may also be required for a patient with a specific diagnosed psychiatric illness. When such services are required, they are covered if the coverage criteria set forth are met. However, if an individual's motivational needs are not related to a specific diagnosed psychiatric illness, the meeting of such needs does not usually require an individualized therapeutic program. Rather, such needs can be met through general activity programs or the efforts of other professional personnel involved in the care of the patient as patient motivation is an appropriate and inherent function of all health disciplines and is interwoven with other functions performed by such personnel for the patient. Accordingly, since the special skills of an occupational therapist or occupational therapy assistant are not required, an occupational therapy program for such individuals is not considered reasonable and necessary for the treatment of an illness or injury. Services furnished under such a program are excluded from coverage.

5. Vocational Services.—As indicated, occupational therapy services include vocational and prevocational assessment and training. When services provided by an occupational therapist and/or an assistant are related solely to specific employment opportunities, work skills, or work settings, they are not reasonable or necessary for the diagnosis or treatment of an illness or injury and are excluded from coverage.

C. Supplies.—Occupational therapy frequently necessitates the use of various supplies, e.g., looms, ceramic tiles, or leather. The cost of such supplies may be included in the occupational therapy cost center.

270. Conditions for Coverage of Outpatient Physical Therapy, Occupational Therapy, and Speech Pathology Services

Outpatient physical therapy (PT), occupational therapy (OT), or speech pathology (SP) services furnished to a beneficiary by a participating provider are covered only when furnished in accordance with the following conditions.

270.1 Physician Certification and Recertification.–

A. Content of Physician Certification.—No payment may be made for outpatient PT, OT, or SP services unless a physician certifies that:

- A plan for furnishing such services is or was established by the physician, physical therapist, occupational therapist, or speech pathologist and periodically reviewed by the physician (see §270.3);
- The services are or were furnished while the patient was under the care of a physician (see §270.2); and
- The services are or were reasonable and necessary to the treatment of the patient's condition.

Since the certification is closely associated with the plan of treatment, the same physician who establishes or reviews the plan must certify the necessity for the services. Obtain the certification at the time the plan of treatment is established or as soon thereafter as possible. A physician is a doctor of medicine, osteopathy, or podiatric medicine if the services are consistent with the function he/she is legally authorized to perform in the State in which he/she performs the function. The services performed by physicians within this definition are subject to any limitations imposed by the State on the scope of practice.

A. Recertification.—When services are continued under the same plan of treatment, the physician must recertify at intervals of at least once every 30 days that there is a continuing need for such services and must estimate how long services are needed. Obtain the recertification at the time the plan of treatment is reviewed since the same interval (at least once every 30 days) is required for the review of the plan. Recertifications are signed by the physician who reviews the plan of treatment. You may choose the form and manner of obtaining timely recertification.

B. Method and Disposition of Certifications.—There is no requirement that the certification or recertification be entered on any specific form or handled in any specific way, as long as the contractor can determine, when necessary, that the certification and recertification requirements are met. Retain certification by the physician and certify on the billing form that the requisite certification and recertifications have been made by the physician and are on file when the request for payment is forwarded.

C. Delayed Certification.—Obtain certifications and recertifications as promptly as possible. Payment is not made unless the necessary certifications have been secured. In addition to complying with the usual content requirements, delayed certifications and recertifications are to include an explanation for the delay and any other evidence necessary in the case. You may choose the form and manner of obtaining delayed certifications and recertifications.

270.2   Outpatient Must Be Under Care of Physician

Outpatient PT, OT, or SP services are furnished only to an individual who is under the care of a physician. There must be evidence in the patient's clinical record that he/she has been seen by a physician at least every 30 days. If the patient has not been seen by the physician within a 30 day period, you are responsible for contacting the physician. This physician may be the patient's private physician, a physician on your staff, a physician associated with an institution which is the patient's residence, or a physician associated with a medical facility in which the patient is an inpatient. The attending physician establishes or reviews the plan of treatment and makes the necessary certifications.

270.3   Outpatient PT, OT, or SP Services Furnished Under a Plan

To be covered, Outpatient PT, OT, or SP services must be provided under a written plan of treatment established by:

- A physician (after any necessary consultation with the physical therapist, occupational therapist, or speech pathologist);
- The physical therapist who provides the physical therapy services;
- The occupational therapist who provides the OT services; or
- The speech pathologist who provides the SP services.

Make sure the plan is established, i.e., it is reduced to writing either by the person who established the plan or by you when you make a written record of that person's oral orders, before treatment begins. The plan must be promptly signed by the ordering physician, therapist, or speech pathologist and incorporated into the patient's clinical record.

Make sure the plan details the type, amount, frequency, and duration of the physical therapy, OT, or SP services to be furnished. The plan must also indicate the diagnosis and anticipated goals. Any changes to this plan must be made in writing and must be signed by the physician, therapist, or pathologist. Changes to the plan may also be made pursuant to oral orders given by the attending physician to a qualified physical therapist, a qualified occupational therapist, a qualified speech pathologist, a registered professional nurse, or a physician on your staff.

Changes to such plans also may be made pursuant to oral orders given by the speech pathologist to another qualified speech pathologist, by the occupational therapist to another qualified occupational therapist, by the physical therapist to another qualified physical therapist, or by the therapist or pathologist to a registered professional nurse on your staff. Such changes must be immediately recorded in the patient's record and must be signed by the individual receiving the orders. While the physician may change a plan of treatment established by the pathologist or therapist providing such services, the therapist or pathologist may not alter a plan of treatment established by a physician.

The patient's plan normally need not be forwarded with the claim but is retained in the provider's file. The provider must certify on the billing form that the plan is on file.

270.4 Outpatient Requirement

PT, OT, and SP services are covered when furnished by a provider to its outpatients, i.e., to patients in their homes, to patients who come to the facility's outpatient department, or to inpatients of other health facilities. In addition, coverage includes PT, OT, and SP services furnished by participating hospitals and SNFs to inpatients who have exhausted their Part A inpatient benefits or who are otherwise not eligible for Part A benefits. Providers of outpatient PT, OT, and SP services that have inpatient facilities (other than participating hospitals and SNFs) may not furnish covered outpatient services to their own inpatients. However, an inpatient of one institution may be considered an outpatient of another institution. Thus, all providers of outpatient PT, OT, and SP services may furnish such services to inpatients of another health facility.

▼ FORMS HCFA-700/701, OUTPATIENT REHABILITATION SERVICES FORMS – (REV. 3, 11-22-00) ▼

The outpatient rehabilitation services forms, Forms HCFA-700/701, are combined MR, certification/re-certification, plan of treatment forms for outpatient Part B, PT, OT and SLP. The forms' design promotes national consistency in reporting and reducing unnecessary requests for additional medical records. HCFA will not mandate use of the hard copy Forms HCFA 700/701. However, some providers have made significant investments in the use of these forms. Therefore, intermediaries must accept hard copy versions of the Forms HCFA-700/701 if the provider chooses to use them. Providers complete the Form HCFA-700 only for initial bills. For interim-to-discharge bills, the provider completes the Form HCFA-701.

Intermediaries use the forms as a source of supporting medical information. They request forms HCFA-700/701 when the reviewers need supporting medical information to help determine whether services are reasonable and necessary.

Intermediaries base payment and denial decisions on information contained in these forms. However, they request additional information when additional medical information is needed to support a decision. A denial determination may not be made solely on the reviewer's general inferences about beneficiaries with similar diagnoses or on data related to utilization.

Instead, reviewers must make determinations based upon clear objective clinical evidence concerning the beneficiary's unique medical condition and individual need for care.

They do not routinely require providers to submit the Forms HCFA-700/701. They request only the Form HCFA-700 for initial bills and obtain the Form HCFA-701 for subsequent bills. They obtain photocopies of prior months forms HCFA-700/701 only when needed for coverage determinations.

If the intermediary standard system can retrieve previously submitted Forms HCFA-700/701 information/data, intermediaries inform providers not to send copies.

Providers must complete all applicable items on the forms. However, if an item is blank and a coverage determination can be made, intermediaries should process the claim. Providers may complete items with "N/A," not applicable, when the item does not apply (e.g., no hospitalization occurred). If information is needed for a coverage decision in an item marked as "N/A" (or left blank), they request the information from the provider.

Intermediaries obtain completed forms HCFA-700/701 from acute hospitals, skilled nursing facilities (SNFs), home health agencies (HHAs), comprehensive outpatient rehabilitation facilities (CORFs), rehabilitation agencies, public health agencies, and clinics (bill types 12X, 13X, 22X, 23X, 34X, 74X, and 75X). They obtain a separate form for each therapy discipline (revenue code) billed.

For example, if a patient received treatment for two services (i.e., PT and OT), the provider must submit two forms. These forms may also be used for outpatient hospital cardiac rehabilitation, respiratory therapy, or psychiatric services. CORFs may also use the forms for SN and MSS.

8.1 Electronic Attachments

Providers submitting batch attachments must use the current version of the UB-92 flat file record type 77. This information may be sent with claim data or independent of claim data. See MIM Addenda A, B, and D and PIM Chapter 9 for further instructions. Intermediaries require the provider to maintain the information to support the electronic format in the beneficiary's medical record, whether hard copy, or electronic. They request additional information to support a decision only as necessary.

8.1.1 Instructions for Completion of Form HCFA-700, Plan of Treatment for Outpatient Rehabilitation - (Rev. 3, 11-22-00)

The provider submits the following information on the Form HCFA-700:

1	Patient's Name	This item indicates the patient's last name, first name, and middle initial as shown on the health insurance card.
2	Provider Number	This item indicates the six digit number issued by Medicare to the provider. The number contains two digits, a hyphen, and four digits (e.g., 00-7000).
3	HICN	This item indicates the numeric plus alpha indicator(s) as shown on the patient's health insurance card, certification award, utilization notice, temporary eligibility notice, or as reported by the Social Security Office.
4	Provider Name	This item indicates the name of the Medicare billing provider.
5	Medical Record Number	This item indicates the patient's medical/clinical record number issued by the billing provider.
6	Onset Date	This item indicates either the onset date of the primary medical diagnosis (if it is a new diagnosis) or the date of the most recent exacerbation of a previous diagnosis. If the exact day is not known, "01" is

used for the day (e.g., 020199). This date must match Occurrence Code 11 on the UB-92.

7	SOC Date	This item indicates the six digit month, day, and year on which rehabilitation services began at the billing provider, i.e., MMDDYY (021599). **The SOC date is the first Medicare billable visit (normally the date of initial evaluation). This date remains the same on subsequent claims until the patient is discharged or the claim is denied.** A provider may suspend services and later resume them under the same SOC date in accordance with its internal procedures. The SOC date may also reflect a re-initiation after discharge or denial if for an exacerbation. For PT, the SOC date must correspond to Occurrence Code 35 on the UB-92, for OT code 44, for SLP code 45, and for CR code 46.
8	Type	The provider checks this item for the type of therapy furnished, i.e., PT, OT, SLP, for outpatient hospital cardiac rehabilitation, respiratory therapy, or psychiatric services. CORFs may also check SN and/or MSS.
9	Primary Diagnosis	This item indicates the medical DX that has resulted in the therapy disorder and which is most closely related to the current plan of care for therapy. The diagnosis may or may not be related to the patient's most recent hospital stay but must relate to the services furnished by the provider. If more than one diagnosis is treated concurrently, the provider enters the diagnosis that represents the most intensive services (over 50 percent of rehabilitation effort for the revenue code billed). The primary DX may change on subsequent forms if the patient develops an acute condition or an exacerbation of a secondary diagnosis requiring intensive services different than established on the initial plan of treatment. In all such instances, the date treatment started at the billing provider remains the same until the patient is discharged.
10	Treatment Diagnosis	This item indicates the DX for which rehabilitative services were furnished (e.g., for SLP the treatment DX is a communication disorder). For example, while cerebrovascular accident (CVA) may be the primary medical DX, aphasia might be the SLP treatment DX. If the treatment DX is the same as the medical DX, the word "same" is used in this item.
11	Visits From Start of Care	This item indicates the cumulative total visits that were completed since the start of services at the billing provider for the treated DX through the last visit on the bill. This total corresponds to the UB-92 Value Code 50 for PT, 51 for OT, 52 for SLP, or 53 for CR.

12	Plan of Treatment Functional Goals	
	A. Functional goals	This item indicates the initial short and long-term goals in measurable, objective, and functional terms. Included are the functional levels (or safety levels) the patient is expected to achieve upon discharge as a result of therapy services. Also, indicated are the levels the patient is to achieve outside of the therapeutic environment. Time-oriented goals are entered when applicable. For example, communicate basic physical needs and emotional status within weeks (as a functional goal for SLP).
	B. Plan	This item indicates the initial overall plan of care, type, and specific nature of rehabilitation procedures that are to be furnished (i.e., treatment the therapist is using: procedures or modalities used).
13	Signature	The signature (or name) and professional designation of the professional who established the plan of treatment is entered in this item. A qualified therapist or speech/language pathologist may establish the plan of treatment for PT, OT, or SLP.
14	Frequency Duration	This item indicates the frequency of treatment the provider expects to furnish per day, week, or month. Also, projected is the length of time the provider expects to furnish services. This is to be expressed in days, weeks, or months (e.g., 3/Wk x 4 Wks).
15	Physician's Signature	The physician signs and dates this item if the Form HCFA-700 is to be used as the physician's certification. If you use an alternative signed certification form, the "On File" box should be checked (Item 18). Identify the period of certification in Item 17 on the HFCA-700. When certification is not required, the provider uses "N/A." Rubber signature stamps are not acceptable as the physician signature. The provider must keep the form containing the physician's original signature on file at the provider site.
16	Date	This item indicates the date the physician signed the form in 6 digits (i.e., month, day, and year).
17	Certification	This item indicates the six digit month, day, and year (i.e., MMDDYY 021599-041599) which identifies the period covered by the plan of treatment. The "From" date for the initial certification must match the SOC date. The "Through" date can be up to, but never exceed, 30 days (60 days for CORFs). The "Through" date is repeated on a subsequent re-certification as the next sequential "From" date. Services delivered on the "Through" date are covered in the next re-certification period.

18	On File	This box is checked if the provider uses the form for certification. The provider is to enter the name of the physician who certified the plan of treatment that is on file at the billing provider. If certification is not required for the type of service checked in Item 8, the name of the physician who referred or ordered the service should be entered, but the "On File" box is not to be checked.
19	Prior Hospitalization	This item indicates the six digit month, day, and year (inclusive dates) of the most recent hospitalization that is pertinent to the patient's condition or primary DX billed (date from 1st day of admission through discharge day). The provider enters "N/A" if this is not applicable. If the period is not known, they enter "N/A."
20	Initial Assessment	This item indicates a brief historical narrative of the injury or illness and the reason(s) for referral as they relate to the primary or treatment DX. The providers use the following guidelines when constructing their narrative: Describe pertinent *functional deficits* and clinical findings and problems found on the initial assessment. Use objective, measurable terminology such as tests and measurements; Assess the patient's ADL, ROM, strength, functional abilities, psychological status, level of assistance required, and pertinent speech-language functional deficit findings. Include tests administered with scores; Relate pertinent safety precautions and medical complications which require skilled intervention that may affect a patient's progress or attainment of goals; List the patient's rehabilitation potential, cognitive status that affects functional ability, and psychological, respiratory, cardiac tests and measurements, as appropriate; and Document audiologic results, vision status, and use or status of amplification for patients receiving speech reading services.
21	Functional Level	This item indicates the patient's functional physical, cardiac, respiratory, or psychological status reached **at the end of the claim period.** The provider is to compare results to that shown on the initial assessment (Item 20). Record functional levels and progress in objective terminology. Include test results and measurements as appropriate. Record information about any change in functional level related to the goal(s) of treatment. When only a few visits have been made (e.g., evaluation) and

when there is no change in function, the training/treatment furnished and the patient's response to the visit(s) are recorded. The provider checks the box titled "Continue Services" if services were continued. The provider checks the box titled "DC Services" if services were discontinued (e.g., if the patient was discharged).

| 22 | Service Dates | This item indicates the "From/Through" dates that represent this billing period. If the provider uses this form for certification (with the exception of CORFs), this billing period should be monthly. The "From/Through" dates in field 22 on the UB-92 must match the dates in this item. Providers may not use "00" in the date, e.g., 042799 for April 27,1999. |

8.1.2 Instructions for Completion of Form HCFA-701, Updated Plan Progress for Outpatient Rehabilitation - (Rev. 3, 11-22-00)

Fields 1 through 11 are the same on forms HCFA 700 and HCFA 701. The provider submits the following information for the remaining fields on the Form HCFA-701:

12	Current Frequency Duration	This item indicates the frequency of treatment the provider expects to furnish per day, week or month. Also, projected is the length of time the services are expected to be furnished per days, weeks, or months (e.g., 3/Wk $\times$ 4 Wks).
13	Current Plan Update, Functional Goals	This item indicates the functional treatment goals for the patient for this billing period. The provider is to state the goals in measurable, objective terms. They are to stress functional short-term goals to reach overall long-term outcomes that the patient is expected to achieve upon discharge (Item 12, HCFA-700). They are to document changes to the initial plan of treatment and effective date(s). Providers must estimate time-frames to reach goals when possible. They are to record procedures or modalities used. If appropriate, they are to describe justification of intensity or any changes to the initial plan in Item 18.
14	Re-certification	This code indicates the six digit month, day, and year, i.e., MMDDYY (061598-071598), that identifies the period covered by the plan of treatment. The "From" date for the initial certification must match the SOC date. The "Through" date can be up to, but never exceed 30 days (60 days for CORFs). The provider is to repeat the "Through" date on a subsequent recertification as the next sequential "From" date. Services delivered on the "Through" date are covered in the next recertification period. On interim CORF claims, "N/A" is used.

EXAMPLE: Initial certification "From" date 051599. Initial certification "Through" date 061599. Re-certification "From" date 061599. Re-certification "Through" date 071599. Certification/re-certification is **required for outpatient PT, OT, and SLP and CORF plans of care. Certification is required for partial hospitalization PS.** When certification/re-certification is not required, the provider uses "N/A."

There is no requirement that the provider enter the certification on the Forms HCFA-700/701 or handle it in any specific way as long as the reviewer can determine, where necessary, that certification/re-certification requirements are met.

15	Physician Signature	If the provider uses the Form HCFA-701 as the physician's recertification, the physician must sign and date the statements. If not, when appropriate, the "On File" box in Item 17 must be checked. Identify the period of recertification in Item 14 on the form. For interim CORF claims and when re-certification is not required, the provider must use the "N/A" box. If the physician established the plan of treatment, the physician must sign both Items 15 and 19. If the plan of treatment is established by a physical therapist, occupational therapist, or speech-language pathologist, that therapist or speech-language pathologist must sign the plan (Item 19). A physician who has knowledge of the care signs the certification/re-certification.
16	Date	This item indicates the date the physician signs the certification/re-certification in six digits (month, date, and year). The date must be shown even if the provider checks the "On File" box in Item 18.
17	On File	When the "On File" box is checked, request the certification/re-certification in accordance with your internal procedures, that are approved by your Regional Office (RO).
18	Reason(s) for Continuing Treatment This Billing Period	This item indicates the major reason(s) justifying continued therapy and the need for additional rehabilitation. Safety/medical complications are to be stated when further applicable. In the event of discharge, the provider is to provide the reason.
19	Signature	The professional who furnishes care or supervises services must enter his/her signature and professional designation.
20	Date	This item indicates the date of the signature in 6 digits (month, day, and year).
21	Continued or Discontinued	The provider checks this box to identify whether services are continued, or discontinued (last bill).
22	Functional Level (end of claim period)	This item indicates the functional level(s) and progress made at the **end of the billing period.** Obtain objective tests and measurements when practical.

The providers are to date specific short-term gains **when practical** (e.g., when the patient is able to consistently perform them in this billing period). Providers are to document pertinent safety problems and/or precautions needed. They are to update the patient's current functional level(s) and progress (or lack of progress with an explanation) achieved as compared to the previous month and/or initial assessment. They are to document assistive devices used. Providers are to submit concise, quality, objective documentation and restrict subjective quantity. They should avoid such terms as "improved strength" or "improved communication." Providers billing 5 or more visits per week should use this space to update progress at 2 weeks and at the end of the claim period.

NOTE: When relating functional level(s) and progress made, the reviewer considers that a patient might not progress (or progress little) during a part of a claim period and the patient notes will reflect that fact. This should not be interpreted so stringently to result in an impulsive termination of coverage at that point. Medically review the entire period (including the prior month in relation to the full month in question) to determine coverage.

23   Service Dates

This item indicates the "From and Through" dates which represent the billing period. If the Provider uses the form for certification/re-certification, with the exception of CORFs, the provider bills monthly. The "From and Through" dates in field 23 are to match the dates on UB-92. Providers should not use "00" in the date, e.g., 042799 for April 27, 1999.

Reproducible Forms

OCCUPATIONAL THERAPY EVALUATION REPORT AND INITIAL INTERVENTION PLAN

BACKGROUND INFORMATION

Date of report: Client's name or initials:

Date of birth &/or age: Date of referral: M   F

Primary intervention diagnosis/concern:

Secondary diagnosis/concern:

Reason for referral to OT: *(or questions to be answered)*

Therapist: *(Print or type your name, sign and date the report at the end.)*

Assessments performed: *(Give a brief description of the method(s) used to gather evaluation data; i.e. interview, informal observation, name of formal assessments, etc.)*

FINDINGS

Occupational Profile: *(Describe the client's occupational history and experience, patterns of living, interests, values and needs that are relevant to the current situation.)*

OCCUPATIONAL ANALYSIS:

    Areas of occupation:

    Performance skills:

    Performance patterns:

    Client factors:

    Activity demands:

    Contexts:

INTERPRETATION

Supports and hindrances to occupational performance

Prioritization of need areas:

PLAN

    Mutually agreed on long-term goals:

    Mutually agreed on short-term goals:

    Recommended intervention methods and approaches:

    Expected frequency, duration and intensity:

    Location of intervention:

    Anticipated D/C environment:

_____

Signature   **Date**

OCCUPATIONAL THERAPY EVALUATION REPORT

BACKGROUND INFORMATION
Date of report: Client's name or initials:
Date of birth &/or age: Date of referral: M   F
Primary intervention diagnosis/concern:
Secondary diagnosis/concern:

Reason for referral to OT: *(or questions to be answered)*

Therapist: *(Print or type your name, sign and date the report at the end.)*

Assessments performed: *(Give a brief description of the method(s) used to gather evaluation data; i.e. interview, informal observation, name of formal assessments, etc.)*

FINDINGS
Occupational Profile: *(Describe the client's occupational history and experience, patterns of living, interests, values and needs that are relevant to the current situation.)*

OCCUPATIONAL ANALYSIS:
      Areas of occupation:

      Performance skills:

      Performance patterns:

      Client factors:

      Activity demands:

      Contexts:

OCCUPATIONAL THERAPY EVALUATION REPORT (PAGE 2)

INTERPRETATION
Supports and hindrances to occupational performance

Prioritization of need areas:

PLAN

Mutually agreed on long-term goal	Mutually agreed on short-term goal	Intervention methods/approaches

Expected frequency, duration and intensity:

Location of intervention:

Anticipated D/C environment:

_____
Signature   Date

OCCUPATIONAL THERAPY INTERVENTION PLAN

BACKGROUND INFORMATION:

Date of report: **Client's name or initials:**

Date of birth &/or age: **Date of referral:**   M   F

Primary intervention diagnosis/concern:

Secondary diagnoses/concerns:

Reason for referral to OT: *(or questions to be answered)*

Therapist: *(Print or type your name and credential, you will sign and date the report at the end.)*

FINDINGS

Occupational profile: *(Describe the client's occupational history and experience, patterns of living, interests, values and needs that are relevant to the current situation.)*

Progress toward goals so far; reasons for progress or lack thereof in:

   Areas of occupation:

   Performance skills:

   Performance patterns:

   Activity demands:

   Client factors:

   Contexts:

Equipment/orthotics issued:

Home programs/training:

OCCUPATIONAL THERAPY INTERVENTION PLAN (PAGE 2)

INTERPRETATION

Analysis of occupational performance: *(Describe the barriers and challenges, supports and strengths.)*

PLAN

Long-term Goal	Short-term Goal	Methods/Approaches

Expected frequency, duration and intensity:

Location of intervention:

Anticipated discontinuation environment:

_____

Signature   *Date*

Occupational Therapy Evaluation Plan (page 2)

PROGRESS NOTES

DATE: NOTE:

____   _____

____   _____

____   _____

____   _____

____   _____

____   _____

____   _____

____   _____

____   _____

____   _____

____   _____

____   _____

____   _____

____   _____

____   _____

____   _____

____   _____

____   _____

____   _____

____   _____

____   _____

____   _____

____   _____

Client name:
Record number:
Physician name:
Diagnosis/condition:

SOAP NOTES

S:

O:

A:

P:

S:

O:

A:

P:

```
Client name:
Record number:
Physician name:
Diagnosis/condition:
```

SAMPLE DISCONTINUATION SUMMARY REPORT

Date of report: Name:
Date of birth &/or age: Date of initial referral: M   F
Primary intervention diagnosis/concern:
Secondary diagnosis/concern:
Precautions/contraindications:
Reason for referral to OT:
Reason for OT discontinuation:

Therapist: *(print or type your name and credential, you will sign and date the report at the end.)*

Description of OT intervention: *(Include service delivery model, duration/frequency of interventions, # of intervention sessions or beginning and end dates of interventions, location of interventions and types of interventions provided.)*

Brief summary of progress toward goals: *(Statements of progress toward or achievement of long-term goals or reasons why goals were not met.)*

Occupational therapy outcomes:
   Initial performance in areas of occupation:
   (Concise summary of changes in the client's performance in the areas of activities of daily living, instrumental activities of daily living, education, work, play, leisure, and social participation.)

   Current level of performance in areas of occupation:
   (Concise summary of current performance and expectations for performance within the contexts of the client's anticipated environments following discontinuation.)

Contextual aspects related to discontinuation:
   (Concise summary of the cultural, physical, social, personal, spiritual, temporal and/or virtual contexts.)

Discontinuation recommendations:
   (Concise description of discontinuation plans other referrals, follow-up, home program suggestions, support systems, and caregiver suggestions.)

_____
Signature   Date

SAMPLE IEP GOAL PAGE

<u>Individualized Education Program for:</u> _____

IEP Dates: from _____ **to** _____   **DOB:** _____

Current Level of Performance/Measurable Annual Goals/Benchmarks

Goal # _____
Educational need area: _____ Academic/cognitive   _____ Behavior   _____ Communication
_____ Motor   _____ Self-help   _____ Social   _____ Vocational

<u>Current Level of Performance</u>:

Measurable Annual Goal:

Benchmark/Objectives:

Goal # _____
Educational need area: _____ Academic/cognitive   _____ Behavior   _____ Communication
_____ Motor   _____ Self-help   _____ Social   _____ Vocational

<u>Current Level of Performance</u>:

Measurable Annual Goal:

Benchmark/Objectives:

DEPARTMENT OF HEALTH AND HUMAN SERVICES
CENTERS FOR MEDICARE & MEDICAID SERVICES

PLAN OF TREATMENT FOR OUTPATIENT REHABILITATION
(COMPLETE FOR INITIAL CLAIMS ONLY)

1. PATIENT'S LAST NAME	FIRST NAME	M.I.	2. PROVIDER NO.	3. HICN
4. PROVIDER NAME	5. MEDICAL RECORD NO. (Optional)		6. ONSET DATE	7. SOC. DATE

8. TYPE	9. PRIMARY DIAGNOSIS (Pertinent Medical D.X.)	10. TREATMENT DIAGNOSIS	11. VISITS FROM SOC.
☐ PT ☐ OT ☐ SLP ☐ CR ☐ RT ☐ PS ☐ SN ☐ SW			

12. PLAN OF TREATMENT FUNCTIONAL GOALS	PLAN
GOALS *(Short Term)* OUTCOME *(Long Term)*	

13. SIGNATURE *(professional establishing POC including prof. designation)*	14. FREQ/DURATION *(e.g., 3/Wk. x 4 Wk.)*

I CERTIFY THE NEED FOR THESE SERVICES FURNISHED UNDER THIS PLAN OF TREATMENT AND WHILE UNDER MY CARE ☐ N/A	17. CERTIFICATION
15. PHYSICIAN SIGNATURE	16. DATE	FROM THROUGH N/A

18. ON FILE *(Print/type physician's name)*
☐

20. INITIAL ASSESSMENT *(History, medical complications, level of function at start of care. Reason for referral.)*	19. PRIOR HOSPITALIZATION
	FROM TO N/A

21. FUNCTIONAL LEVEL *(End of billing period)* PROGRESS REPORT   ☐ CONTINUE SERVICES OR   ☐ DC SERVICES

22. SERVICE DATES
FROM   THROUGH

Form CMS-700-(11-91)

INSTRUCTIONS FOR COMPLETION OF FORM CMS-700

(Enter dates as 6 digits, month, day, year)

1. **Patient's Name** - Enter the patient's last name, first name and middle initial as shown on the health insurance Medicare card.

2. **Provider Number** - Enter the number issued by Medicare to the billing provider *(i.e., 00–7000)*.

3. **HICN** - Enter the patient's health insurance number as shown on the health insurance Medicare card, certification award, utilization notice, temporary eligibility notice, or as reported by SSO.

4. **Provider Name** - Enter the name of the Medicare billing provider.

5. **Medical Record No.** - *(optional)* Enter the patient's medical/ clinical record number used by the billing provider.

6. **Onset Date** - Enter the date of onset for the patient's primary medical diagnosis, if it is a new diagnosis, or the date of the most recent exacerbation of a previous diagnosis. If the exact date is not known enter 01 for the day *(i.e., 120191)*. The date matches occurrence code 11 on the UB-92.

7. **SOC** *(start of care)* **Date** - Enter the date services began at the billing provider (the date of the first Medicare billable visit which **remains the same on subsequent claims** until discharge or denial corresponds to occurrence code 35 for PT, 44 for OT, 45 for SLP and 46 for CR on the UB-92).

8. **Type** - Check the type therapy billed; i.e., physical therapy (PT), occupational therapy (OT), speech-language pathology (SLP), cardiac rehabilitation (CR), respiratory therapy (RT), psychological services (PS), skilled nursing services (SN), or social services (SW).

9. **Primary Diagnosis** - Enter the pertinent written medical diagnosis resulting in the therapy disorder and relating to 50% or more of effort in the plan of treatment.

10. **Treatment Diagnosis** - Enter the written treatment diagnosis for which services are rendered. For example, for PT the primary medical diagnosis might be Degeneration of Cervical Intervertebral Disc while the PT treatment DX might be Frozen R Shoulder or, for SLP, while CVA might be the primary medical DX, the treatment DX might be Aphasia. If the same as the primary DX enter SAME.

11. **Visits From Start of Care** - Enter the **cumulative total** visits *(sessions)* completed since services were started at the billing provider for the diagnosis treated, through the last visit on this bill. *(Corresponds to UB-92 value code 50 for PT, 51 for OT, 52 for SLP, or 53 for cardiac rehab.)*

12. **Plan of Treatment/Functional Goals** - Enter brief current plan of treatment goals for the patient for this billing period. Enter the major short-term goals to reach overall long-term outcome. Enter the major plan of treatment to reach stated goals and outcome. Estimate time-frames to reach goals, when possible.

13. **Signature** - Enter the signature *(or name)* and the professional designation of the professional establishing the plan of treatment.

14. **Frequency/Duration** - Enter the current frequency and duration of your treatment; e.g., 3 times per week for 4 weeks is entered 3/Wk x 4Wk.

15. **Physician's Signature** - If the form CMS-700 is used for certification, the physician enters his/her signature. If **certification is required and the form is not being used for certification, check the ON FILE box in item 18.** If the certification is not required for the type service rendered, check the N/A box.

16. **Date** - Enter the date of the physician's signature only if the form is used for certification.

17. **Certification** - Enter the inclusive dates of the certification, **even if the ON FILE box is checked in item 18.** Check the N/A box if certification is not required.

18. **ON FILE** (Means certification signature and date) - Enter the **typed/printed name of the physician** who certified the plan of treatment that is on file at the billing provider. If certification is not required for the type of service checked in item 8, type/print the name of the physician who referred or ordered the service, **but do not check the ON FILE box.**

19. **Prior Hospitalization** - Enter the inclusive dates of recent hospitalization *(1st to DC day)* **pertinent** to the patient's current plan of treatment. Enter N/A if the hospital stay does not relate to the rehabilitation being rendered.

20. **Initial Assessment** - Enter only **current relevant history** from records or patient interview. Enter the major functional limitations stated, if possible, in objective measurable terms. Include only relevant surgical procedures, prior hospitalization and/or therapy for the same condition. Include only pertinent baseline tests and measurements from which to judge future progress or lack of progress.

21. **Functional Level** (end of billing period) - Enter the pertinent progress made and functional levels obtained at the end of the billing period compared to levels shown on initial assessment. Use objective terminology. Date progress when function can be consistently performed. When only a few visits have been made, enter a note indicating the training/treatment rendered and the patient's response if there is no change in function.

22. **Service Dates** - Enter the From and Through dates which represent this billing period *(should be monthly)*. Match the From and Through dates in field 6 on the UB-92. DO NOT use 00 in the date. Example: 01 08 91 for January 8, 1991.

DEPARTMENT OF HEALTH AND HUMAN SERVICES
CENTERS FOR MEDICARE & MEDICAID SERVICES

UPDATED PLAN OF PROGRESS FOR OUTPATIENT REHABILITATION

(Complete for Interim to Discharge Claims. Photocopy of CMS-700 or 701 is required.)

1. PATIENT'S LAST NAME	FIRST NAME	M.I.	2. PROVIDER NO.	3. HICN

4. PROVIDER NAME	5. MEDICAL RECORD NO. *(Optional)*	6. ONSET DATE	7. SOC. DATE

8. TYPE ☐ PT ☐ OT ☐ SLP ☐ CR ☐ RT ☐ PS ☐ SN ☐ SW	9. PRIMARY DIAGNOSIS *(Pertinent Medical D.X.)* 12. FREQ/DURATION *(e.g., 3/Wk. x 4 Wk.)*	10. TREATMENT DIAGNOSIS	11. VISITS FROM SOC.

13. CURRENT PLAN UPDATE, FUNCTIONAL GOALS *(Specify changes to goals and plan.)*

GOALS *(Short Term)*

OUTCOME *(Long Term)*

PLAN

I HAVE REVIEWED THIS PLAN OF TREATMENT AND RECERTIFY A CONTINUING NEED FOR SERVICES. ☐ N/A ☐ DC	14. RECERTIFICATION FROM THROUGH N/A
15. PHYSICIAN'S SIGNATURE 16. DATE	17. ON FILE *(Print/type physician's name)* ☐

18. REASON(S) FOR CONTINUING TREATMENT THIS BILLING PERIOD *(Clarify goals and necessity for continued skilled care.)*

19. SIGNATURE *(or name of professional, including prof. designation)*	20. DATE	21. ☐ CONTINUE SERVICES OR ☐ DC SERVICES

22. FUNCTIONAL LEVEL *(At end of billing period — Relate your documentation to functional outcomes and list problems still present.)*

22. SERVICE DATES FROM   THROUGH

Form CMS-701(11-91)

INSTRUCTIONS FOR COMPLETION OF FORM CMS-701

(Enter dates as 6 digits, month, day, year)

1. **Patient's Name** - Enter the patient's last name, first name and middle initial as shown on the health insurance Medicare card.

2. **Provider Number** - Enter the number issued by Medicare to the billing provider *(i.e., 00–7000).*

3. **HICN** - Enter the patient's health insurance number as shown on the health insurance Medicare card, certification award, utilization notice, temporary eligibility notice, or as reported by SSO.

4. **Provider Name** - Enter the name of the Medicare billing provider.

5. **Medical Record No.** - *(optional)* Enter the patient's medical/clinical record number used by the billing provider. *(This is an item which you may enter for your own records.)*

6. **Onset Date** - Enter the date of onset for the patient's primary medical diagnosis, if it is a new diagnosis, or the date of the most recent exacerbation of a previous diagnosis. If the exact date is not known enter 01 for the day *(i.e., 120191).* The date matches occurrence code 11 on the UB-92.

7. **SOC** *(start of care)* **Date** - Enter the date services began at the billing provider (the date of the first Medicare billable visit which **remains the same on subsequent claims** until discharge or denial corresponds to occurrence code 35 for PT, 44 for OT, 45 for SLP and 46 for CR on the UB-92).

8. **Type** - Check the type therapy billed; i.e., physical therapy (PT), occupational therapy (OT), speech-language pathology (SLP), cardiac rehabilitation (CR), respiratory therapy (RT), psychological services (PS), skilled nursing services (SN), or social services (SW).

9. **Primary Diagnosis** - Enter the pertinent written medical diagnosis resulting in the therapy disorder and relating to 50% or more of effort in the plan of treatment.

10. **Treatment Diagnosis** - Enter the written treatment diagnosis for which services are rendered. For example, for PT the primary medical diagnosis might be Degeneration of Cervical Intervertebral Disc while the PT treatment DX might be Frozen R Shoulder or, for SLP, while CVA might be the primary medical DX, the treatment DX might be Aphasia. If the same as the primary DX enter SAMPLE.

11. **Visits From Start of Care** - Enter the **cumulative total** visits *(sessions)* completed since services were started at the billing provider for the diagnosis treated, through the last visit on this bill. *(Corresponds to UB-92 value code 50 for PT, 51 for OT, 52 for SLP, or 53 for cardiac rehab.)*

12. **Current Frequency/Duration** - Enter the current frequency and duration of your treatment; e.g., 3 times per week for 4 weeks is entered 3/Wk x 4Wk.

13. **Current Plan Update, Functional Goals** - Enter the current plan of treatment goals for the patient for this billing period. *(If the same as shown on the CMS-700 or previous 701 enter "same".)* Enter the short-term goals to reach overall long-term outcome. Justify intensity if appropriate. Estimate time-frames to meet goals, when possible.

14. **Recertification** - Enter the inclusive dates when recertification is required, **even if the ON FILE box is checked in item 17.** Check the N/A box if recertification is not required for the type of service rendered.

15. **Physician's Signature** - If the form CMS-701 is used for recertification, the physician enters his/her signature. If recertification is not required for the type of service rendered, check N/A box. **If the form CMS-701 is not being used for recertification, check the ON FILE box - item 17.** If discharge is ordered, check DC box.

16. **Date** - Enter the date of the physician's signature only if the form is used for recertification.

17. **On File** *(Means certification signature and date)* - Enter the **typed/printed name of the physician** who certified the plan of treatment that is on file at the billing provider. If recertification is not required for the type of service checked in item 8, type/print the name of the physician who referred or ordered the service, **but do not check the ON FILE box.**

18. **Reason(s) For Continuing Treatment This Billing Period** - Enter the **major reasons** why the patient needs to continue skilled rehabilitation **for this billing period** (e.g., briefly state the patient's need for specific functional improvement, skilled training, reduction in complication or improvement in safety and how long you believe this will take, if possible or state your reasons for recommending discontinuance). Complete by the rehab specialist prior to physician's recertification.

19. **Signature** - Enter the signature *(or name)* and the professional designation of the individual justifying or recommending need for care *(or discontinuance)* for this billing period.

20. **Date** - Enter the date of the rehabilitation professional's signature.

21. Check the box if services are continuing or discontinuing at end of this billing period.

22. **Functional Level** *(end of billing period)* - Enter the pertinent progress made through the end of this billing period. Use objective terminology. Compare progress made to that shown on the previous CMS-701, item 22, or the CMS-700, items 20 and 21. Date progress when function can be consistently performed or when meaningful functional improvement is made or when significant regression in function occurs. Your intermediary reviews this progress compared to that on the prior CMS-701 or 700 to determine coverage for this billing period. Send a photocopy of the form covering the previous billing period.

23. **Service Dates** - Enter the From and Through dates which represent this billing period *(should be monthly).* Match the From and Through dates in field 6 on the UB-92. DO NOT use 00 in the date. Example: 01 08 91 for January 8, 1991.

REQUEST FOR REVIEW OF PART B MEDICARE CLAIM
Medical Insurance Benefits – Social Security Act

NOTICE – Anyone who misrepresents or falsifies essential information requested by this form may upon conviction be subject to fine and imprisonment under Federal Law.

1. Carrier's Name and Address	2. Name of Patient
	3. Health Insurance Claim Number

4. I do not agree with the determination you made on my claim as described on my Explanation of Medicare Benefits dated:

5. MY REASONS ARE: (Attach a copy of the Explanation of Medicare Benefits, or describe the service, date of service, and physician's name. NOTE: If the date on the Explanation of Medicare Benefits mentioned in Item 4 is more than six months ago, include your reason for not making this request earlier.)

6. Describe illness or injury:

7. ☐ I have additional evidence to submit. (Attach such evidence to this form.)
☐ I do not have additional evidence.

COMPLETE ALL OF THE INFORMATION REQUESTED. SIGN AND RETURN THE FIRST COPY AND ANY ATTACHMENTS TO THE CARRIER NAMED ABOVE. IF YOU NEED HELP, TAKE THIS AND YOUR NOTICE FROM THE CARRIER TO A SOCIAL SECURITY OFFICE, OR TO THE CARRIER. KEEP THE DUPLICATE COPY OF THIS FORM FOR YOUR RECORDS.

8. SIGNATURE OF *EITHER* THE CLAIMANT *OR* HIS REPRESENTATIVE

Claimant		Representative	
Address		Address	
City, State and ZIP Code		City, State and ZIP Code	
Telephone Number	Date	Telephone Number	Date

Form CMS-1964 (9/91)

Carrier's Copy

REQUEST FOR REVIEW OF PART B MEDICARE CLAIM
Medical Insurance Benefits – Social Security Act

NOTICE – Anyone who misrepresents or falsifies essential information requested by this form may upon conviction be subject to fine and imprisonment under Federal Law.

1. Carrier's Name and Address	2. Name of Patient
	3. Health Insurance Claim Number

4. I do not agree with the determination you made on my claim as described on my Explanation of Medicare Benefits dated:

5. MY REASONS ARE: (Attach a copy of the Explanation of Medicare Benefits, or describe the service, date of service, and physician's name. NOTE: If the date on the Explanation of Medicare Benefits mentioned in Item 4 is more than six months ago, include your reason for not making this request earlier.)

6. Describe illness or injury:

7. ☐ I have additional evidence to submit. (Attach such evidence to this form.)
   ☐ I do not have additional evidence.

COMPLETE ALL OF THE INFORMATION REQUESTED. SIGN AND RETURN THE FIRST COPY AND ANY ATTACHMENTS TO THE CARRIER NAMED ABOVE. IF YOU NEED HELP, TAKE THIS AND YOUR NOTICE FROM THE CARRIER TO A SOCIAL SECURITY OFFICE, OR TO THE CARRIER. KEEP THE DUPLICATE COPY OF THIS FORM FOR YOUR RECORDS.

8. SIGNATURE OF *EITHER* THE CLAIMANT *OR* HIS REPRESENTATIVE

Claimant		Representative	
Address		Address	
City, State and ZIP Code		City, State and ZIP Code	
Telephone Number	Date	Telephone Number	Date

Form CMS-1964 (9/91)

Claimant's Copy

PRIVACY ACT ADVISORY STATEMENT

COLLECTION AND USE OF MEDICARE INFORMATION

We are authorized by the CENTERS FOR MEDICARE & MEDICAID SERVICES to ask you for information needed in the administration of the Medicare program. Social Security's authority to collect information is in section 205(a), 1872 and 1875 of the Social Security Act, as amended.

The information we obtain to complete your Medicare claim is used to identify you and to determine your eligibility. It is also used to decide if the services and supplies you received are covered by Medicare and to insure that proper payment is made.

The information may also be given to other providers of services, carriers, intermediaries, medical review boards, and other organizations as necessary to administer the Medicare program. For example, it may be necessary to disclose information about the Medicare benefits you have used to a hospital or doctor.

Additional disclosures are made through routine uses for information contained in systems of records. Disclosures of this information via routine uses may be made to: a congressional office from the record of an individual in response to an inquiry from the congressional office made at the request of that individual; the Department of Justice, to a court or other tribunal, or to another party before such tribunal, when HHS is a party to litigation or has an interest in such

litigation; or a contractor for the purpose of collating, analyzing, aggregating or otherwise refining or processing records in this system for developing, modifying and/or manipulating ADP Software. See the notice for system No. 09-70-0512, titled "Review and Fair Hearing Case Files," as last published in the *Federal Register*, Privacy Act Issuances 1989 Comp., Vol. 1, page 413.

You should be aware that P.L. 100-503, the "Computer Matching and Privacy Protection Act of 1988," permits the government to verify information by way of computer matches.

With one exception, which is discussed below, there are no penalties under social security law for refusing to supply information. However, failure to furnish information regarding the medical services rendered or the amount charged would prevent payment of the claim. Failure to furnish any other information, such as name or claim number, would delay payment of the claim.

It is mandatory that you tell us if you are being treated for a work related injury so we can determine whether worker's compensation will pay for the treatment. Section 1877(a)(3) of the Social Security Act provides criminal penalties for withholding this information.

According to the Paperwork Reduction Act of 1995, no persons are required to respond to a collection of information unless it displays a valid OMB control number. The valid OMB control number for this information collection is 0938-0033. The time required to complete this information collection is estimated to average 15 minutes per response, including the time to review instructions, search existing data resources, gather the data needed, and complete and review the information collection. If you have any comments concerning the accuracy of the time estimate(s) or suggestions for improving this form, please write to: CMS, Mailstop N2-14-26, 7500 Security Boulevard, Baltimore, Maryland 21244-1850.

Summary of the Occupational Therapy Practice Framework

Areas of Occupation	Performance Skills	Performance Patterns	Contexts	Activity Demands	Client Factors

Activities of Daily Living
• Bathing, showering
• Bowel and bladder management
• Dressing
• Eating
• Feeding
• Functional mobility
• Personal device care
• Personal hygiene and grooming
• Sexual activity
• Sleep/rest
• Toilet hygiene
Instrumental Activities of Daily Living
• Care of others
• Care of pets
• Child rearing
• Communication device use
• Community mobility
• Financial management
• Health management and maintenance
• Home establishment and management
• Meal preparation and cleanup
• Safety procedures and emergency responses
• Shopping
Education
• Formal educational participation
• Exploration of informal personal education needs or interests
	Motor
	• Posture
	  ○ Stabilizes
	  ○ Aligns
	  ○ Positions
	• Mobility
	  ○ Walks
	  ○ Reaches
	  ○ Bends
	• Coordination
	  ○ Coordinates
	  ○ Manipulates
	  ○ Flows
	• Strength and effort
	  ○ Moves
	  ○ Transports
	  ○ Lifts
	  ○ Calibrates
	  ○ Grips
	Process
	• Energy
	  ○ Paces
	  ○ Attends
	• Knowledge
	  ○ Chooses
	  ○ Uses
	  ○ Handles
	  ○ Heeds
	  ○ Inquires
	• Temporal organization
	  ○ Continues
	  ○ Sequences
	  ○ Terminates
	• Organizing space and objects
	  ○ Searches/locates
	  ○ Gathers
		Habits
		• Useful
		• Impoverished
		• Dominating
		Routines
		Roles
			Cultural
			Physical
			Social
			Personal
			Spiritual
			Temporal
			Virtual
				Objects and Their Properties
				Space demands
				Social demands
				Required Actions
				Required Body Functions
				Required Body Structures
					Body functions
					• Mental functions
					  ○ Global
					    ▪ Consciousness
					    ▪ Orientation
					    ▪ Sleep
					    ▪ Temperament and personality
					    ▪ Energy and drive
					  ○ Specific
					    ▪ Attention
					    ▪ Memory
					    ▪ Perceptual
					    ▪ Thought
					    ▪ Higher-level cognitive functions
					    ▪ Mental functions of language
					    ▪ Calculation
					    ▪ Mental functions of sequencing complex movement
					    ▪ Psychomotor
					    ▪ Emotional
					    ▪ Experience of self and time functions
					• Sensory functions and pain
					  ○ Seeing and related functions
					  ○ Hearing and vestibular functions
					  ○ Additional sensory functions
					  ○ Pain
					• Neuromusculoskeletal and movement-related functions
					  ○ Functions of joints and bondes
					    ▪ Mobility of joints
					    ▪ Stability of joints
					    ▪ Mobility of bone functions
					  ○ Muscle functions
					    ▪ Muscle power
					    ▪ Muscle tone
					    ▪ Muscle endurance

○ Movement functions
  ■ Motor reflex
  ■ Involuntary movement reactions
  ■ Control of voluntary movement
  ■ Involuntary movement
  ■ Gait pattern
• Cardiovascular, hematological, immunological and respiratory function
  ○ Cardiovascular system
  ○ Hematological and immuno-logical systems
  ○ Respiratory system
  ○ Additional functions and sensations of the CV and Respiratory systems
• Voice and speech functions
• Digestive, metabolic, and endocrine system functions
• Genitourinary and reproductive functions
• Skin and related structure functions
  ○ Skin
  ○ Hair and nails

Body Structure
• Nervous system
• Eye, ear and related
• Voice and speech
• Cardiovascular, immunological, and respiratory
• Digestive
• Genitourinary and reproductive
• Structures related to movement
• Skin and related structures

○ Organizes
○ Restores
○ Navigates
• Adaptation
  ○ Notices/responds
  ○ Accommodates
  ○ Adjusts
  ○ Benefits

Communicates
• Physicality
  ○ Contacts
  ○ Gazes
  ○ Gestures
  ○ Maneuvers
  ○ Orients
  ○ Postures
• Information exchange
  ○ Articulates
  ○ Asserts
  ○ Asks
  ○ Engages
  ○ Expresses
  ○ Modulates
  ○ Shares
  ○ Speaks
  ○ Sustains
  • Relations
    ○ Collaborates
    ○ Conforms
    ○ Focuses
    ○ Relates
    ○ Responds

• Informal personal educational participation

Work
• Employment interests and pursuits
• Employment seeking and acquisition
• Job performance
• Retirement preparation and adjustment
• Volunteer exploration
• Volunteer participation

Play
• Play exploration
• Play participation

Leisure
• Leisure exploration
• Leisure participation

Social Participation
• Community
• Family
• Peer, friend

Adapted from: American Occupational Therapy Association. (2002). Occupational therapy practice framework: Domain and process. *American Journal of Occupational Therapy 56*, 609–639.

Index